THE MOST
EFFECTIVE WAYS TO Live
LONGER

THE MOST EFFECTIVE WAYS TO Live LONGER

THE SURPRISING, UNBIASED TRUTH ABOUT WHAT YOU SHOULD DO TO PREVENT DISEASE, FEEL GREAT, AND HAVE OPTIMUM HEALTH AND LONGEVITY

Jonny Bowden, Ph.D., C.N.S.

FAIR WINDS
PRESS
BEVERLY, MASSACHUSETTS

The secret to a long life, from Frank Cuckles, 108, the last surviving veteran of World War I: *"When you start to die, don't."*

Text © 2010 Jonny Bowden

First published in the USA in 2010 by
Fair Winds Press, a member of
Quayside Publishing Group
100 Cummings Center
Suite 406-L
Beverly, MA 01915-6101
www.fairwindspress.com

14 13 12 11 10   2 3 4 5

ISBN-13: 978-1-59233-340-0
ISBN-10: 1-59233-340-0

Library of Congress Cataloging-in-Publication Data
Bowden, Jonny.
 The most effective ways to live longer : the surprising, unbiased truth about what you should do to prevent disease, feel great, and have optimum health and longevity / Jonny Bowden.
     p. cm.
 Includes bibliographical references and index.
 ISBN-13: 978-1-59233-340 0
 ISBN-10: 1-59233-340-0
 1. Dietary supplements. 2. Longevity. 3. Health. I. Title.

RM258.5.B695 2010
613.2—dc22

                                        2009031146

Cover design + book design: Luke Herriott
Layout: doublemranch.com

Printed and bound in China

The information in this book is for educational purposes only. It is not intended to replace the advice of a physician or medical practitioner. Please see your health-care provider before beginning any new health program.

To Anja

"You are the butter to my bread
and the breath to my life"

Contents

Rein in the Four Horsemen of Aging

·····································

Don Wildman is a personal trainer who lives in Malibu, California. Which is kind of like saying, "Babe Ruth is a baseball player from New York."

Wildman has completed the Ironman triathlon nine times; the Aspen, Colorado, downhill ski race; a three-thousand-mile bike race called the "Race across America"; and the Los Angeles and New York City marathons. In his spare time, he snowboards the Alaskan backcountry and competes in sailing events—he's in the record books for winning all three of the Chicago Yacht Club's Mackinac races in a single season.

At his private gym in Paradise Cove, California, he leads a legendary workout known as "The Circuit," which features more than 3,000—yes, *thousand*—repetitions of weight lifting mixed with abdominal and balancing exercises. Participants cycle through twenty multipart exercises six times. There's only one rule: You can't stop until it's done. Not surprisingly, few people can do it, so classes are small. Those who *do* manage to finish it can barely drive home afterward—Wildman usually spends the rest of the day mountain biking.

Oh, one more thing. Don Wildman is seventy-five years old.

ACTIVE AND AGING

Now maybe you don't aspire to be exactly like Don, and truth be told, few of us could, even if we wanted to. But Don Wildman is one of the thousands of people who are changing the way we look at aging in the twenty-first century. They're showing us what's possible. And they're demonstrating, time and again, that aging doesn't have to look like what it looked like back in your grandmother's day.

There are shepherds in their seventies who right now climb punishing hills each day in Sardinia and glow with good health. There are folks in Okinawa who tend vegetable gardens and hoe fields well into their nineties. Explorer and writer Dan Buettner recently met a lovely hundred-year-old woman named Panchita in the Nicoya peninsula off Costa Rica, who spends her days cooking, splitting logs, and clearing brush with a machete. He wrote about her and her eighty-year-old son Tommy, who bicycles to see her every day, in his book, *The Blue Zones*. Closer to home, Thomas Perls, M.D., director of the New England Centenarian Study, told *Time* magazine about a man who was repairing roofs in his nineties (he lived to be 103 years old).

Then there's Bill Finch, who, at ninety-six, is a champion badminton player and the world record holder for the 1,500-meter run among ninety-five- to ninety-nine-year-olds (astonishingly, they have enough athletes in that age group to create an entire competitive class of runners). By the way, Bill still dates. And as of this writing, the mountain climbing world is all in a dither as professional climbers all over the globe vie for the privilege of accompanying legendary mountain climber Fred Beckey, who is about to depart for uncharted territories in Northern Spain. Beckey is eighty-five.

WHAT AGING WELL LOOKS LIKE

So maybe you don't aspire to be an elite runner at ninety, or the world's fittest man at seventy-five, or conquering mountains at eighty-five. But I'm betting you wouldn't be reading this book if you weren't interested in living long and living vigorously. Think about it: Would you like to wake up in the morning with energy and enthusiasm, with all your faculties intact, able to take care of yourself physically and free of any major aches, pains, and disabilities? Would you like to live well into your nineties feeling basically happy, content, fulfilled, and healthy?

Let me guess: The answer is "yes."

And here's the thing: It's totally possible.

There's been a major paradigm shift in the study of aging and longevity. By observing societies that have unusual numbers of centenarians, we've been able to discover patterns of living that are associated with long life and good health. By experimenting in the lab we've been able to discover not only the genes that have an impact on life and health, but also, more important, what you can do to "turn those genes on" (more on that later). Scientists now have a pretty good idea of what behaviors are linked to longevity and why. And there's a ton of research showing just what people actually die of, and what factors influence those deaths.

Take, for example, the ten top causes of death in the United States.[1] Heart disease, cancer, and stroke top the list, and those three diseases—out of the more than 100,000 diseases listed in the World Health Organization's *International Statistical Classification of Diseases and Related Health Problems*—account for a whopping 60 percent of the deaths in the United States! Genetics are a factor in 10 percent of your risk for heart disease, while lifestyle choices contribute to the other 90 percent![2] The two single biggest culprits when it comes to causing cancer are diet and tobacco, according to a 1981 landmark study in the *Journal of the National Cancer Institute*.[3] One 1996 study from the Harvard School of Public Health attributed a full 30 percent of cancer deaths specifically to diet (the same percentage attributed to smoking)![4] And data from the National Cancer Institute suggests that the percentage of cancer cases in which diet and lifestyle play major roles ranges from 35 percent to an unbelievable 60 percent![5]

Then there's diabetes, which comes in at number six on the top ten list. But that doesn't begin to give you the full story of the diabetes connection to longevity, because diabetes—and its relative, metabolic syndrome (or pre-diabetes)—puts you at enormous risk for heart disease. As many as 80 percent of diabetics die from vascular problems like stroke or heart disease.[6] And, as you'll learn in this book, diabetes is *almost 100 percent preventable, or reversible,* if you make the right lifestyle choices. Which, by the way, are not all that difficult.

The payoff, in terms of extra healthy years, is absolutely amazing. The Nurses Health Study, which has been going on since 1976 and involves more than 84,000 women, found that just five attainable strategies resulted in an astonishing 83 percent reduction in risk for major coronary events (including those that typically result in death).[7] Are you ready for those five strategies? They are:

1. Not smoking
2. Consuming alcohol moderately
3. Exercising moderately
4. Eating a healthy diet
5. Keeping your weight under control

The take-home point is simple: Your future is in large measure determined by your own choices. Your life is in *your* hands. And while not everybody who makes all the right choices will live to be one hundred in great health, there's an awful lot you can do to increase the odds that you'll be one of the growing number of folks who will. Living well, living long, and living with a high degree of function up to the very (peaceful) end is the goal of everyone reading this book— and it's completely doable.

Which brings us to a concept I call "the functionality curve."

THE FUNCTIONALITY CURVE

If you drew a graph showing age on one axis and function on the other (function meaning everything from how well your heart performs to your ability to have passionate sex), you'd see a depressing slope in which function decreases as age increases. It would look like Figure A, below. Notice how the slope goes down?

Well, it doesn't have to. "The goal of anti-aging medicine is to rectangularize the functionality curve," says Ron Rothenberg, M.D., author of *Forever Ageless*. "That is, to maintain all functions—heart, brain, muscle, lungs, etc.—at a high level to the end and then fall apart quickly all at once."

A "rectangularized" functionality curve might look like Figure B.

"Isn't that what everyone wants?" asks Rothenberg.

Let me guess again: The answer is a resounding "yes."

"For most of us, death will be preceded by a decline in function and we would all like that period of decline to be as brief as possible," write David Jones, M.D., Jeffrey Bland, Ph.D., and Shelia Quinn in an article on healthy aging.[8]

In labs all over the country, scientists like David Sinclair at Harvard University (more on him later) labor tirelessly to discover the secrets of unlocking longevity genes and engage in experiments that—at least in animals—have extended life in every species tested and slowed aging by 35 percent. Cynthia Kenyon, director of the Hillblom Center for the Biology of Aging at the University of California, San Francisco, has found a way to lengthen the life span of worms from a normal 18 days to 144 days—an increase of 800 percent! No one thinks that these discoveries won't eventually translate into useful strategies for humans. Many of us think they already do (more on that throughout this book).

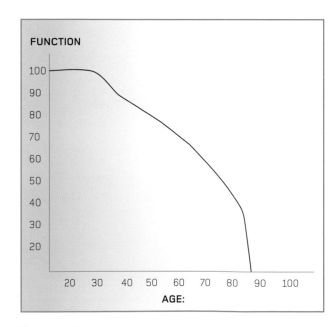

Figure A: Function over age

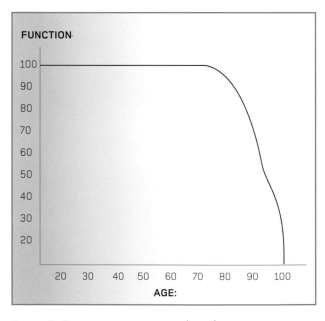

Figure B: Function over age, rectangularized

And here's the good news: An enormous amount of research has shown that healthful lifestyle activities are associated with less disability, less loss of function, and fewer chronic illnesses during the life span. This is empowering news that should make everyone happy. There are things you can do right now on a daily basis that will make all the difference in how long you live and how well you live.

One study on more than 1,700 University of Pennsylvania alumni followed for more than thirty years showed that just three factors accounted for major differences in the length of disability at the end of life, and for the severity of that disability. In other words, by manipulating just three factors you could go a long way toward "rectangularizing" the functionality curve. Those three factors are (1) smoking, (2) weight, and (3) patterns of exercise.[9]

Later research at Harvard[10] corroborated the importance of the same three factors and added a couple more, including "a stable marriage," which I discuss under "Section III: The Secrets of Emotional Intelligence." We'll refine, flesh out, and add to that list of things you can actually do to "rectangularize" the curve throughout this book.

The take-home point is this: What you do *matters*. Very much. How long you live—and how *well* you live—is largely in your own hands. "Research is making it increasingly clear that there are many behaviors (diet, exercise, stress reduction) and treatments (antioxidants, essential fatty acids, minerals, certain amino acids, the B vitamins, and much more) that can counteract the functional decline that leaves us vulnerable to disease and disability as we age," writes Jones.

WHAT IS AGING ANYWAY?

If you think computers are complex, welcome to the world of aging. There are so many interconnected parts in that collection of 100 trillion cells we call our bodies that the number of possible places where things can break down is almost infinite.

Think of the Internet, which in some ways is a good model for the body. Connections can get lost, systems can crash, servers can go down, viruses and spyware can lurk, and because of the interconnectedness of everything, something that happens in one part of the system can have deep consequences in another. Although your body isn't as large as the Internet, it's certainly as complex.

Your computer can crash because of things that go wrong inside your actual desktop, but malfunctions can *also* happen because of outside influences (think virus and spyware, or electrical surges). On the simplest level, your computer won't work if there's an electrical outage in your neighborhood; it needs a steady supply of current just to get up and running. Similarly, we humans need a steady supply of outside energy to keep functioning at our best. At the most basic level, we need food, especially the right kind of food (which you'll read a lot about in this book).

On a more global level, we need social contacts and connections (see section III). Without them, we literally wither away and die no matter how good our "hardware" performs.

Although there are many theories of aging, and though scientists continue to debate the many metabolic pathways, organs, and genes that are undoubtedly involved, there are four specific processes that are unquestionably linked to the breakdown of systems within the body and that contribute not only to aging but also to virtually every degenerative disease known. When these processes wreak havoc on the eyes, you have dimming vision. When they work their mischief on the brain, you have memory loss. When they turn their collective attention to the circulatory system, you have heart disease. Understanding that these four processes have a hand in virtually every disease of aging can help us really get to the core of the issue and yield a much more productive approach than concentrating on the symptoms.

I'll give you an example.

Just as this was being written, I was interviewed by one of the biggest Internet portals in the world for an article on anti-aging. The reporter asked me typical questions that are on the mind of so many of us: "What can I do to protect my brain?" "Are there specific nutrients I can take or foods I can eat that will help protect my aging eyes?" and "What can I do/take/eat to keep my heart healthy?"

These are reasonable questions, and ones to which we'd all like some answers.

After all, heart disease and Alzheimer's are both in the top ten list of things that kill us, so who wouldn't want to protect the organs that are affected by them? But what disturbed me was that the questions were being framed as if the events that happen in the eyes or the brain or the heart are fundamentally *different* and require *different* interventions. Although there are undoubtedly issues that are specific to each body system—and we'll discuss those in section II—the bigger issue is *what all these age-related breakdowns have in common*!

And that's where the Four Horsemen of Aging come in.

THE FOUR HORSEMEN OF AGING

I've nicknamed the four dangerous processes that age our bodies "the Four Horsemen of Aging." Wherever something breaks down in the body—be it the brain, muscles, circulatory or immune system, you name it—you don't have to dig too deeply to find the handiwork of one or more of the Four Horsemen. These Four Horsemen *together* are probably responsible for the *bulk* of what happens to our bodies when they break down.

By now you're probably asking yourself, "What exactly are these horsemen he's talking about anyway?" Or, more to the point, "Why should I care?" And here's the answer: Anything that's happening in your body that you wish were not happening, from the beginnings of disease to the breakdown of systems to the loss of functionality, is being driven by the engine of these four processes.

The names of these processes may not yet be familiar to you, but guaranteed, they are behind the scenes of every disease of aging ever experienced by the human species.

So without further ado, allow me to introduce them to you:

1. Oxidative damage
2. Inflammation
3. Glycation
4. Stress

Many of the strategies I talk about in this book pertain to preventing or combating the damaging effects of these four processes. The four of them, collectively, can damage cells and DNA, wear down organs and systems, deeply damage the vascular pathways that deliver blood and oxygen to your entire body, and even shrink the size of your brain. They're involved in heart disease, cancer, diabetes, obesity, Alzheimer's, and cognitive decline, not to mention a host of "less serious" diseases that can vastly diminish the quality of your well-being.

Even though these four processes often overlap and work together to cause serious damage to both your physical health and your mental well-being, let's break them down into manageable chunks and tackle them one by one. In a short time it will be apparent how each contributes to the damage the other does, and how the same weapons—whole foods, nutrients, stress reduction, exercise, detoxification, relationship improvement, and the many other things we'll be discussing in this book— actually do double duty, effectively battling more than one of the four processes that effectively shorten your life.

So let's get started.

1

Fight the First Horseman of Aging: Free Radicals

I magine leaving your car outdoors in the rain for years without any protection. What would it look like? I'd say "junkyard ready."

If you looked underneath that car you'd probably find many areas that had rusted. That rusting is caused by *oxidative damage*. Preventing—or combating—oxidative damage (also known as *oxidative stress* or *oxidation* for short) is one of the major anti-aging strategies under your control, and you're more likely to do it if you understand why it's so important.

Here's how oxidative damage works in your body. You may remember from Chemistry 101 that every atom and molecule has electrons circling around it. These electrons like to fly around in pairs, which keeps the atoms and molecules nice and stable and balanced. But once in a while, one of those electrons breaks free—and that's when all the trouble starts.

Once one of the paired electrons breaks off, the molecule or atom where it *used* to reside is now running around with an unpaired single electron. The presence of that "unpaired" electron turns our formerly stable molecule into what is known as a *free radical*—the raging bull of molecules. It's not a happy camper. In fact, the free radical acts like a college kid on spring break without adult supervision—it literally goes wild looking for a "mate" for its newly separated electron.

If you're a man, you can think of a free radical as the obnoxious drunk single guy at your high school reunion who keeps trying to pick up your wife. (Women, just reverse the image!) The free radical starts "hitting" on every molecule it encounters, looking for another electron to steal away from a normal, stable molecule that still has all its electrons neatly paired up.

THE FIRST HORSEMAN OF AGING: FREE RADICALS

What they are:
Free radicals are dangerous molecules created from oxygen (sometimes called *oxygen free radicals* or *reactive oxygen species*).

Why they're bad for you:
These nasty rogue molecules attack your cells and damage your DNA and slowly "wear you down," aging you from within. This insidious damage is called *oxidation* and is similar to the *rusting* that happens when you leave metal out in the rain or the browning that happens when you leave apple slices out in the sun.

What you can do about them:
Eat plenty of vegetables and fruits, all high in antioxidants, and consider adding antioxidant supplements such as vitamin C, vitamin E, selenium, zinc, alpha-lipoic acid, and coenzyme Q10 to your diet.

The irony, of course, is that when it *does* finally steal an electron away from a stable molecule, that molecule becomes unstable itself and turns into a *free radical* (because it's now left with an unpaired electron). And the process begins again. The whole process is kind of like having a vampire on the loose: Each time a new victim gets bitten, it turns into a vampire and the whole sequence repeats. Anti-aging expert Ron Rothenberg, M.D., has a clever name for the sequence: He calls it "Cellular World War lll."

Every time these free radicals "hit" on your cells looking for a mate for their unpaired electron, they damage the cells. This cumulative damage is a huge part of aging. "If the DNA is damaged when the cell divides to make new cells, the copies will be wrong and whatever function that cell performs will not be done correctly," Rothenberg says.

If "aging" is another name for "breakdown," then you can see immediately why free radicals age us. Cells break down, organ systems don't function as well, DNA becomes damaged, DNA replication—an incredibly complex and delicate, enzyme-dependent process—doesn't happen efficiently, and DNA can become mutated. When this kind of damage accumulates in the body it contributes to all sorts of disorders typical of aging. For example, when it accumulates in the heart or vascular system, you have heart disease. When it accumulates in the skin, you have aging skin.

There's not a disease of aging in which free radical damage is not an important component. That's why fighting free radical damage is such a running theme throughout this book, and why you'll be hearing the term "antioxidants" in virtually every chapter.

THE FREE RADICAL THEORY OF AGING

The role of free radicals in aging has been recognized at least since the 1950s, when an innovative scientist (and 1995 Nobel Prize nominee) named Denham Harman, M.D., Ph.D., proposed the *free radical theory of aging*. Harman believed that as go the cells, so goes the body; if our cells age, our whole body ages (which makes perfect sense because we are, after all, made up of nothing but cells). Harman saw aging as the cellular accumulation of free radical damage over time—that our bodies are essentially "rusting from within."

Years later, the free radical theory of aging was expanded to include not just aging, but degenerative diseases in general. We now know that oxidative damage plays a major role in every degenerative disease of aging, from Alzheimer's and cancer to heart disease and diabetes and even immune dysfunction.[1, 2, 3, 4, 5, 6]

AVOID ENVIRONMENTAL FREE RADICALS BY GOING ORGANIC

There are several sources of free radicals, including the environment. Tobacco smoke, air pollution, pesticides, herbicides, contaminants in our water; all of these form free radicals—which we then take into our body by breathing, drinking, and eating—that contribute to the aging process and the diseases that kill us. This is what we mean when we talk of a "toxic environment" (and this is why I consider *detoxification* one of the "Seven Pillars of Longevity"—more on this later).

People who are constantly assaulted by these environmental free radicals—and who don't have good defenses against them—tend to age badly. The free radicals come into our body and attack our cells. They destroy genetic material, damage and mutate DNA, burden the immune system, and virtually destroy a cell's identity. The damage is enormous, and it's a huge part of what ages us.

Some of the obvious sources of free radicals—tobacco smoke, pesticides, and certain chemicals—are also sources of cancer-causing chemicals called *carcinogens*. The combination is lethal to anyone wanting to live in optimal health for nine or more decades. Smoking, for example, creates free radicals that damage the lungs *and* just for good measure, exposes us to carcinogenic chemicals. Tobacco smoke is literally a turbo-charged free radical factory on steroids.

Then there are the pesticides sprayed on crops. "Pesticides kill the pest by *creating* free radicals," says Hari Sharma, M.D., a fellow of the Royal College of Physicians and Surgeons and a consultant to the National Institutes of Health. "If you consume them, you will be damaged by those free radicals, also." At least fifty-three carcinogenic (cancer-causing) pesticides are applied in large amounts to

the major food crops, according to a study by the U.S. Food and Drug Administration. In 2005, for example, 73 percent of fresh vegetables and fruits contained pesticide residues, as did 61 percent of processed fruits and vegetables, 22 percent of soybeans, 75 percent of wheat, a whopping 99 percent of milk and cream, and 16 percent of bottled water. [7]

It gets worse. The Centers for Disease Control and Prevention tested for 116 pesticides and other artificial chemicals in the blood and urine of 2,500 volunteers and found detectable levels of 89 chemicals, including pesticides, phthalates, herbicides, pest repellants, and disinfectants.[8,9] And a 2006 study by the Environmental Working Group uncovered the "dirty dozen" of fruits and vegetables that it assessed to be the most contaminated of all. (See the sidebar on page 20 for a list of the dirty dozen.)[10] "The effects of these chemicals may be difficult to separate from normally mildly debilitating aspects of the aging process," says professor Harvey Blatt of the Institute of Earth Sciences at Hebrew University of Jerusalem.

Go Organic to Fight Environmental Free Radicals

Choosing organic foods is especially important with foods that are known to have a high level of contamination. The following foods, according to the Environmental Working Group (EWG), have the highest level of contaminants of forty-seven tested fruits and vegetables. They're known as "the dirty dozen."

→ Peaches

→ Apples

→ Bell peppers

→ Celery

→ Nectarines

→ Strawberries

→ Cherries

→ Pears

→ Grapes

→ Spinach

→ Lettuce

→ Potatoes

Although the following aren't in the EWG's list, which deals only with produce, I'd personally add the following three items to my "should buy organic" list. Meat and milk can be heavily laced with antibiotics, steroids, and growth hormone, and coffee is a widely sprayed crop.

→ Meat

→ Milk

→ Coffee

This is the primary reason for recommending organic foods as part of an anti-aging lifestyle. Although studies have been mixed about whether the nutritional content of organic food is any greater than that of conventionally grown food, the primary reason for eating organic food is to avoid the intake of the chemicals used in nonorganic farming.

AGING FREE RADICALS FROM OUR OWN BODIES

The environment isn't the only source of these toxic free radicals. Our bodies are a virtual free radical *factory*. Now why in the world would you produce free radicals in your body, you might ask, especially because these are such dangerous and health-robbing compounds?

Good question, and the answer is simple: All free radicals aren't bad.

Our immune system, for example, produces free radicals to help protect us from harmful microorganisms and fight infections. The very process of creating energy—respiratory metabolism, or in simpler terms, *breathing*—creates free radicals. Free radicals can help activate enzymes and produce hormones. The problem arises when the *amount* of free radicals in our body is excessive and out of control. Then the damage significantly outweighs the benefits.

Although free radicals can search for that extra electron anywhere, they cause the most damage when they are derived from oxygen. Yup, oxygen—the stuff you breathe and without which you couldn't live for more than a few moments. But oxygen has a dark side. Oxygen free radicals are actually one of the most damaging kinds on the planet. When oxygen molecules are the ones that give up their electrons, we're in big trouble. It's like those wild unpaired electrons decided to pick on the biggest, toughest guy in the schoolyard—and mayhem ensues. (To use the earlier analogy, imagine that drunk guy at the high school reunion hitting on Mike Tyson's date!) Free radicals derived from oxygen are known collectively as *reactive oxygen species*, and they are a virtual aging factory.

Oxygen-derived radicals are a normal part of aerobic metabolism, so they're constantly being formed. In fact, anywhere there's oxygen, there are oxygen free radicals. Doing some aerobic exercise? You're making oxygen free radicals! Just breathing? Oxygen free radicals! White blood cells are especially talented at producing oxygen free radicals, which they then use as a defense against invading microbes. But all those toxins from the environment that we spoke about earlier also have oxidizing effects on cells

and produce tons of oxygen free radicals. So does radiation, which actually produces the most damage in tissues that have a heavy concentration of oxygen (we call these heavily oxidized tissues).

Another way free radicals age us is through their effect on DNA. You may remember from high school biology that your DNA is kind of like your own individual genetic instruction manual. It's found in every cell and it's like a set of master blueprints that tell every *other* cell what to do. When free radicals attack the DNA in your cells, they screw up their ability to replicate properly and pass on their instructions. This kind of DNA damage eventually shortens your DNA strands and triggers a process called *apoptosis*, or "programmed cell death." It's as if you were passing on a repair manual that constantly got dropped in the dirt, burned at the edges, or dropped in the water and finally became so worn that anyone trying to use it couldn't read the words anymore and had to guess what was written on the page. A mechanic relying on a manual like that couldn't be counted on to do a good job with your car, and DNA that's been damaged like that doesn't do a good job of repairing and rebuilding your cells, tissues, and organs. The result? What we know as aging!

But wait, there's more!

Protect Your Cells with the Best Fats

I recommend that you consume healthy oils every day to strengthen cells so they can fight off free radicals. In addition to fish oil, use oils such as walnut oil, flaxseed oil, macadamia nut oil or almond oil as part of salad dressings. Macadamia oil and coconut oil are particularly good for cooking. Remember that oils are high in calories, so if you're looking to lose weight, keep it down to 1–2 tablespoons per use.

Oils

→ Fish oil (in capsules or liquid): 1,000–4,000 mg a day

→ For the remaining oils, see portion recommendations above.

→ Flaxseed oil (do not cook with it)

→ Extra-virgin olive oil

→ Walnut oil

→ Almond oil

→ Macadamia nut oil

→ Coconut oil

Anti-Aging Foods High in Fat

→ All nuts: ½ ounce–1 ounce, up to five times a week, is great!

→ Avocado: Use in salads or guacamole.

→ Cold-water fish, such as wild Alaskan salmon, tuna, mackerel, and sardines: Eat at least twice a week, more if you can!

→ Yogurt: A good "daily" food. Avoid the no-fat kind because it contains too much sugar.

Do Not Fear Saturated Fats from Whole Foods

→ Eggs

→ Butter

→ Grass-fed meat

→ Coconut and coconut oil

→ Raw, organic milk

EAT THE RIGHT FATS FOR FLEXIBILITY

One of the best-known toxic effects of oxygen free radicals is the damage to cellular membranes. Nothing will age you faster than an assault on your cell membranes, even though it takes place under the radar and even though you can't see it (except with a microscope). Why? *Because the membranes are critical to cell health*—they're what hold the cell together. Cell membranes have to be flexible enough to allow information to pass in and out, but stiff enough so that they don't collapse. They're delicate structures. (One of the reasons trans fats are so harmful is that they damage the cell membrane.)

Cell membranes are made up largely of fats (lipids) called *phospholipids*, and the oxidative damage done to cell membranes is called *lipid peroxidation*. The fats that are most vulnerable to this kind of oxidative damage are the very fats we've been told to eat *more* of—unsaturated fats like vegetable oil. (Check out the box at left for the best fats to eat for anti-aging.) Those fats are much more susceptible to oxidative damage than the more stable (and stiffer) saturated fats. A paradox, but it's completely true. Does that mean we shouldn't eat unsaturated fats? No. But it *does* mean they need special protection in the form of antioxidants if we're going to get their full benefit.

The vulnerability of unstable fats to oxidative damage is actually the reason why health practitioners always recommend a little vitamin E with your fish oil. Fish oil, one of the healthiest, most anti-aging compounds on the planet, is nonetheless made up of delicate fatty acids extremely vulnerable to damage from both heat and oxygen (that's why you can't cook with either fish oil or flaxseed oil). Vitamin E is a powerful antioxidant and will protect the delicate structures of the omega-3 fatty acids in fish (and flax). We'll discuss this at greater length later on.

Lipid peroxidation—the damage to cell membranes caused by oxygen free radicals—can have a number of effects, none of them good. It can make the membranes stiffer. It can decrease the activity of enzymes that are bound in the membranes. It can alter the activity of membrane receptors. Ultimately, on the cellular level, lipid peroxidation ages you from the inside out.

To me, one of the most God-awful missteps made by conventional medicine and conventional public health policy has been to focus on cholesterol lowering as an anti-aging strategy when in fact the big risk factors for disease are oxidative damage and inflammation. Cholesterol itself doesn't do any damage in the body at all—until it's *oxidized*. When cholesterol just sits there minding its own business, it is perfectly harmless. Only when it gets attacked by oxygen free radicals does it become a problem.

If we could prevent the oxidation of cholesterol by fighting off free radical damage, as well as preventing or reversing the inflammation that nearly always accompanies this oxidative damage, we'd be sitting pretty. Oxidized cholesterol is indeed a health risk, but blaming poor cholesterol is like blaming the St. Bernard for the avalanche.

FREE THE RADICALS FROM YOUR BODY

By now it should be pretty apparent that there's no aging without free radical damage, and there's no way to fight the effects of aging without a strong army to fight off that damage. If your body didn't have any built-in defenses against the constant assault of free radicals, you probably wouldn't be here reading this book. In fact, you'd be quite dead.

Fortunately, nature hardwired into our DNA the ability to make chemicals that help protect the cells against

When a cook slices up some apples, she'll often squeeze some lemon juice over them. Left alone without that protection, the apple slices will turn brown—that's oxidation (or oxidative damage) in action. But the lemon juice contains powerful antioxidants, including vitamin C, and thus apple slices "protected" with this antioxidant will survive in the air a lot longer without changing color. You can try this for yourself. It's the perfect home science project for demonstrating the protective power of antioxidants in the real world.

Your body has some powerful antioxidants of its own. At the top of the list is one called *coenzyme Q10*, which is found in every cell (and discussed in greater length in chapter 7, on the heart). Another is called *superoxide dismutase* (SOD), an enzyme that repairs cells and reduces damage done by one of the most common (and damaging) oxygen free radicals in the body—*superoxide*. (If you're interested, SOD works its magic by breaking down the harmful superoxide into two harmless components—oxygen and hydrogen peroxide. Now you know.) Rounding out this native superstar trio is *glutathione,* arguably the most important antioxidant in the body.

oxidative damage. These chemicals are called—can you guess?—*anti*oxidants.

An antioxidant works by exactly the mechanism you might imagine from its name—by fighting oxidation. It donates one of its own electrons to the rogue molecule, essentially rendering it impotent and unable to do any damage. You've probably used the power of antioxidants yourself without realizing it.

When cholesterol just sits there minding its own business, it is perfectly harmless.
Only when it gets attacked by oxygen free radicals does it become a problem.

"These built-in antioxidants keep us alive through the reproductive age," explains Rothenberg.

But there's one big problem. They can't keep up with the workload. Our internal antioxidants become less effective as we age, especially when we live in an environment that assaults us with free radicals on a daily basis.[11] "After 30, these *built-in* antioxidants cannot keep up with the cellular damage that has been produced by free radicals," says Rothenberg.

But fortunately, there's help out there.

ANTIOXIDANTS IN FOOD AND PILLS

If you've read my book, *The 150 Healthiest Foods on Earth*, you probably know that one of the biggest benefits of many of the foods I consider to be among the healthiest in the world is that they are absolutely loaded with antioxidants (and natural anti-inflammatories). Plants have their own built-in protection against the oxidative damage of the sun, and these built-in protectors function as cell protectors in our bodies. The very pigments that make blueberries blue and raspberries red protect those berries from oxidative

ANTI-AGING ACTION PLAN:
How to Get Your Antioxidants— and Get Rid of Your Free Radicals

Take Antioxidant Supplements
→ Vitamin C: 500–2,000 mg
→ Gamma-tocopherol vitamin E (or mixed tocopherols): 400 IUs
→ Pycnogenol: 100 mg
→ Grapeseed extract: 100–200 mg
→ Alpha-lipoic acid: 100 mg or more
→ Selenium: 100–200 mcg
→ Zinc: 15–50 mg

Eat Antioxidant and Anti-Inflammatory- Rich Foods
→ Berries (wild blueberries, raspberries, blackberries, strawberries, cranberries, etc.): Consume daily. A serving is ½–1 cup.
→ Apples: True to the old saying, one a day.
→ Prunes: Three times a week or as part of your morning meal.

→ Green leafy vegetables: As often as possible.
→ Brassica vegetables (broccoli, Brussels sprouts, cabbage): As often as possible.
→ Beans (red beans, kidney beans, pinto beans): Three times a week.
→ Wild salmon (especially sockeye): At least twice a week.
→ Tea (all kinds): Daily.
→ Pomegranate juice: Drink 4–8 ounces daily.
→ Spices (ginger, turmeric, cinnamon, cloves, oregano). Use as often as possible.
→ Herbs: Use as often as possible.
→ Cocoa (or dark chocolate with 60–80 percent cocoa content): Weekly.

Avoid These Foods
→ Sugar and high-sugar foods
→ Trans-fatty acids (trans fats)

WHICH FOODS CONTAIN ANTIOXIDANTS

CLASS/COMPONENTS	REPRESENTATIVE SOURCES	POTENTIAL ANTI-AGING BENEFIT
Carotenoids		
Beta-carotene	Carrots, red pepper, sweet potato, kale, spinach	Neutralizes aging free radicals
Lutein, zeaxanthin	Kale, spinach, turnip greens, collard greens	Helps protect aging eyes and may help vision
Lycopene	Tomatoes, guava, watermelon	Helps protect against prostate cancer
Flavonoids		
Anthocyanidins	Berries, dark grapes, cherries	Boosts antioxidant defenses and may help protect aging brain
Flavonols: catechins, epicatechins, procyanidins	Tea, chocolate, cocoa, apples, grapes	Helps protect aging heart
Flavanones	Citrus fruits	Neutralizes aging-related free radicals
Flavonols	Onions, apples, tea, broccoli	Neutralizes aging-related free radicals
Proanthocyanidins	Cranberries, peanuts, wine, grapes, strawberries, apples, cocoa	Helps protect urinary tract and heart from damage
Isothiocyanates		
Sulforaphane	Broccoli, broccoli sprouts, cabbage, kale, cauliflower	Enhances detoxification of toxins, boosts antioxidant defenses
Phenols		
Caffeic acid, ferulic acid	Apples, pears, citrus fruits, coffee (caffeic acid)	Powerful antioxidants; caffeic acid is a carcinogenic (cancer) inhibitor
Sulfides/Thiols		
Diallyl sulfide, allyl methyl trisulfide	Garlic, leeks, scallions, onions	Enhances detoxification of toxins, supports heart and immune function in aging body
Dithiolthiones	Cruciferous vegetables: broccoli, cabbage, collards, bok choy	Supports immune system

Adapted from the International Food Information Council Foundation:
Media Guide on Food Safety and Nutrition: 2004–2006.

damage, and they do the same for you once inside your body. This is probably one of the many reasons for the greater health and longevity of people who regularly consume tons of fruits and vegetables.

The most famous of the powerhouse antioxidants are vitamin C and vitamin E, but that's only the beginning of the list. Vitamin A is an antioxidant. Minerals like zinc and selenium are powerful antioxidants, as are dozens, perhaps hundreds, of plant compounds known as *phytochemicals*. Quercetin, for example, a member of the flavonoid family, is found in apples and onions and has tremendous antioxidant activity. So does curcumin, a phytochemical found in turmeric, the spice that makes Indian food yellow. Spices in general are a tremendous source of antioxidants, as we'll see later. And nutrients rarely found in any appreciable amount in food, such as alpha-lipoic acid, are also tremendous weapons in the battle against oxidative damage.

One study of healthy centenarians from four different geographical areas found that in at least three of them, blood levels of vitamin A and vitamin E seemed to be important for longevity.[12] Another study, published in *Free Radical Biological Medicine* in April 2000 concluded that "it is evident that healthy centenarians show a particular profile in which high levels of vitamin A and vitamin E seem to be important in guaranteeing their extreme longevity."[13] While these studies, and others like them, don't mean that you can stave off aging just by popping a couple of supplements, they do strongly suggest that optimizing your antioxidant stores —propping up your internal defenses against the aging effects of free radical damage—is a big part of any strategy for living longer. It's no accident that every anti-aging clinic in the world routinely recommends high levels of antioxidant supplementation in its programs.

TEAM PLAYERS

Scientists have discovered a novel way to assess the antioxidant "power" of foods. It's called the ORAC test. Usually, when I write articles about the ORAC test I don't bother to tell people what it stands for because it's complicated and hard to explain in a short magazine article. But it's going to make complete sense to you because of the material we've already covered. Ready?

ORAC stands for *oxygen radical absorbance capacity*. Sure, it's a mouthful, but we already know what oxygen free radicals are—those really bad actors also known as free radicals. So the ORAC test basically looks to see how effective foods are at mopping up these suckers, hence the "absorbance capacity." The ORAC test is similar to what you see in those television commercials for paper towels—the best performers are the ones that soak up the junk more effectively!

Why, you might ask, don't the scientists just measure vitamins C and E and all those other antioxidants in the food and be done with it? Good question, and the answer is an important key to anti-aging eating strategies in general.

Number one, there are probably hundreds of antioxidants we don't even know about. The plant chemicals called *flavonoids*, for example, have more than 4,000 members, and many of these act as antioxidants. Sure, we could measure the best-known antioxidants, but that wouldn't necessarily present a complete picture of the food's true age-fighting potential, because it might miss many of the most important antioxidants not being tested. (Not to mention that a specific test for each individual antioxidant is expensive!)

Number two, and even more important, is a mysterious thing called *synergy*. Vitamins, minerals, phytochemicals, and nutrients in general work in mysterious ways, which is one reason hard-nosed scientists sometimes have trouble isolating and "proving" their effects. Actually, it's not really mysterious at all when you think about it. There is something about *groups* that's different than the individual members, and there is something in a *food* that's different from the sum total of its individual components.

Sometimes a particular nutrient only becomes beneficial when it's in the presence of *another* nutrient on which it depends to do its job. Recent research, for example, has shown that vitamin D protects against colon cancer—unless your levels of vitamin A are too high, in which case the protective effect of vitamin D disappears. Sometimes two (or three) nutrients work together synergistically, like calcium, magnesium, and vitamin D, which, together, offer a substantial measure of protection for aging bones.

Sometimes a nutrient's "good deeds" depends on being in an environment provided by the rest of the components in the food, and without these, the isolated nutrient doesn't "perform" as well. (An example: The vision-enhancing carotenoids *lutein* and *zeaxanthin* are only absorbed properly when they're consumed with some fat.)

Because of this synergistic effect, it's much more useful to look at the food itself and see how it performs, with all its components, in fighting free radicals. The best example of this is a rock and roll band. I'll bet most of you can name at least one great album by the Rolling Stones. A Mick Jagger solo album? Not so much. Same thing with a championship basketball team, a superb doubles team in tennis, or even a pair of figure skaters. The team may have the ability to perform together better than the individuals can perform alone.

So in the ORAC test, scientists take whole foods and test them against various oxygen free radicals of the nastiest kind. They look to see which foods mop up those unfriendly, age-robbing, cell-destroying free radicals the most effectively, and rate those foods, giving them a number that is, not surprisingly, called their ORAC value.

Here are the ORAC values and rankings for the top-scoring antioxidant-containing fruits as tested by scientists at the U.S. Department of Agriculture[14] (all values are for about 3½ ounces):

1.	Prunes	5770
2.	Raisins	2830
3.	Blueberries	2400
4.	Blackberries	2036
5.	Kale	1770
6.	Strawberries	1540
7.	Spinach	1290
8.	Raspberries	1220

9.	Yellow squash	1159
10.	Brussels sprouts	980
11.	Plums	949
12.	Alfalfa sprouts	930
13.	Broccoli florets	890
14.	Beets	840
15.	Oranges	750
16.	Red grapes	739
17.	Red bell pepper	710
18.	Cherries	670
19.	Kiwifruit	610
20.	Pink grapefruit	495
21.	Kidney beans	460
22.	Onion	450
23.	Corn	400
24.	Eggplant	390

No big surprise, right? And nothing you need to memorize. In fact, you'll pretty much cover all the antioxidant bases by simply following one of the smartest overall pieces of nutritional advice for anti-aging I ever heard, all the more elegant because of its utter simplicity: *Shop so your grocery basket looks colorful.* In fact, if your pile on the checkout counter at the market looks like one of those gorgeous postcards of a European outdoor farmers' market, you're in good shape. You will automatically be eating a ton of high-antioxidant (high-ORAC) foods that will help protect you from a virtual encyclopedia of syndromes and diseases associated with aging.

RATINGS, RATINGS, WHO'S GOT RATINGS?

Of course, the ORAC rating is not the only way scientists assess the anti-aging power of foods. After all, there are lots of different oxygen free radicals to test foods with, and other aging compounds as well, leading to a whole host of complicated lab tests that put foods and beverages in the ring with the enemies of aging and see who survives the best.

One popular lab test is called TAC*, or total antioxidant capacity. Look at the results for the top twenty foods in TAC and see whether you notice any interesting similarities to the ORAC test:

1.	Small red bean (dried)	½ cup	13727
2.	Wild blueberry	1 cup	13427
3.	Red kidney bean (dried)	½ cup	13259
4.	Pinto bean	½ cup	11864
5.	Blueberry (cultivated)	1 cup	9019
6.	Cranberry	1 cup (whole)	8983
7.	Artichoke (cooked)	1 cup (hearts)	7904
8.	Blackberry	1 cup	7701
9.	Dried prune	½ cup	7291
10.	Raspberry	1 cup	6058
11.	Strawberry	1 cup	5938
12.	Red Delicious apple	1	5900
13.	Granny Smith apple	1	5381
14.	Pecan	1 ounce	5095
15.	Sweet cherry	1 cup	4873
16.	Black plum	1	4844
17.	Russet potato (cooked)	1	4649
18.	Black bean (dried)	½ cup	4181
19.	Plum	1	4118
20.	Gala apple	1	3903

* Source: *Journal of Agriculture and Food Chemistry*, June 9, 2004. Also *Newswise Science News*: www.newswise.com/articles/view/505608/

ANTI–AGING ACTION PLAN:

Eat Wild Salmon to Fight Oxidative Damage

Wild Alaskan salmon is the perfect anti-aging food. It's not only loaded with anti-inflammatory omega-3 properties, but it also contains a powerful and little-known antioxidant called *astaxanthin*, which is what gives salmon its natural red color. (Farmed salmon get their color from artificial coloring and chemicals.)

Wild Alaskan salmon from pristine sources is remarkably free of mercury as well as PCBs, a particularly nasty chemical that has been found in high amounts in farmed salmon. Farmed salmon eat a diet of grains, which makes their fat content much higher in inflammatory omega-6s—not so for the wild kind. Plus, wild Alaskan salmon is free of the antibiotics that are routinely fed to salmon raised in crowded pens on a salmon farm.

Like many health professionals, including Andrew Weil, M.D., Nicholas Perricone, M.D., Joseph Mercola, D.O., and Christiane Northrup, M.D., I recommend the absolute best source in the world for salmon and fish: Vital Choice. I have a link to this terrific company, located in Alaska, on my website, www.jonnybowden.com, and the company even has a *Dr. Jonny Starter Pack*, consisting of my personal favorites. Once you've tasted real pristine Alaskan salmon you'll never settle for the average kind again.

Check out the following recipe for salmon from my book *The Healthiest Meals on Earth*, cowritten by my friend Jeanette Bessinger.

BROILED SALMON WITH TAMARI-ORANGE MARINADE

Prep Time: 10 minutes, then marinate for 4 to 6 hours
Cook Time: 10 to 15 minutes

Ingredients

1½ pounds (680 g) wild Alaskan salmon fillet, cut into 4 equal portions,
or four 6-ounce (186-g) salmon steaks

⅓ cup (80 ml) high-quality dry white wine, such as Chardonnay,
or medium sweet wine, such as Riesling

2 tablespoons (30 ml) low-sodium tamari

⅓ cup (80 ml) orange juice (fresh squeezed is best; about 1 large juice orange)

3 tablespoons (24 g) peeled and fnely grated ginger

¼ cup (25 g) finely chopped green onions

1 teaspoon raw honey

½ teaspoon extra virgin olive oil

Rinse the salmon gently in water and pat to dry.

In a small bowl, combine the wine, tamari, orange juice, ginger, scallions, and honey, and whisk to combine well.

Place the salmon in a shallow glass baking pan, skin side down If fillet, and pour the marinade evenly on top.

Cover the baking pan with plastic wrap and refrigerate for 4 to 6 hours or overnight, tipping the dish occasionally to recoat the salmon.

Remove the baking pan from the refrigerator and let it stand at room temperature for 30 minutes. Preheat the broiler.

Lift the salmon out of the baking pan and remove any ginger or scallions to prevent burning. Rub the oil on the skin/bottom side of the salmon and place it on the broiling pan, oiled side down.

Broil the salmon under high heat for 10 to 15 minutes, until the salmon flakes easily with a fork and the flesh inside is firm and light pink. The top should lightly brown and caramelize. (If the salmon browns within the first 5 minutes, move the broiling pan down 1 rack in your oven.)

Yield: 4 servings

From *The Healthiest Meals on Earth* by Jonny Bowden and Jeannette Bessinger (Fair Wisnds Press, 2008)

It's worth pointing out that there are several different versions of these tests for antioxidant power, depending on exactly which of the bad guys the scientists decide to throw into the pit. In other scientific tests, spinach, peppers, and asparagus have come out on top, while in almost any version of the test berries score at or near the top of the heap for fruits. In one test of "soft beverages," grapefruit juice came out the winner, and—good news for Starbucks lovers—coffee scored at the top of the heap in antioxidant capacity among alcohol, teas, and coffee (though tea was definitely in the top ten).[15]

If you're confused by the difference in the numbers and ratings between the two tests, don't be. These tests use completely different rating systems, and the actual numbers don't matter as much as the *rankings*. The ratings of the foods will also vary depending on where they were grown and at what time of year. The point is that the same foods tend to show up on everyone's list. You can't go wrong eating a diet rich in foods from the top ten to twenty of either of these lists, regardless of which particular test was used to generate it.

So what's interesting about all this—and what the takeaway message should be—is that these lists of foods look as similar as the "ten best" lists of different movie

critics at the end of any given year. Sure, there's some differences depending on the test, but the top winners show up on everyone's list (or in this case, on every version of the test). It's a safe bet that *any* of the foods from the leafy green vegetable family, the brassica family (Brussels sprouts, cabbage, broccoli), *any* beans and legumes, or *any* brightly colored vegetables and fruits are going to contain a whopping number of antioxidants that will help your body fight off the damaging, aging effects of free radical attacks.

Recent research from the Agricultural Research Service[16] investigated the effects of antioxidants on after-meal "oxidative stress." In it, volunteers first drank a shake containing carbohydrates, protein, and fat, but no antioxidants. Sure enough, they produced blood samples with a reduced ability to counter noxious free radicals.

Not good.

"We're learning that antioxidants should be consumed with every meal," says Ronald Prior, a chemist who was the lead researcher on the study. "And if you routinely skip antioxidants in your diet, over time, the excess number of free radicals being produced may begin damaging cellular components, ultimately leading to atherosclerosis, cancer, and other diseases." In other words, all the diseases of aging.

But here's where it gets interesting. The researchers also found something that absolutely qualifies as usable information that you can apply right now in your fight against aging and disease: Consuming *grapes* with that same test meal *prevented* the decline in antioxidant capacity.

Of course, it's not just grapes, though they're high in antioxidants and were used in this research. It can be any antioxidant-rich food or foods—vegetables and fruits being the most obvious. In other research, Prior found that grapes, kiwi, and wild blueberries were high performers when it came to raising blood levels of important antioxidants. Adding high-antioxidant foods, whether a portion of grapes or a couple of servings of vegetables, seems to act as a kind of damage control button even when you eat a bad meal. When you eat those foods as part of a *good* meal, it's even better.

Bottom line: If you can pluck it or gather it—if it's a food you could eat straight from the ground or right off a tree or a bush—it's probably good for you. These are the foods that make up a large part of the diet of virtually every one of the longest-lived and healthiest populations on the planet.

OH, MY AGING SKIN

Much of what we consider "aging" skin is really the accumulation of oxidative (free radical) damage.

"The unstable free radical molecules vibrate in the skin, literally poking holes in the collagen fibers of the dermis," explains Michael N. Chang, Ph.D., the former deputy director of medical chemistry at Merck. Collagen is the main protein in connective tissue, and over the years, under continuous assault from free radicals, it basically becomes weaker and weaker, eventually causing the skin to wrinkle.

"Every day each skin cell can be exposed to more than 73,000 damaging assaults," says Chang. And it doesn't help that the skin is an external organ. As the first line of defense against any environmental elements, it's often the first and most visually obvious place that we age. In fact, you can think of the skin, especially the face, as a marker for the kind of damage that free radicals are doing inside the body. (Not always a pretty picture, is it?)

I can tell you about free radical damage on a cellular level from now to doomsday, but because you can't see it, it doesn't seem real. So think of your face as a kind of "visual aid" in this lesson. If you find yourself noticing wrinkles, scars, lines, and the like, consider that the exact same thing is happening inside, where you can't see it. And free radical damage is aging you inside just as sure as it's aging your face—only sometimes with much worse consequences. (A wrinkle on your face may hurt your vanity, but free radical damage to the heart and vascular system will shorten your life.)

It's no coincidence that the hottest thing in skin care products are antioxidant-rich creams. Antioxidants can easily be absorbed through the skin, which is why the best of these creams can actually help you look better. Antioxidants in the diet and on the skin are a great defense against damage, inside *and* out.

OH, MY AGING EYES

There's not a baby boomer alive who doesn't know this feeling—all of a sudden you can't see items on the menu, or read the movie times in the paper or the ingredients on a bottle. Boomers everywhere nod understandingly when a fellow boomer says, "Hold on, I can't see it without my glasses."

Everybody winds up needing reading glasses eventually (at least if he or she wants to read). That's a fact of life that no diet or exercise or lifestyle program can change. Here's why: As they die, all cells are carried away by the bloodstream (or sloughed off in the skin or cut off in the hair). But in the eyes, these cells have nowhere to go, because the lens is in a capsule. As you live longer, more and more cells get trapped inside there and the capsule gets more crowded and stiff. By the time you're forty or forty-five, you can't "flex" the lens, or focus it enough, for close reading. So you need glasses.

The condition just described is called *presbyopia*, and truth be told, it's no big deal. That's not the aspect of aging eyes we're concerned with. After all, you just whip out a pair of those cool drugstore glasses that every boomer carries around, and you're good to go. There's a far more serious kind of aging disease that affects the eyes—it's called *macular degeneration*.

The reason I'm bringing this up now will be clear in a moment. Read on.

Macular degeneration is the leading cause of vision loss and blindness in Americans aged sixty-five and older. It produces a slow, or rarely, sudden, painless loss of vision. Symptoms include seeing shadowy areas in your central vision or experiencing unusual fuzzy or distorted vision. When it comes to "aging eyes," macular degeneration is the real problem, much more serious than a minor problem that can be addressed with some fashionable reading glasses.

In 2001, the National Eye Institute conducted the Age-Related Eye Disease Study (AREDS) involving more than 3,600 people. The researchers found that *supplementation with certain nutrients* reduced the risk of progressing to advanced macular degeneration by 28 percent. What you eat profoundly affects the macula, that small sensitive part of the retina responsible for detailed vision. Many experts feel strongly that diet and supplements can be used to treat or prevent its degeneration.

Want to know what those nutrients are? I'm sure you can guess by now: *antioxidants*.

The specific daily amounts of antioxidants and zinc used by the study researchers were 500 milligrams of vitamin C, 400 IU of vitamin E, 15 milligrams of beta-carotene (often labeled as equivalent to 25,000 IU of vitamin A), 80 milligrams of zinc, and 2 milligrams of copper. (Copper was added to the AREDS formulations containing zinc to prevent copper deficiency anemia, a condition associated with high levels of zinc intake.) Since the time of the study, experts now consider the carotenoids lutein and zeaxanthin to be essential to the protection of the eyes, largely through their ability to fight free radical damage in that area.

"Lutein and zeaxanthin were not used in the original AREDS study, but have since been found to be among the most effective supplements for eye health," E. Michael Geiger, O.D., author of *Eye Care Naturally* told me recently. Both are powerful antioxidants.

Since the ARED study came out, published research has shown that omega-3 fatty acids also help prevent macular degeneration. At the same time, consumption of omega-6 fatty acids, prevalent in vegetable oils, was associated with an *increased* risk of developing the condition. The reason for this finding brings us to the second major component of every single disease of aging and the focus of the next chapter: *inflammation*.

2

Put out the Fire of the Second Horseman of Aging: Inflammation

If you've ever stubbed your toe, banged your head against a beam, or gotten a splinter or an abscess on your skin, you know what inflammation is. The affected area gets red and swollen. Why? Because the body immediately sends blood and fluid into the area. White blood cells—also known as *leukocytes*—mobilize to the injury site, surrounding it like an army blocking off an invading force. Specialized white blood cells called *macrophages* (from the Greek, meaning "big eaters") act like little Pac Men, initiating defense mechanisms and literally swallowing up and immobilizing any invading pathogens.

All these activities, which your body does automatically as part of its immune defenses, are collectively called *inflammation*. (The Cleveland Clinic offers a great definition of inflammation: "[The] process by which the body's white blood cells and chemicals protect us from infection and foreign substances such as bacteria and viruses.") So inflammation isn't really a bad thing; we actually *need* inflammatory chemicals in our body, and the ability to mobilize them effectively is an integral part of the body's inborn healing responses.

"Inflammation is one of the things that keeps us alive in a hostile world," writes my great friend Barry Sears, Ph.D., creator of the world-famous Zone diet and author of *The Anti-Inflammation Zone*. "Without inflammation we would be sitting ducks in a very hostile world, with no way to repair the damage constantly being inflicted on us. Our internal inflammatory responses let us attack (the) invaders, surround them, and ultimately kill them before they kill us."

The problem is that our inflammatory army is in overdrive.

A WORLD OUT OF BALANCE

Imagine, for example, that your blood clotted too easily. You'd be at increased risk for a stroke, because blood clots can easily travel to the brain and cut off the supply of oxygen. (This is the reason why so many older adults are on anti-clotting meds such as Coumadin, and why their clotting factors are monitored so closely.) But consider if you *didn't* have the ability to clot *at all*—you'd hemorrhage every time you cut your finger!

Clearly, a healthy body is able to *balance* the ability to clot blood effectively and appropriately and enable blood to run effortlessly through the vascular system, producing so-called "good circulation." If either of these processes, clotting or blood flow, were unnaturally weighted in one direction, you'd be in trouble.

It's exactly the same with inflammation. We need inflammation to heal—we want those white blood cells rushing to the site of injury. But we *also* need *anti-inflammatory* compounds to act as correctives when there's *too much* inflammation. We need our body's anti-inflammatory army to be just as strong and active and robust as our inflammatory army. "It's the internal anti-inflammatory response that not only turns off the attack phase of inflammation but also generates the repair processes that lead to cellular rejuvenation," says Sears. Bottom line: Inflammation and anti-inflammation forces need to be in a constant balance, or else we're in trouble.

Now here's the problem: The inflammatory army doesn't *just* get mobilized whenever there's an obvious injury, such as a kick to the shins. It *also* gets mobilized whenever there's damage to cells.

Readers will immediately remember from the previous chapter that *damaging the cells is exactly what free radicals do*!

Is it all starting to make sense?

On the one hand, we have a constant assault from free radicals doing oxidative damage to the cells. On the other, we have the constant response of inflammation to this cellular injury. These processes are going on all the time, slowly wearing down our bodies, contributing to disease, aging, and breakdown. Problem is, the kind of injury and inflammation we're talking about here flies beneath the radar. It happens every day and is happening right now in your body, but you're unaware of it. You will certainly notice the pain of inflammation in your knee or hip or joints, but you will probably *not* notice it in your vascular system, where it is doing incalculable damage on

Inflammation and anti-inflammation forces need to be in a constant balance, or else we're in trouble.

a daily basis. Chronic inflammation (about which more in a moment) is a part of diseases as diverse as cancer, Alzheimer's, obesity, congestive heart failure, diabetes, and digestive system diseases. That "silent inflammation" is literally a stealth bomber, reducing your odds of long life just as effectively, and as silently, as breathing an invisible, odorless poison gas.

CHRONIC INFLAMMATION: THE SLOW KILLER

Inflammation comes in two flavors—acute and chronic. We're all familiar with the acute kind; it's what we see when we stub our toe or get a splinter. But the chronic kind, well, that's a whole different animal. And from an anti-aging perspective, this is where everything gets dicey.

"By definition, chronic inflammation lasts for more than two weeks, occurs when the invading organism is not totally destroyed, a foreign body or an ongoing irritant is still present, an autoimmune response continues, and/or there is a very significant amount of tissue destruction," says J.P. Saleeby, M.D., founder of the Saleeby Longevity Institute in Savannah, Georgia. Many practitioners in the field of anti-aging health believe that most of us are walking around in a state of chronic inflammation. Sears puts it beautifully: "Classic (acute) inflammation hurts," he says. "Silent (chronic) inflammation slowly kills."

Chronic inflammation is a part of every degenerative disease known to humankind. We're familiar with its role in allergies, acne, and asthma (what is asthma but inflamed airway passages?), but what you might *not* be aware of is inflammation's role in obesity, cancer, diabetes, Alzheimer's, and cognitive decline—all the diseases of aging.

Instead of being a transient event, the inflammatory response persists over time, "like an ornery child who can't resist picking at a scab," says science writer Christine Gorman. Eventually, chronic inflammation can and will destroy tissue. And it can absolutely cut off any chances you have for a long, disease-free life. Not for nothing did *Time* magazine presciently title a cover article back in 2004 "Inflammation: The Silent Killer."

GET THIS MEDICAL TEST

Here's another place where we've missed the boat in our obsessive focus on cholesterol lowering as a life-extending, disease-preventing strategy. A much publicized 2008 study called the JUPITER study[1] illustrates the point perfectly. It showed that a cholesterol-lowering drug (Crestor) reduced the risk for heart disease by 40 percent. Not terribly interesting, you might think, but consider this: *None of the 17,000 participants in the study had high cholesterol in the first place.*

"Classic (acute) inflammation hurts.
Silent (chronic) inflammation slowly kills."

—Barry Sears, Ph.D.

What they *did* have were elevated levels of inflammation, as measured by a blood test for an inflammatory compound called *C-reactive protein* (much more on this below). And the cholesterol-lowering drugs, known collectively as *statin drugs*, lower inflammation. For years, I, and many of my colleagues, have argued that the benefit of statin drugs has little to do with lowering cholesterol. It's *inflammation* that attacks oxidized cholesterol deposits in the arteries, causing the problems that are blamed on cholesterol. Saying statin drugs lower heart disease because they reduce cholesterol is like saying aspirin prevents clotting because it's white.

Any benefit statin drugs may have—and believe me, their benefit is a lot more hotly debated than you might imagine from reading the press releases of the drug companies—comes because they lower inflammation, a far more serious risk for the diseases of aging than cholesterol ever was. Trying to prevent heart disease by lowering cholesterol is like trying to prevent avalanches by outlawing St. Bernard dogs. I'm not at all sure we need to worry about lowering cholesterol if we want to live longer. I'm *very* sure we need to worry about lowering inflammation.* "Chronic inflammation" writes Gorman, "may be the engine that drives many of the most feared illnesses of middle and old age."

And drug companies are taking notice. "Virtually our entire research and development effort is focused on inflammation and cancer," said Robert Tepper, M.D., a former clinical professor of medicine at New York University School of Medicine and now president of research and development at Millennium Pharmaceuticals

in Cambridge, Massachusetts. "The whole field of inflammation research is about to explode," adds Paul Ridker, M.D., a cardiologist at Brigham and Women's Hospital in Boston.

Just as free radicals come from both internal and external sources, so do inflammatory chemicals. Nearly everything that's an irritant to the system—the air pollution we breathe, the tobacco smoke we inhale directly or indirectly, the some 80,000 chemicals we're exposed to in our environment—has the potential to produce some level of inflammation.

For instance, the food we eat can produce an inflammatory reaction—and frequently does, when you think of food allergies or sensitivities. "The standard American diet, commonly referred to as SAD, is inherently pro-inflammatory due to its excess of sugars … and its insufficiency of omega-3 fatty acids and phytonutrients," writes Alex Vasquez, D.C., N.D., in *Textbook of Functional Medicine*. In other words, some foods, such as certain sugars, have the effect of turbo-charging our inflammatory production pathways, while some foods have the opposite effect. And here's where the situation gets interesting.

Our bodies make both inflammatory and anti-inflammatory compounds called *eicosanoids* from raw materials that come from our diet. And the raw materials for both sets of compounds come from one source only: fat. The *type* of fat you consume affects the eicosanoid production factory. Omega-6 fatty acids, the kind found in vegetable oils such as corn oil, safflower oil, sunflower oil, and the like, are the precursors for the inflammatory chemicals in the body: They're known as *pro-inflammatory*.

* It's worth pointing out that fully half the people who have heart attacks have normal cholesterol. The drug that lowers the risk of heart attack the most is aspirin, and it doesn't do a thing to cholesterol levels. It does, however, lower inflammation. Something to think about.

Omega-3 fatty acids, the kind found in fish, and fish oil, are the exact opposite. They're the precursors for the *anti-inflammatory* compounds in the body.

Now if you go back and look at the diet of all the hunter-gatherer societies, the "natural" diet of Paleolithic man, and the basic diet of any civilization that lived off the land, eating unprocessed and unrefined foods, you find an interesting relationship between the consumption of these two types of fatty acids: It was always in balance. Most researchers agree that the ideal relationship of omega-6 (pro-inflammatory fatty acids) to omega-3 (anti-inflammatory fatty acids) fats is about 1:1, which is exactly the ratio you find in the diet of the hunter-gatherer

societies that were so remarkably free of the diseases of aging.[*] This ratio keeps the eicosanoid production factories in harmony, with the body producing a nice balance of pro-inflammatory and anti-inflammatory chemicals.

The importance of this balance to good health and anti-aging can't be overstated. "It is the balance of eicosanoids in your body that is the ultimate key to wellness," Sears says. So when both factories are being adequately fueled— omega-6 fats for the "pro-inflammatory" eicosanoids and omega-3s for the "anti-inflammatory" ones—everything hums along really well.

Would you like to know the ratio of pro-inflammatory fats to anti-inflammatory fats in the typical Western diet?

Fifteen to one[†].

Think it doesn't matter? Think again. "A high omega-6/omega-3 ratio, as is found in today's Western diet, promotes the pathogenesis of many diseases, including cardiovascular disease, cancer, osteoporosis, and inflammatory and autoimmune diseases," writes Artemis P. Simopoulos, M.D., founder and president of the Center for Genetics, Nutrition, and Health in Washington, DC.[2] "A lower ratio of omega-6/omega-3 fatty acids is needed for the prevention and management of chronic diseases."

In other words, inflammation is killing us.[†] It's arguably the most significant "engine" driving premature aging. And we're helping it along by overfueling our inflammation factories and undernourishing our anti-inflammatory ones. You couldn't come up with a more perfect prescription for aging badly.

---

[*] Yes, you might say, but they died so much younger. True, but they died from exposure, violence, and attacks from wild animals, and all the anthropological evidence suggests that they did not have any early signs of the degenerative diseases that kill most of us in the twenty-first century.

[†] That's a conservative estimate that has been demonstrated in research, but many scientists suspect that estimate is low, and it probably is.

This is one reason why it's impossible to put together a serious or an effective anti-aging program without dealing with inflammation (and oxidation).[34] Our food choices make it easier for our tissues to become inflamed, as does lack of exercise and many other aspects of our lifestyle. Our diet is a huge factor in promoting inflammation, as is our method of cooking (more on that in a moment). But this is actually *good* news because it means there's a lot we can do to slow or prevent inflammation, just like there's a lot we can do to slow or prevent oxidative damage. In practical terms, that's further evidence that there's a lot we can do to slow aging.

The imbalance in our intake of fats adds fuel to the proverbial fire, literally as well as figuratively. Not the least of the reasons that you'll hear so much about omega-3 fats (such as fish oil) throughout this book is their amazing ability to calm inflammation and provide raw materials for the body's anti-inflammatory factories.

INFLAMMATION: HOW DO WE MEASURE IT?

The body releases many biochemicals in an inflammatory response, and a fair amount of research has attempted to link elevated levels of these different biochemicals with increased risk for heart disease (and death). These biochemicals have long and technical names, and your eyes would glaze over if I listed them (but okay, if you insist, here they are: serum amyloid A, IL-6, tumor necrosis factor, a class of compounds called adhesion molecules, and a family of enzymes called phospholipase A2 (PLA2). (Aren't you sorry you asked?)

Although small studies have attempted to link elevated measures of these inflammatory chemicals with increased risk of heart disease, it is not always clear whether measuring these individual components of inflammation has great predictive value for telling us who is at risk for dying, or even for developing heart disease. But before you despair, there's good news: One marker has consistently shown predictive value in determining the risk for heart disease and even death. And that marker is so important and its effect so clear, that many of the smaller markers mentioned above tend to move in tandem with it.

Let me explain by using the stock market as an analogy. A bunch of small, independent stocks might go up or down as the overall market rises or falls, but none of them by itself might predict the Dow Jones Industrial Average very well. However, one or two huge stocks, such as Wal-Mart, might predict it *very* well, and the little stocks tend to move in the same direction as the Wal-Mart ones. So if you're trying to predict the Dow, you're better off looking at the Wal-Marts of the world as markers for the overall condition of the market. (It's not a perfect analogy, but it will have to do.) And if you're trying to measure inflammation, you're better off measuring this one important compound that I'm about to tell you about and, at least for the time being, not worrying about the other ones so much.

So what's this Wal-Mart of the inflammatory measures?

It's something called *C-reactive protein* (CRP). CRP is a protein that's produced by the liver as part of the immune response to infection or injury. It's also produced by muscle

[†] It's worth mentioning that more than 30 million people worldwide take NSAIDs (non-steroidal anti-inflammatory drugs) on a daily basis. NSAIDs include aspirin and ibuprofen. In the United States, annual sales of NSAIDs and COX-2 inhibitors (another class of anti-inflammatories) exceed $6 billion. And this is just for the inflammation we notice!

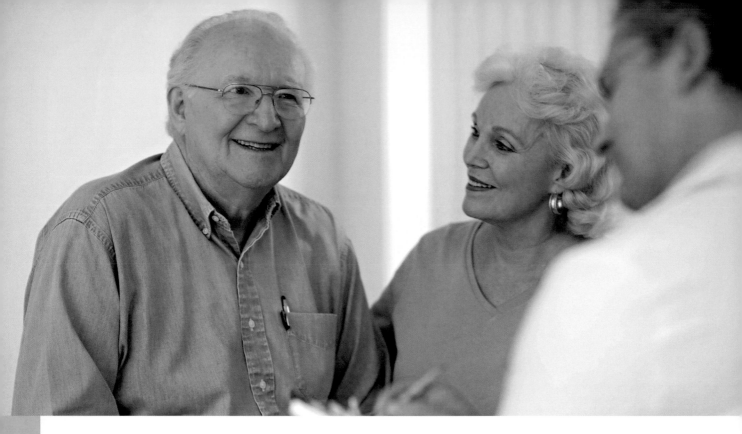

ANTI-AGING ACTION PLAN:

Get an hs-CRP Test to Assess Your Risk of Heart Disease

The liver produces c-reactive protein (CRP) as part of the immune response to infection or injury. It's also produced by muscle cells in the coronary arteries.

Levels of CRP in the blood increase dramatically in response to bacterial infections, trauma, and other inflammatory conditions. Studies show that in the majority of healthy individuals, circulating levels of CRP were found to be below the detection threshold for most standard blood tests, but a new "high-sensitivity" CRP test has fixed the problem. It's the hs-CRP (high-sensitivity CRP) test you should demand from your doctor.

So get an hs-CRP test the next time you have blood work done. If your hs-CRP is lower than 1.0mg/L, you have a low risk of developing cardiovascular disease. Lower than 1.0 mg/L is the ideal level.

If your hs-CRP is between 1.0 and 3.0 mg/L, you have an average risk. If your hs-CRP is higher than 3.0 mg/L, you are at high risk for developing heart disease. What can you do? Consult your doctor and start eating an anti-inflammatory diet (see page 43).

cells in the coronary arteries. Levels of CRP in the blood increase dramatically, a hundredfold or more, in response to bacterial infections, trauma, and other inflammatory conditions.[5] In the majority of healthy individuals, circulating levels of CRP were found to be below the detection threshold for most standard blood tests, but a new "*high-sensitivity*" CRP test has fixed the problem.[6] It's the hs-CRP (high-sensitivity CRP) test you should demand from your doctor.

You'll remember that I mentioned the JUPITER study, in which a statin drug lowered the risk for heart disease but didn't have a whit of effect on cholesterol. You may also remember that the people in the JUPITER study had high levels of inflammation. How did the researchers know about this inflammation? Simple. They measured the participants' levels of CRP, the most reliable measure of inflammation now available. The study participants all had elevated CRP, and their risk for heart disease was lowered *not* because their cholesterol went down (it was normal to begin with) but because their *inflammation* went down. Though experts will continue to debate the true meaning of this study, I'd argue that it's further proof that inflammation is a far greater risk to your health and longevity than cholesterol ever was.

In many large-scale prospective studies as well as a number of meta-analyses (studies *of* studies), knowing your hs-CRP significantly improves the predictive value of a blood test when it comes to determining who is at risk for heart disease, the number one life-shortening disease in the United States.

A number of studies have found that the higher your hs-CRP levels, the higher the risk of a heart attack. Not a good thing for longevity! In fact, according to the American Heart Association, the risk for heart attack in people in the upper third of hs-CRP levels is *twice* that of those whose

hs-CRP level is in the lower third.[7] These studies have also shown an association between high hs-CRP and sudden cardiac death as well as the incidence of stroke.

If you want to live long and well, one thing you absolutely have to do is reduce your systemic inflammation. And if you want to see how successful you are at it, get your CRP measured.

WHAT YOU CAN DO ABOUT INFLAMMATION

Fortunately, a great deal of inflammation is under our control. If you can control the "fire within," you'll be well ahead of the game when it comes to extending your life as well as improving the quality of the years you have.

Once again, it all starts with food.

As with antioxidants, the plant kingdom is absolutely loaded with natural anti-inflammatory properties. Some of the superstars that you should include in your diet are:

- Onions and leeks
- Garlic
- Leafy greens (e.g., spinach, chard, kale)
- Tomatoes
- Bell peppers
- Brassica vegetables (e.g., brussels sprouts, cabbage, broccoli, cauliflower)
- Beans: all types
- Nuts and seeds
- Spices: ginger, turmeric, cinnamon, cloves
- Herbs: parsley, rosemary, thyme, oregano, mint, tarragon, dill
- Tea: all types
- Red wine
- Cocoa/chocolate (minimum sugar, maximum chocolate)
- Flaxseeds and flaxseed oil

ANTI-AGING ACTION PLAN:
Lower Inflammation with These Supplements

Take These Supplements:

- Omega-3 fatty acids with DHA and EPA: 2–4 g per day
- GLA (found in evening primrose oil, borage oil, and black currant oil): 250-500 mg per day
- MSM (methyl-sulfonyl-methane): 1,000–2,000 mg twice a day

And of course, wild salmon, which is not a member of the plant kingdom, but a great source of the two most important omega-3s found in food, as well the superstar antioxidant astaxanthin. Grass-fed beef also has omega-3 fats, as do sardines, mackerel, herring, and tuna.

Put this all together and we start to notice an interesting and inescapable conclusion: Many of the foods that are high in anti-inflammatory properties are *also* high in antioxidants, thus providing a double whammy of a weapon against two of the most significant processes involved in every disease of aging: oxidation and inflammation. It's hardly coincidental that these foods form the bulk of the diets of the longest-lived people on the planet. (At the risk of pointing out the obvious, I've been unable to find a single long-lived society, where the "functionality curve is rectangularized," where there are a high number of centenarians, where people live robustly into their ninth decade, and where the main source of calories comes from McDonald's.)

As discussed in detail above, one of the most anti-inflammatory compounds on the planet is the class of fats known as omega-3 fatty acids, which are found in fish and flaxseeds. But remember that it's not just the fish oil you want—it's the stuff that's in it. The two fatty acids of greatest importance for the human body are EPA (*eicosapentanoic acid*) and DHA (*docosahexanoic acid*); these are like the golden nuggets in the prospector's tin of sand. So it's not enough to just "take 1,000 milligrams of fish oil"; you want to pay attention to how much EPA and DHA is in that fish oil. That's the stuff you care about, not the rest of the oil. Look on the label for how much EPA and DHA the fish oil actually contains, and try to take at least 2 (preferably 3 to 4) grams of total EPA and DHA for the best anti-inflammatory results.

When you take large doses of EPA and DHA it's a good idea to "balance" them with another fat called gamma-linolenic acid (GLA). That name may be unfamiliar to you, but it's the reason people take supplements such as evening primrose oil, which is an excellent source of GLA. GLA is actually an omega-6 fat, but it's one of the good ones, and it converts in the body to "good" prostaglandins (anti-inflammatory eicosanoids). I suggest taking about 1 gram of evening primrose oil (with GLA) for every 2 to 4 grams of fish oil.

Another supplement that's recommended is MSM (methyl-sulfonyl-methane). I discussed MSM at length in my book, *The Most Effective Natural Cures on Earth*, because of its fantastic effect on pain and inflammation caused by arthritis, but it's equally good as an all-around anti-inflammatory compound. My friend Mark Houston, M.D., M.S., clinical professor of medicine at Vanderbilt University Medical School, recommends 1,000 to 2,000 milligrams of MSM twice a day as part of a supplemental program to reduce inflammation in the body. Remember, the better you are at reducing inflammation, the better your chances of living longer and living well!

When it comes to fighting the negative effects of aging with food, it's not just *what* we eat that matters, but also what we *don't* eat. Some of the biggest enemies of a long and healthy life are sugar and foods cooked at very high temperatures.

And this leads us neatly into a discussion of the third of the "Four Horsemen of Aging," an insidious factor called *glycation*.

3

Avoid the Damage of the Third Horseman of Aging: Glycation

I magine, if you will, a nice, fluid substance such as almond oil. Imagine the liquid flowing from the amber brown glass container, clear and golden, as you pour it into a cooking pan or drizzle it on a salad, or even as you might use it as a wonderful, fragrant massage oil.

Now imagine what happens if you drop some sticky, pink cotton candy into that lovely, fluid oil.

Not a very appealing picture, is it? But there's no better visual analogy for what happens in your body when proteins—fluid substances just like almond oil—get dirtied up by sugar. The sugar molecules glom onto those formerly glistening, sleek, slippery protein molecules, gumming up the works, jamming up the flow, and generally making a big mess.

And aging your body—and all its systems—like nobody's business.

There's more bad news. Once the sugar is in the mix, you can't get it back out. It's like trying to shove the toothpaste back into the tube.

The process of sugar "gumming up the works," attaching to formerly sleek proteins and making them sticky, is called *glycation*. It's happening in your body every single day. And it ages you just like the hot noonday sun ages unprotected skin.

Take diabetes, for example, a condition in which the damage from glycation can be seen in clear relief. Type II diabetes is a disease in which blood sugar typically rises higher than it should, which is why diabetics need to constantly monitor their blood sugar levels. Because diabetics often have uncontrolled blood sugar, they are at greater risk for the aging effects of glycation. All that excess sugar floating around the bloodstream where it doesn't belong is like a crowd of unruly teenagers staying out after curfew—you just know they're going to get into trouble!

THE THIRD HORSEMAN OF AGING: GLYCATION

What it is:

Glycation is what happens when sugar molecules glom onto protein (or fat) molecules.

Why it's bad for you:

These sticky proteins gum up the works like cotton candy, and eventually create AGEs (advanced glycation end products), which are implicated in many of the diseases of aging, including diabetes, cardiovascular disease, Alzheimer's, and cancer.

What you can do about it:

Take carnosine, which is one of the most effective weapons against glycation. Just for good measure, it's also a powerful antioxidant.

capillaries and create the problems in circulation that often lead, for diabetics, to blindness, foot amputations, and kidney problems. In large measure, the problems of diabetics can be seen as the problems of *glycation on steroids*—and can serve as a lesson for what we need to do to reduce the less dramatic (but still severely aging) effects of this third horseman of aging.

You can measure that amount of glycated hemoglobin in a blood test called hemoglobin A1c, which is a much more accurate measure of the damage high blood sugar is doing over time than a blood sugar level test is. See, when you prick your finger and measure your blood sugar, you're just getting a *snapshot* of where your blood sugar is at the exact moment you pricked your finger. It's like knowing what a batter is doing during one single inning of one baseball game. Blood sugar could be high on Tuesday morning, but totally normal by Wednesday afternoon.

But knowing your A1c is like getting a batting average for the season, instead of knowing how many hits a player got today. Because hemoglobin sticks around for the life of the red blood cell, any A1c test is going to tell you how much damage sugar has done *over time*, how much damaged hemoglobin is still hanging around. It's like surveying the wreckage after the floodwaters have receded.

Diabetics have high A1c levels (higher than 6 percent)—in fact, an unexpectedly high measurement on an A1c test is often the first way someone finds out he or she has diabetes in the first place. Because of the fact that once sugar has "linked up" with a hemoglobin molecule it stays bonded, the A1c test is a far more accurate measure of what the long-term aging (glycation) effects of high blood sugar are.

Now at this point, if you're not diabetic, you might be saying, "What does this have to do with me?" And the

Even in nondiabetics, some of the glucose (sugar) in the bloodstream enters the red blood cells and "hooks up" (glycates) with a protein called *hemoglobin*. Okay, a small amount of "hooking up" can't be helped, and if only a small percentage of hemoglobin is "gummed up," it's no big deal. (Much like unwanted pregnancy, we want to keep it as low as possible, but a certain amount is probably unavoidable.) And remember, once a hemoglobin molecule gets "stuck" by sugar, it stays stuck! For the life of that red blood cell, about 120 days, that hemoglobin remains "glycated."

In diabetics, because there's so much more sugar hanging around just waiting to get into trouble, there's much more wreckage: more sugar, more glycation. Those sticky proteins can't flow freely through the smaller answer is, *a lot*. Although their uncontrolled blood sugar certainly makes them easier targets, diabetics are hardly the only ones at risk for the aging effects of glycation. Even in nondiabetics, about 5 percent of hemoglobin is glycated. And glycation, with its damaging consequences on all systems in the body, has myriad effects on aging and comes from far-ranging sources in the diet and environment, many of which you can actually *do* something about.

TURN DOWN THE HEAT

One of the ways you can lower the amount of glycated proteins in your body is to be careful about the way you cook food.

When you cook foods at really high temperatures like those needed for frying, it results in what's been called a "browning" effect, which is simply another term for glycation. You can see the browning effect in action when you heat sugar and butter together in a frying pan or when you brown a chicken in the oven. When you eat that stuff, delicious as it may taste, you're basically eating glycated proteins. Not for nothing are the resulting combinations of sugar and protein known as *glycotoxins* (*glyco* meaning sugar, and *toxins* meaning . . . well, toxins!).

Foods cooked at high temperatures are virtual glycation factories, and when you eat those foods you are ingesting nasty compounds called AGEs, which are basically the *end result* of glycation. The aptly named acronym AGE stands for *advanced glycation end products*. Your body will make these AGEs, or you can eat them ready-made right out of your frying pan. Let's review how it works:

1. The proteins in your body (or your frying pan) get gummed up by cross-linking with sugars, forming glycated proteins, or glycotoxins.

2. These damaged proteins lose their elasticity and become difficult for the body to break down—they literally become old and inflexible.

3. Damaged glycated proteins then hook up with *other* damaged glycated proteins (think: Losers attract each other!).

4. When these damaged glycated proteins link together, they form insoluble masses, which in turn generate more free radicals!

And these rather disgusting insoluble masses of linked, damaged proteins—these free radical–generating factories—are what we call AGEs.

AGEs accumulate everywhere—in the skin, the brain, the nervous system, the vital organs, the vascular system—and they do exactly what their name implies. They age you. AGEs play a big role in diabetes, and, whether you're diabetic or not, high levels of sugar intake (or foods that convert quickly into sugar, such as most breads and commercial cereals) make it all the more likely that *some* of that excess sugar will wind up binding with proteins and causing glycation, contributing to a whole cascade of aging effects.

The fact that you can ingest fully formed AGEs by eating foods that have been cooked at high temperatures is no longer in doubt. A recent study published in the *Proceedings of the National Academy of Sciences* strongly

ANTI–AGING ACTION PLAN:

Slow Down the Aging Process by Slowing Down Your Cooking

Cooking foods at high temperatures results in what's called a browning effect, another term for glycation, The Third Horseman of Aging.

Here are some good ways to avoid it:

→ Use slow-cooking cookware (such as Crock-Pots).

→ Cook foods in general at lower temperatures, such as simmering at low heat.

→ Don't blacken and don't grill over a high flame.

→ Avoid caramelization.

suggests that eating foods cooked at high temperatures will increase the rate at which we age, largely due to the fact that such foods cause both chronic inflammation and the formation of AGEs.[1]

You may have figured out that *glycation* and *oxidation* are two sides of the same coin. Glycated proteins generate the very agents of oxidative damage—free radicals—which in turn create *more* damaged proteins, which then hook up with one another and become AGEs, producing more free radicals, and continuing this awful cycle of

destruction and aging. Glycation and oxidation reinforce themselves in the nastiest of vicious circles.

Glycation can occur even *without* oxidation, which is why antioxidants alone aren't enough to battle this enemy of a long, youthful life. And the aging effects of glycation are irreversible. "Since we cannot yet reverse the pathological effects of glycation, it becomes critical for those seeking to prevent premature aging to at least slow this lethal process," says anti-aging expert Paul Wand, M.D.[2] Enter carnosine.

THE ULTIMATE ANTI–AGING NUTRIENT?

Carnosine's claim to fame is that it helps prevent glycation. For that reason alone, it has a seat at the head of the table when it comes to "ultimate anti-aging nutrients." Certain cells that live a long time, including muscle cells and neurons, already contain a fairly high amount of this naturally occurring compound (technically called a *dipeptide*, just in case you're interested). But given the amount of age-damaging free radicals, AGEs, and lipid peroxidation that we have to deal with on a daily basis, both from inside and outside our bodies, our natural carnosine stores aren't enough to handle the workload. This is where carnosine supplementation comes in. Many anti-aging specialists and health professionals consider carnosine to be one of the premier anti-aging supplements.

In addition to helping to prevent glycation, carnosine is also a powerful antioxidant in its own right. Carnosine has been shown to protect DNA. It "quenches" some of the nastiest of the reactive oxygen species, rendering them inactive. And remember *lipid peroxidation* from our discussion about how fats can be damaged or oxidized? Carnosine helps suppress it. It's been shown to sharply reduce lipid peroxidation in the brains of aging mice, extending their life span by 20 percent. It's been shown to restore youthful appearance and growth patterns to aging human cells as well!

"A substance that protects and extends the functional life of the body's key building blocks—cells, proteins, DNA, lipids—can be fairly called an agent of longevity," says Swedish physician Karin Granstrom Jordan, M.D., who has written extensively on longevity.[3] "When that

agent is safe, naturally present in the body and in food, and has demonstrated prolongation of life span in animals and cultured human cells, it is fundamental to any life extension program. Mounting research suggests that carnosine has just such anti-aging potential."

We've now looked at three of the four agents of destruction when it comes to aging, and time and again throughout this book we'll see how each of these agents leaves its respective fingerprints all over the aging process. So far, all of these agents of destruction have had very physical descriptions—oxidative damage by free radicals, inflammatory damage by pro-inflammatory chemicals in the body, and the damage that occurs when sugar "hooks up" with proteins (glycation).

Now we're going to turn to the fourth horseman of aging, one that, at first glance, appears to be in a different category. But we'll soon see that although this fourth horseman may have more mental, spiritual, and psychological components than the other three, it is no less destructive and damaging to the body on a physical level than the others are.

And what is this mysterious fourth horseman of aging? Read on.

ANTI–AGING ACTION PLAN:
Take Carnosine to Prevent Glycation

Add 1,000 mg of carnosine to your daily anti-aging regime. Carnosine helps prevent glycation, the Third Horseman of Aging, from happening in the first place. It's also a powerful antioxidant. However, our natural stores of carnosine aren't sufficient, so we need supplementation.

4

Calm The Silent Killing of the Fourth Horseman of Aging: Stress

....

There's an old saying that goes, "If a fish could think, the last thing it'd think about is water." The point of the saying is that water is a fact of life for the fish—it takes water for granted, and as long as it's there, the fish would no more spend time thinking about it than we would about air.

Well, unfortunately, the same thing could be said for modern humans and stress.

It's popular to complain, "Oh, I'm so stressed out." Indeed, stress has become a buzzword to signal the standard reaction to anything mildly annoying in your life. It's almost a badge of honor these days. When you're "stressed" you're in good company, sharing marquee space with type A personalities, movers and shakers, masters of the universe, having-it-all moms, and other busy and productive types.

But stress is a lot more than a mild annoyance. It's a true life shortener.

Stress is probably the single most potent enemy of longevity and health on the planet. It's hard to understate how important it is that you understand what stress actually *is* and why it contributes to every single disease of aging. Stress can and will shorten your life. If longevity is something you want, you need to have a plan of action when it comes to dealing with stress.

If you're like many folks who don't spend a lot of time reading biochemistry textbooks, you can be forgiven for buying into the common myth that "stress is all in your mind." Fact is, the complicated stress response does *begin* in the brain, often out of conscious awareness, but it doesn't *stay* there. The stress response is a complicated, multidimensional set of biochemical and hormonal responses and signals that affect virtually the entire body. You can measure blood (and saliva) levels of specific

THE FOURTH HORSEMAN OF AGING: STRESS

What it is:

Any physical, mental, or emotional factor that causes mental tension or bodily harm.

Why it's bad for you:

Stress produces hormonal reactions in the body that can shrink parts of the brain, damage your vascular system, and increase blood sugar levels, heart rate, and blood pressure. Stress can exacerbate less deadly but nonetheless important conditions such as skin problems, asthma, and allergies, and it makes recovery from illness much more difficult.

What you can do about it:

Meditation, deep breathing, and/or relaxing are the best antidotes to stress. A full night of restful, recuperative sleep helps correct some of the imbalances created by stress. Remove the conditions that create stress—toxic relationships, for example—or at least balance them with rewarding interpersonal connections, volunteering, time with friends, and gentle exercise such as yoga or qi gong.

stress hormones—they have a concrete reality—it's not "all in your head"! And their effect over time can shorten your life if you don't know how to manage them. It's not a coincidence that the longest-lived and healthiest people on the planet either have relatively stress-free existences or have in place a number of useful ways of dealing with stress so it doesn't shorten their lives (see section III on emotional intelligence, page 228).

Like many things we wish we didn't have—cravings for sugar, for example—the stress response plays an important role in our survival. In fact, if we weren't wired to respond to stressors, we'd be dead because our physiology wouldn't react any differently to a Mozart concerto than it would to a raging lion that thinks we'd make a tasty lunch. Clearly, God, Mother Nature, or the G.O.D. (Geonome Organizing Device) decided to give us some built-in mechanisms to respond to threats that were designed to save our life in an emergency. The problem with these mechanisms is not the mechanisms themselves, but the fact that we are no longer following the manual that says "use as directed."

Let me explain.

OUR CAVEMAN HERITAGE

Assume for a moment that you are a calm, happy caveman, resting peacefully on the African Serengeti. All of a sudden, an enraged wildebeest comes charging at you. What do you do?

Well, obviously, you run like hell. Or you pick up a stick, or the nearest object you can use as a weapon, and prepare to do battle for your life. But even before your conscious brain registers the "get butt in gear" command, a number of important physiological events occur that prepare you for action. A tiny section deep in the brain called the *amygdala* registers danger even before you're consciously aware of it and sends an instant message to the air-traffic controller of hormones in your brain called the *hypothalamus*. The hypothalamus shoots a hormonal signal to the pituitary gland, which in turn sends a hormonal signal of its own to the intended target of all this rapid-fire communication: a pair of walnut-shaped glands perched atop the kidneys called the *adrenals*. All this happens faster than you can press "send" on an email.

The adrenals send out powerful hormones, cortisol and adrenaline, which accomplish a number of things. They get your heart racing. They shut off other metabolic operations that might interfere with the energy needed to fight or run (for example, digestion). In some cases of extreme fear, your body will evacuate your bowels and bladder, because your primitive brain knows you don't need any extra weight while you're trying to scale a tree. Cortisol and adrenaline are known as the *fight or flight* hormones, precisely because that is what they prepare your body to do. If they weren't onboard, you'd continue to lounge lazily on your way to becoming a tasty dinner for the wildebeest.

Stress is a lot more than a mild annoyance. It's a true life shortener.

So far, so good. This is how nature intended it. The stress hormones are like a first gear for the body, turbocharging the engine to prepare for an emergency. You're instantly alert, primed for action. Your blood is coursing through your veins. Your blood pressure has gone up and your heart is racing, all good things if you're about to run for your life.

But nature meant for the stress response to be used in emergencies. It's like the nuclear option for the body—a special gas pedal to be used only when there's an important threat to survival. Nature did *not* mean for that pedal to be pressed to the metal all day long.

And here's why: A quick burst of cortisol (and adrenaline) will get your heart racing (so you can run quicker), increase your lung and heart function (same reason), dilate your pupils (so you can see where you're going and what you're running from!), and raise your blood sugar (you'll need it for energy!), all the while turning down the metabolic "volume" on bodily systems that are temporarily superfluous, such as the reproductive and immune systems. But in the long term, cortisol is a big problem.

Although cortisol is always described as a stress hormone, it's actually more of an antidote, or *anti*stress, hormone (which is why your doctor will give you a shot of cortisone, a cortisol mimic, when you have a lot of inflammation). After adrenaline has moved out of the way, cortisol hangs around, trying to put out some of the fires and quench some of the damage that happens as a result of all the hormonal and metabolic changes your body goes through in a state of emergency. It's like the fire department rushing to a scene of a fire and aiming a big fat hose with high-pressure water at everything in sight. It eventually puts out the fire, but boy does it leave a mess!

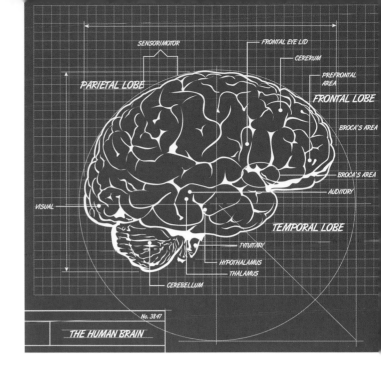

And so it is with cortisol. Make no mistake—you need cortisol for survival—it's one of your most important hormones. Problem is, it has a number of nasty side effects, or collateral damage, which you really don't want. The effects are okay for the short term, but long term, they're an aging nightmare. And when you're in a continual state of stress, cortisol is *always* elevated—not a good thing from a longevity point of view.

For example, high levels of cortisol shrink an important portion of the brain called the *hippocampus*, which is essential to memory and thinking (we'll discuss the role of stress on the brain in more detail in chapter 8).

In addition, high levels of cortisol also increase insulin resistance, metabolic syndrome, and heart disease, all well-known longevity robbers. Stress hormones lower immunity (which is why marathoners, who put their body through enormous physical stress during an event, for instance, often get sick the week after competing). And cortisol breaks down muscle and causes your body to gain weight, and not just *any* old weight gain, but weight gain around the middle. Abdominal weight (the well-

ANTI-AGING ACTION PLAN:

Practice Deep Breathing to Reduce Stress

Take ten minutes out of each day for a deep-breathing exercise. Here's how:

1. Sit quietly in a comfortable position.

2. Close your eyes.

3. Slowly and gradually relax all your muscles one by one, beginning at the feet and moving up to the face.

4. Breathe deeply in through your nose and out through your mouth, concentrating only on your breath.

5. As you breathe out, silently say a calming word to yourself. It can be as simple as "joy," "peace," "calm," or even "one."

6. Continue for at least ten minutes.

Nature meant for the stress response to be used in emergencies. It's like the nuclear option for the body—a special gas pedal to be used only when there's an important threat to survival. Nature did *not* mean for that pedal to be pressed to the metal all day long.

known "apple shape") is the most metabolically active and dangerous fat on your body, greatly increasing the risk of a whole host of life shorteners, such as heart disease. That's quite a bit of collateral damage if you're trying to live longer and healthier. The bottom line: Continuous, relentless stress shortens your life.

If you've read my book, *The Most Effective Natural Cures on Earth*, you know that for virtually every disease and condition I discussed, stress was a factor. Now I am not of the belief that stress *causes* cancer, for example, or even that it *causes* any disease or condition directly (although there are interesting exceptions: dying of fright, for example, from a voodoo curse that you believe in, is really dying from stress).

Although stress may not directly *cause* diseases, it *contributes* to many of them, and makes almost all of them worse. Simple examples you may be aware of include acne and asthma, all of which are commonly triggered by stress. Herpes outbreaks can be brought on by stress, as can allergies. And even more insidiously, stress hormones produce metabolic activities that are *direct* contributors to hypertension, high blood pressure, and heart disease.

I tell you all this now, because it's important that you understand how essential it is to have a system in place for dealing with, moderating, or eliminating stress if you really want to live long and well. You'll see many subjects discussed in the following pages, such as community, family, contribution, and group membership, which have a demonstrated relationship to living longer and living well. It's a good bet that these activities exert their anti-aging magic largely because they are ways of balancing and managing the aging effects of stress hormones.

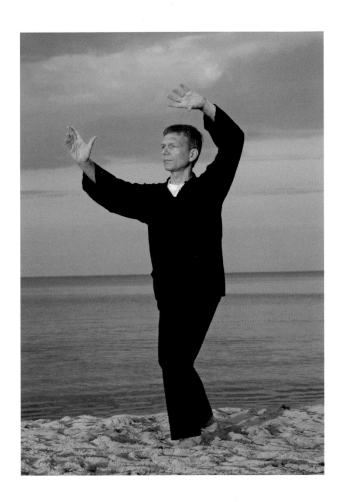

HOW TO AGE YOUR BODY IN ONE EASY LESSON

Nothing ages the body (and the mind) like imbalance, and perhaps the most serious imbalance of all is between the two parts of your autonomic nervous system.

Let me explain.

The nervous system is one huge interconnected matrix of organs (such as the brain), nerves, and muscles. The *voluntary nervous system* is what you depend on when you decide to put your foot on the brake to avoid colliding with the idiotic driver text messaging in the car next to you.

Your brain sends a lightning-fast message down to your foot and you promptly hit the brake. Because we usually have control over actions such as braking, or tossing a ball, or dancing the mambo, the part of the nervous system responsible for executing them is called *voluntary*.

But there's another part of the brain that's responsible for the thousands of responses that you *don't* have control over (or at least not easily, or at least not without a course in biofeedback), such as blushing, sweating, digesting, or even having an orgasm. These responses are not under conscious control and more or less happen automatically. The name of the nervous system responsible for these mostly unconscious activities is the *autonomic nervous system*. And understanding how it works is the key to understanding how stress ages you.

The autonomic nervous system is divided into two parts, the *sympathetic* nervous system and the *parasympathetic* nervous system. When you get excited—when your heart races, your skin flushes, and you start to sweat—that's the good old sympathetic nervous system in action. When you calm down and relax—when your breathing deepens, your heartbeat slows, and you digest your food—that's the work of the parasympathetic nervous system. When these two are nicely balanced, everything is hunky-dory. When the sympathetic nervous system is in overdrive and the parasympathetic nervous system never gets a chance to calm things down, you're in deep trouble.

Every medical student has heard the joke that the sympathetic nervous system is responsible for the four Fs of behavior—flight, fight, fright, and sex. The parasympathetic system is responsible for everything else.

It's hard to imagine a single aging process that doesn't *over-engage* the sympathetic nervous system and *under-engage* the parasympathetic one.

Stress turns on the sympathetic nervous system. Big time. And nothing ages you like "sympathetic overdrive."

Those stress hormones you release when you're in overdrive are *signals* to the body. They mean, quite simply, *something is wrong*. Your body thinks that those stress hormones carousing through your body mean that you're about to be eaten by a woolly mammoth—it doesn't know that all that's happened is that you're stuck on the freeway. The body takes those stress hormones as seriously as an airport security officer takes a "joke" about a bomb. The airport cop treats the threat like it's a real emergency, and your body treats the stress you feel when you're about to be late for lunch just as seriously as it would the stress you feel when you're about to *be* lunch. It can't tell the difference. Stress hormones activate the sympathetic nervous system no matter what their original cause.

WHAT TYPE ARE YOU?

In the history of healing, there have been more than a few systems of thought based on identifying people as being *sympathetic dominant* or *parasympathetic dominant*. Give it a moment's thought and you'll see why. That sweet, slightly heavy, grandmotherly woman who moves slowly and always has a kind word and a cookie for the neighbor? Parasympathetic dominant. A business tycoon always flying around, screaming into the phone, running late for meetings, and barking orders to subordinates while wolfing down a few Big Macs at his desk? Sympathetic dominant, baby. What else?

Who do you think is going to live longer?

We may not be able to do much about it if we are kind of "hardwired" to be sympathetic dominant. But we can certainly learn to modify the behaviors that send our sympathetic nervous system into overdrive.

This is where meditation, deep breathing, and calming exercises such as yoga and qi gong come in, and why they are such profound anti-aging strategies. Maybe you wondered why all those people doing tai chi in the park appear to be over seventy and fit as a fiddle. Now you know why. Deep breathing, yoga, tai chi, and all the myriad things we're going to discuss in the section on emotional intelligence all engage the parasympathetic nervous system, and help rehabilitate the body. They are like replenishing food for the soul, and they calm down the systems that send out the very messages that cause breakdown in your body and age you from the inside out.

It's this engagement of the parasympathetic nervous system and its calming effect on the body (and mind) that helps counter the aging effects of stress. Think of your parasympathetic nervous system as your inner grandmother. When you let her speak, words of wisdom and solace often pour forth. These messages temper the frantic shouting of the sympathetic nervous system and help you live longer and better.

Listen to them. And when they're not talking loudly enough on their own, help them out with activities that turn up their volume—meditating, breathing, relaxing, unwinding, and de-stressing.

That balancing act could not only extend your life— it could also save it.

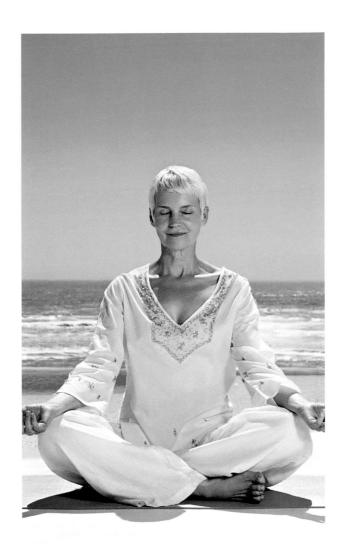

How Much Influence Do Genes Have on the Four Horsemen of Aging?

Most people know of at least one person who lived well into his or her ninth decade or beyond, sometimes in defiance of the odds (e.g., Uncle Ralph who drank a fifth of bourbon every day until he died at 106). We tend to say about these people, "They had great genes." And look, there's no doubt that genes play a role in longevity, just as they do in many diseases. But to explain a long (and healthy) life solely on the basis of genes is to miss a huge portion of the picture.

Truth be told, genes are misunderstood. Many people think genes are inflexible blueprints for what's going to happen to you, regardless of what you do. There's almost nothing that could be further from the truth. The vast majority of our 30,000-plus genes are dependent upon some *interaction* with the environment (which includes our diet) to *express* themselves. (You can think of the average gene as a light switch; it's capable of creating light in the living room, but only if you switch it on. Ignore that switch and you're sitting in darkness. Turning it on is known in gene language as *expressing* it.)

So rather than being fixed entities with only one outcome possible, genes are what is called *plastic*—able to be turned on *or* turned off. They work in conjunction with other genes, literally talking to one another. Their ultimate expression depends on complex interactions, both among themselves and, more important for our purposes, with the outside world. Genes respond to dozens, perhaps hundreds, of outside cues that switch them on or off, and many of those cues are firmly within our control.

Consider a bear that hibernates. Obviously, there are hibernation genes that come with the bear's hardwiring, much like Windows comes with your PC. But those genes are only *turned on* when the temperature changes; they're programmed to respond to an external cue (cold). No

external cue, no gene expression. Bears in a zoo in a warm climate don't hibernate, even though they have the same genes as their wild brethren.

Other genes are turned on or turned off by nutrients. The emerging field of *nutrigenomics* is an exciting area of research that investigates just what effects nutrients and overall dietary practices, such as the number of calories we eat, have on turning on the genes we want to express (such as those for longevity) and turning off the ones we don't (such as those that predispose us to disease). Many of the nutrients we'll discuss throughout this book may exert their anti-aging effects precisely in this way.

Now don't misunderstand me. Genes undoubtedly play a role in longevity. In a study of fifty-two Italian centenarians, scientists found one particular gene variation to be much more prevalent in people who lived past one hundred than in people who did not. Possessing this gene increases the chances of living beyond one hundred by 400 percent, according to the researchers.[1] But the interesting thing about it is that you can get this gene either by inheriting it *or* by "creating" it as a mutation that arises during the course of your life. "This introduces the intriguing idea that there may be specific things you can

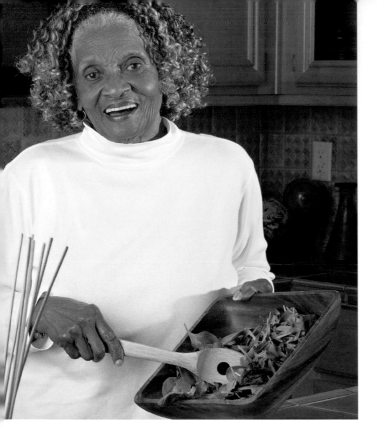

do to *induce* this beneficial mutation, increasing your own chances of living past 100," report scientist Ray Kurzweil and anti-aging pioneer Terry Grossman, M.D., in their terrific book *Fantastic Journey: The Science Behind Radical Life Extension*.

In other words, genes are not destiny.

THE GUN AND THE TRIGGER

In nutrition we have a saying: Genetics load the gun, but environment pulls the trigger. Except in very few cases (such as the genes for Huntington's cholera or cystic fibrosis), what we *do* probably makes way more difference than what we were born with.* And in any case, we can't control what we were born with, but we *certainly* can control what we do with it.

One of the people in the forefront of the emerging research on what exactly we can do to *turn on* our longevity genes is David Sinclair, Ph.D.

In the world of anti-aging research, Sinclair is a rock star. A professor of pathology and codirector of the Paul F. Glenn Laboratories for the Biological Mechanisms of Aging at Harvard Medical School, Sinclair has investigated a set of genes called the *sirtuin genes*, which are considered to be major influencers of how long we live. "The sirtuin genes are the holy grail of medicine and nutrition," says my good friend Mark Houston, M.D. "When you modulate (influence) these genes, they turn on or turn off different metabolic pathways that are designed to promote longevity and health."

One of these genes, called the SIRT1 gene, appears to have an important, if still not fully understood, role in regulating how long we live. When you increase the activity of the SIRT1 gene in animals, it eliminates, or postpones drastically, the diseases of old age and essentially slows down the aging process itself. Leonard Guarente, Ph.D., a biology professor at the Massachusetts Institute of Technology and the discoverer of the sirtuin genes, believes that SIRT1 is activated by caloric restriction (see sidebar at right). Eating about one-third less food than "normal"** may "turn on" these longevity genes, in some way that is not yet fully understood.

Sinclair and his team discovered another way these genes can be turned on. If his research pans out, which many biotech companies are betting heavily on, he may well have discovered one of the paths to the fountain of youth.

---

* This is why no scientist worth his or her salt talks anymore about the false dichotomy of nature versus nurture. Instead, the discussion is typically framed nature via nurture. It's an interactive model, not an either-or one.

EAT LESS, LIVE LONGER

It's a pretty good bet that a diet high in antioxidants, anti-inflammatory properties, and omega-3 fats will stack the odds in your favor when it comes to longevity. But what about the *amount* of food you eat? Could that make a difference?

In 1982, some inventive research scientists decided to investigate the effect of a calorie-restricted diet on longevity and disease.[2] They divided a few hundred male rats into two groups; one group was allowed to eat all the rat chow they desired, and the other group was allowed to eat about two-thirds of what they would have normally consumed when left to their own devices. The results set the stage for some of the most interesting anti-aging research of the past decade.

Here's what happened to the rats: The ones who received the normal diet lived their normal maximum life span of about 1,000 days. And they usually died from cancer, kidney disease, or the deterioration of their hearts. Pretty typical story for a rat, nothing out of the ordinary. But

for the rats fed the limited calorie diet it was a whole different story. These rats lived for about 1,500 days on average—a whopping 50 percent increase in life span. Even better, they avoided much of what we would consider the accompaniments of aging—feebleness, low energy (sluggish behavior), and a grizzled appearance. For example, their coats, which normally would turn gray after the age of two, stayed shiny and white for three and a half years or even longer! And they performed better, running mazes more successfully than their "normal eating" lab mates. Their immune systems were stronger, their rates of diabetes and cancer were far lower, and they had fewer cataracts. When they did finally die, most of them just expired.

They were living examples of what I referred to earlier as a "rectangularized functionality curve." Said Edward Masoro, Ph.D., a physiologist at the University of Texas Health Science Center in San Antonio: "When we look inside them, they're completely clean."

Calorie restriction, at least in rodents, was shown to be a demonstrable anti-aging strategy.

There have now been more than two thousand animal studies confirming these results across species as varied as yeast cells, fruit flies, monkeys, and mice. Scientists have reproduced these dramatic effects hundreds of times under all sorts of laboratory conditions. Because humans live much longer than, say, rats or fruit flies, and because of ethical and practical considerations, there are no long-term definitive studies on calorie restriction and humans. Nevertheless, some people voluntarily practicing caloric restriction—they even have their own Caloric Restriction Society (www.calorierestriction.org). And those who do practice calorie restriction are showing the same effects as those seen in the animal studies—less disease, fewer "markers" of aging, and much thinner bodies![3]

Cut Back on Calories by 33 Percent to Extend Your Life

Eating one-third fewer than your normal number of calories has been shown to extend life and prevent the normal deterioration that comes with aging in every single species studied.

A good place to start is by simply eyeballing the food on your plate, mentally dividing each dish into three equal sections, and then just eating two of them.

In 2003, Sinclair and his research associates published a now-famous paper reporting that plant compounds known as *polyphenols* could activate the human SIRT1 gene as well as extend the life span of yeast. The polyphenol in question is a substance called *resveratrol*, which is found in red wine and the skins of dark grapes (and to a lesser extent, peanuts). Later, Sinclair demonstrated that even if you fed mice a diet known to shorten their life and make them obese, they would still live 15 percent longer when treated with resveratrol. In other studies, he's shown that resveratrol mimics the effect of calorie restriction, effectively slowing down diabetes, cancer, heart disease, and indeed, the very process of aging itself.

Resveratrol may be the closest thing we have at present to an anti-aging elixir. Science—and business—are taking it very seriously indeed. In 2004, Christoph Westphal, who has an M.D. and a Ph.D. in biology from Harvard Medical School, founded Sirtris, a company designed to commercialize Sinclair's research and develop drugs that work with the body's own defenses against aging. They raised more than $140 million in cash from venture capitalists, were featured on the cover of *Fortune* magazine in January 2007, and were purchased by drug manufacturer GlaxoSmithKline in June 2008 for $720 million.

Obviously, there are some heavy bets being made on the potential of resveratrol to extend healthy life.

"I think the sirtuin genes and the work that's been done on how to modify [their] expression is one of the major medical breakthroughs of the past several years," said Houston. "For the first time we have the ability to modify the aging process in humans."

---

* "Normal" means the appropriate number of calories for your height, weight, and activity level. If you're currently chowing down seven super-sized meals a day, you'll certainly improve your health by reducing your calories by one-third, but it's better still if you reduce them starting from a reasonable baseline! In fact, if you're eating an appropriate number of calories for your height and weight to begin with, you may be able to get anti-aging benefits by cutting calories by only 25 percent. For example, a man eating 2,500 calories a day would lower that to 1,900 and a woman eating 1,800 would lower it to about 1,350.

Take 250–500 Milligrams of Trans-Resveratrol Daily to Slow Down the Aging Process

How much resveratrol you need to take to get the anti-aging and life-extension effects shown in the lab is controversial. Certainly, drinking red wine helps, though that may not be appropriate for all people.

"No one knows the correct dose in humans," says Mark Houston, M.D., "but any amount will have health benefits." The smart money is betting that at least 250 milligrams a day should have an effect on aging, though Houston recommends (and takes) more.

One thing is certain: The most effective kind of resveratrol is the *trans-resveratrol* form. Many of the better products on the market will say "standardized to 20 percent trans-resveratrol." That means a 500 milligram pill delivers 100 milligrams of the potent trans-resveratrol form. You only calculate your dose on the trans-resveratrol component.

How to Keep the Key Players in Your Body Fit

Laguna Woods is a lovely gated community deep in the heart of Orange County, California, located on 2,100 rolling acres of lush greenery just minutes from the Laguna Beach coastline. More than 18,000 people (fifty-five-plus years old) live there, in what the *Orange County Register* has voted the "best retirement community in Orange County."

The average age is seventy-eight.

The residents of Laguna Woods are part of one of the largest ongoing studies on health and mental sharpness in the elderly. Begun in 1981, it's called the *90+ Study*. More than 14,000 men and women age sixty-five or older, including more than one thousand people who have made it to ninety, have had their blood and memory tested, their genetics analyzed, and their activities tracked. Researchers have also performed postmortem analyses on the brains of participants who've died.

"These are the most successful agers on earth, and they're only just beginning to teach us what's important, in their genes, in their routines, in their lives," Claudia Kawas,

M.D., a neurologist at the University of California, Irvine, told *New York Times* columnist Benedict Carey, who wrote a story on the community's fascinating residents.[1]

The 90+ Study is specifically concerned with the aging brain, and researchers are understandably interested in teasing out which factors might be responsible for the fact that, for example, ninety-two-year-old Red Bull–slinging bridge playing Ruth Cummins seems not to have lost a whit of her faculties while many of her contemporaries, at least those who are alive, can't remember their names.

"So far, scientists have found little evidence that diet or exercise affects the risk of dementia in people over 90," writes Carey. "But some researchers argue that mental engagement—doing crossword puzzles, reading books— may delay the arrival of symptoms. And social connections, including interaction with friends, may be very important."

I would argue that Carey is being cautious. It's pretty clear from the research we'll look at in section III, "The Secrets of Emotional Intelligence," that social connections are *very* important and may even be arguably the most important factor in successful, healthy aging.

But there's more to successful aging than just preventing dementia.

STRONG IN MIND AND BODY

Although no one would deny for a second that clarity of mind and preservation of memory are high on the desirability checklist for successful aging, life is even better when such an intact and sharp brain is accompanied by a healthy, disease-free body in which the heart beats strongly, the limbs are creak-free, and the owner of said body is able to function autonomously. The owner gets bonus points for possessing the essential qualities of happiness—a connection to others, social integration, a sense of purpose.

In this section, we will look at some of the key areas of the body that can seriously hamper your ability to live well and long should they break down and falter: the heart, brain, immune system, hormonal system, and, taken together, the muscles, joints, and bones.

The selection of these five areas is somewhat arbitrary, but not completely random. If your heart fails, you stop breathing. If your brain fails, you lose your memory and then—worse—your *self*. If your muscles and joints ache or if your bones weaken, you lose mobility and autonomy. If your immune system weakens, you become susceptible to all sorts of opportunistic viruses and bacteria that can weaken your body, sap your energy, and, worst-case scenario, even kill you. And hormones are drivers of behavior and physiology; a hormonal system that isn't working optimally can have far-reaching implications, with results that range from mood disorders such as depression to obesity, loss of sexual desire, and low energy.

Including the liver and the lungs and all the other important body parts and systems in this book that could possibly break down would have made it too heavy for you to carry anywhere except with a small forklift. So I've limited this section to the five above-mentioned areas, for several reasons. First, I believe they are the most important, the "heavy hitters" in the game of health. Second, they get the lion's share of attention in the press (you can't throw a rock without seeing an article about heart disease, memory loss, or osteoporosis). Third, they are the areas most people are concerned with when they think about what it takes to live successfully over the long haul.

But since I brought it up, let's talk for a moment about the liver, the poor organ that does so much and gets so little attention or respect. The liver is the site of many important metabolic operations. It's where cholesterol is made (and yes, that poor maligned molecule is important for your health). It's where fat is processed (broken down and repackaged into molecules such as *triglycerides*). And—perhaps most important of all—the liver is ground zero for what we call detoxification. The liver breaks down every chemical, pesticide, medication, contaminant, and carcinogen in a two-phase sequence of operations commanded by a critical set of enzymes called the *cytochrome P450 enzymes*.

But here's the thing: Follow all the recommendations in this book and, barring a completely unforeseen event out of your control, the liver (and many of the other areas, including the lungs) will work just fine. Think about it—if your diet is clean and wholesome, you're not taking in a lot of toxins. If you reduce inflammation and oxidation, not to mention stress and glycation, you won't be putting undue stress on your liver. And if you keep your heart, brain, and blood pressure healthy, you'll presumably be taking fewer medications that need neutralizing and elimination. So in many ways, a healthy liver will be a natural and desirable side effect of doing all the things that keep the other parts of your system in tip-top shape.

So in this section, we'll talk about how to keep your heart healthy, your brain working, your hormones balanced, your immune system strong, and your muscles, bones, and joints from wearing out prematurely (prematurely being defined by me as "anytime before you die"). Add to this the information in section I on how to reduce the Four Horsemen of Aging—oxidation, inflammation, glycation, and stress—and the information in section III on social connections and emotional health, and we've got a working game plan for a long and healthy life!

Let's keep going!

Start with the Seven Pillars of Longevity

A s you read through the pages of this book, you'll notice that the anti-aging tips you find throughout fall into some certain specific categories. I call these categories "The Seven Pillars of Youngevity." They're basically seven areas in which you can exert control over your destiny and ultimately increase the odds of living a long and healthy life with a "rectangularized" functionality curve.

These seven areas are *food, supplements, detoxification, exercise, sleep, stress reduction*, and a kind of amorphous category that I've chosen to label *emotional intelligence*. We've already talked a little about stress and will be talking about it a lot more in the pages to come. So let's briefly touch on the other six pillars of youngevity.

FOOD: EAT YOUR WAY TO A LONG LIFE

What Hamlet said to Horatio, "There are more things in heaven and earth than are dreamt of in your philosophy," could easily be said of fruits and vegetables. There are more elements in them that can extend your life than science has been able to put its collective finger on. Some of their value is certainly because of the synergistic action of nutrients I wrote about earlier. Some of their anti-aging value undoubtedly comes from nutrients—antioxidants and anti-inflammatory properties—some of which have not even been identified yet. And other benefits may even be incidental to the fruits and vegetables themselves, because people who eat lots of these foods tend to have other healthy habits as well, such as eating less of the junk foods that shorten life. Regardless, the effect on aging, disease, and health of a diet high in fruits and vegetables is absolutely incontrovertible and noncontroversial. The results of a meta-analysis of nine different studies,

published in the *Journal of Nutrition*, found that fruit and vegetable consumption is inversely associated with coronary heart disease. The authors admitted that the exact causal mechanism wasn't clear but that the relationship was crystal clear nonetheless—the more fruits and vegetables people ate, the fewer heart problems they experienced.[1] The review found a 4 percent decrease in the risk of fatal and nonfatal heart attacks, coronary death, and incident coronary heart disease for *each additional fruit or vegetable portion* consumed per day. That sure makes fruit and vegetable eating look like a powerful anti-aging strategy to me. And by the way, when fruit alone was examined, the risk reduction increased to 7 percent. There was also a 26 percent reduction in coronary deaths with each additional portion of vegetables consumed per day.

ANTI-AGING ACTION PLAN:

Get Your Nine a Day to Prevent Diseases of Aging

Eat nine, not five, servings of fruits and vegetables a day, with emphasis on the vegetables. The U.S. Department of Agriculture now recommends between five and nine servings a day, and the Centers for Disease Control and Prevention's slogan regarding fruits and vegetables says it all: "More matters!" Serving sizes are small—about 1 cup—so it's not nearly as hard as you think to get in nine servings. And potatoes and rice don't count.

For whatever reason—the fiber, the anti-inflammatory agents, the anti-oxidants, the vitamins, the minerals, or some combination thereof—high fruit and vegetable intake consistently correlates with a lower rate of the diseases of aging. In fact, according to *World Health Report* (2002) estimates, up to 2.7 million lives could potentially be saved each year if fruit and vegetable consumption were sufficiently increased. Low fruit and vegetable intake is estimated to cause about 31 percent of ischemic heart disease and 11 percent of strokes worldwide—amazing numbers![2]

And if you want to talk anti-aging strategies, consider this little factoid: The recent Joint Food and Agriculture Organization/World Health Organization Expert Consultation on diet, nutrition, and the prevention of chronic diseases recommended that a minimum intake of 400 grams of fruits and vegetables a day (not counting potatoes!) would dramatically help prevent chronic diseases of aging, such as heart disease, cancer, diabetes, and obesity.[3] If there were a pill that would have that effect on aging, we'd all be lining up to take it at any price!

We've already seen the enormous effect food can have on reducing oxidative damage, inflammation, and glycation. It can also do the same for stress.. How, you ask? Because the wrong food choices stress our bodies. They cause our defenses to go into overdrive, our liver to work extra hard (trying to rid the body of toxins), our hormones to fall out of balance, and our immune system to be weakened. All of these responses contribute to aging.

Ultimately, food is probably the most powerful drug we have in our anti-aging arsenal.

72   THE MOST EFFECTIVE WAYS TO LIVE LONGER

MULTIVITAMINS: THERAPY IN THE PALM OF YOUR HAND

I like to think of supplements as a technology, a kind of modern-day delivery system for nutrients. The more we know about the diseases of aging, the more we understand how specific nutrients can help. Often, the doses of those nutrients needed for a therapeutic effect are simply way more than are going to be available in the average diet, even a diet constructed according to the best longevity principles. Some nutrients are not even found in food in any appreciable amount (coenzyme Q10, alpha-lipoic acid, or the previously mentioned carnosine).

The realization that many nutrients in the ideal dosages have an almost pharmaceutical effect has led to wide use of the term *nutraceuticals* for these beneficial compounds. As we discuss each system in the following chapters, we'll see how therapeutic use of nutraceuticals can help support various systems in the body and protect them from the typical breakdown and malfunction that happens during the diseases of aging.

Food is also the primary delivery system for all those antioxidants and anti-inflammatories we talked about earlier, not to mention nutrients (such as resveratrol) that have the power to influence our "good" genes (and perhaps turn off some of our not-so-good ones). And, as we'll see in chapter 11 on hormones, our food selections have a powerful influence on our hormones, which in turn have a powerful effect on how we age. Ultimately, food is probably the most powerful drug we have in our anti-aging arsenal.

ANTI-AGING ACTION PLAN:

To Reduce Your Risk of Disease, Take More Than an Apple a Day

Take a daily multivitamin and an antioxidant formula (extra vitamin C and E) supplement.

Studies have shown that people who regularly take multivitamins have a reduced risk of cardiovascular and cerebral stroke. Consistent use of multivitamins with minerals and such single-nutrient supplements as calcium and antioxidants (vitamins C and E) helped boost the immune systems of elderly people and played a key role in protecting eye and brain function and maintaining bone mass, according to another study.

Sometimes the most obvious proof that a supplement works is found by looking at a particularly challenged population. For example, a 2003 study found that people with AIDS who took a multivitamin lived longer[4] than those who didn't. Although most responsible scientists would not generalize from this study that multivitamins extend life in all populations, the study nonetheless shows that multivitamins do *something* positive in the body (why else would those people with AIDS who take them experience enhanced survival rates?).*

It's a reasonable assumption that multivitamins probably do some good for those of us who are not sick as well as for those of us who are. In fact, a large study on multivitamin use and mortality published in the *American Journal of Epidemiology* that examined more than 1,063,000 American adults found that people who took a multivitamin *plus* extra vitamins A, C, and E had a cardiovascular and cerebral stroke mortality risk that was 15 percent lower than that of the people who didn't take vitamins.[5]

A comprehensive report released by the Council for Responsible Nutrition (CRN) found that consistent use of multivitamins with minerals and such single-nutrient supplements as calcium and antioxidants (vitamins C and E) demonstrated substantial positive impact on the immune systems of elderly people and played a key role in protecting eye and brain function and maintaining bone mass.[6] Even doctors at Harvard Medical School now recommend that everybody, regardless of age and health status, take a daily multivitamin.[7]

DETOXIFICATION: TAKE THIS AGE-OLD TIME-OUT

The almost ancient practice of detoxification has been around forever, whether as part of religious purification rites or as part of a natural healing program. The ability to give our systems a much-needed rest—a kind of "time-out" from the daily assault on our cells of toxic foods and environmental pathogens—is a deeply valuable asset in our quest for a long and healthy life.

Fortunately, we have a number of ways of detoxifying, from "cleansing diets" (which are usually just very sparse, nutrient-dense programs of whole foods) to infrared sauna (see my book, *The 150 Most Effective Ways to Boost Your Energy*).

Although detoxification isn't discussed in great detail in this book, you should be aware that the *reason* it is a pillar of longevity is because it helps combat every one of the Four Horsemen of Aging: oxidation, inflammation, glycation, and stress.

A ton of stuff has been written in the media in the last few years about detoxification and cleansing, some of it sheer nonsense and some of it sensible. Some critics claim that commercial "detox" products are nothing more than laxatives (sometimes true), while other critics claim that the body is constantly detoxifying anyway (true) and doesn't need any help (false). And finally, some argue that there's no way to effectively measure the toxins we supposedly eliminate through a detox program, and even if there were, there's no way to prove we've actually eliminated them (partially true, partially not).

* One hypothesis is that vitamins may plug the nutritional holes that go along with the disease, but it's reasonable to assume that closing any nutritional gaps may be beneficial—and possibly life extending—for those who aren't seriously ill as well.

Do the SNACC Detox Program and Take a Break from the Chemicals That Age Us

Here's how to do the SNACC (sugar, nicotine, alcohol, caffeine, and chemicals) detoxification program developed by Elson Haas, M.D. One week before beginning, eliminate the following in your diet:

→ Sugar

→ Nicotine

→ Alcohol

→ Caffeine

One or two days before starting, eliminate:

→ Red meat

→ Milk products

→ Eggs

→ Wheat and baked goods

(You eliminate the meat, eggs, and wheat not because they are necessarily bad for you, but because many people have low-grade reactions to them, especially wheat, which contains gluten, a common food allergen. It's a way of starting with an essentially "clean slate.")

Then, for a week, simply follow this program:

Upon rising:

Drink two glasses of filtered water, one glass with half a lemon squeezed into it.

Breakfast:

Eat one piece of fresh fruit, such as an apple, a pear, a banana, a grapefruit, or even some grapes. Don't forget to chew well.

Fifteen to 30 minutes later:

Eat one bowl of cooked whole grains—try millet, amaranth, quinoa, or brown rice. Oatmeal may be okay, but it sometimes contains gluten by cross-contamination, so if you suspect gluten sensitivity, leave it alone for now. You can sweeten the grain with a couple of tablespoons of fruit juice and feel free to use some organic butter (or butter blended with olive or flaxseed oil).

Lunch:

Eat one to two medium-size bowls of steamed vegetables (save the water). Use a variety, including roots, stems, and greens. For example: potatoes or yams, green beans, broccoli, cauliflower, carrots, beets, cabbage, asparagus, chard or kale, and cabbage. Be creative. And feel free to put butter on it; just make it organic.

Dinner:

This is easy. Eat the same thing you did for lunch.

Just in case you feel a little fatigued (there's not a ton of protein in this week-long program), feel free to add 3 to 4 ounces of fish, poultry, or beans to the evening meal, or have it between meals. I recommend wild fish from Vital Choice (available through a link on my website under "healthy foods") and free-range poultry only. Although Haas doesn't mention this, I'd personally feel fine doubling up on the protein (two portions a day instead of one) if you find you have more energy and feel generally better eating a bit more of it.

And one more thing: Remember that water you collected from steaming the vegetables? Drink it all day long. You can flavor it with some garlic salt or sea salt.

You can do Haas's SNACC program for a week or so, and then add back some of the foods you've been without. Some nutritionists, including the legendary Oz Garcia, Ph.D., of New York City, have been doing variations on these programs with their clients for decades, and often recommend that you do this kind of a "clean eating" detox four times a year with the season changes.

Adapted from *The New Detox Diet* by Elson Haas, M.D. and Daniella Chace, M.S.,C.N. (Celestial Arts, 2004)

ANTI–AGING ACTION PLAN:

Eat Crunchy Vegetables to Help Rid Your Body of Toxins

A diet high in cruciferous vegetables (kale, cabbage, broccoli) will help with detoxification. Broccoli contains sulfuraphane, a powerful antioxidant that helps the liver do its job of ridding the body of age-robbing carcinogens and other toxins. Eat these vegetables as often as possible, daily if you can.

For the purposes of this book, let's take a middle ground. We can all agree that our bodies (not to mention our minds and souls!) are assaulted with toxins on a daily basis, including from the air we breathe (especially if you live in Los Angeles, like I do), the water we drink, the chemicals in our soil, the medications in our medicine cabinet, the hormones, antibiotics, and steroids in our meat, and the hundreds of other minor exposures we rack up just in the course of daily living. We can also agree that 1) this is not a good situation and 2) we don't help matters by eating bad food (fried foods, high-fructose corn syrup, and processed meats, the usual suspects). And finally, I hope we can agree that it might be a good thing to give the body (and the mind) an occasional rest from the constant onslaught and perhaps a little help getting rid of the excess garbage that's accumulated.

My friend Elson Haas, M.D., author of *The New Detox Diet* as well as countless other important books on nutrition and health, has been doing detox programs with his patients for three decades. "Detoxification is the missing link in Western nutrition," he told me. "People need to take a break from their substances [SNACC for short: sugar, nicotine, alcohol, caffeine, and chemicals]. A detox can give the body a rest so it can rebalance."

A middle ground indeed. So for those who want to try a sensible, smart, easy-to-do, low-tech detox program that makes sense, I recommend Haas's Basic Detox, which he calls the SNACC program.

Because the liver is the main organ of detoxification for the body, this is a good time to give it a little support. The best supplements for the liver are milk thistle, alpha-lipoic acid, and selenium. I recommend 400 to 900 milligrams of milk thistle, 100 to 300 milligrams of alpha-lipoic acid, and 200 micrograms of selenium as a basic "liver support" formula. There are many good nutritional supplements (such as Liver Support by Vital Nutrients, available on my website, www.jonnybowden.com) that combine different herbs and nutrients that are liver-friendly (such as artichoke heart) and make a good addition to the program.

For more information on some other simple detox programs you can do, see my book, *The 150 Most Effective Ways to Boost Your Energy*.

EXERCISE: AN ACTIVITY FOR THE AGES

There isn't a long-lived society on earth in which the members are not active. They may not go to gyms, but they shepherd goats, climb mountains, tend gardens, milk cows, walk, and do all the other active things that people have done for eons.

We'll discuss the effects of exercise later on, specifically in the sections on hormone systems, the heart, the brain, and the musculoskeletal system. Exercise can help you control blood sugar, weight, and blood pressure. It can elevate your "good" cholesterol and reduce your risk of heart disease. It can lower your risk for Alzheimer's disease.[8] A single thirty-minute bout of aerobic exercise can improve mood, measures of positive well-being, and vigor, even in people with major depressive disorder![9] It can certainly lower stress, and recent research shows that exercise actually helps you grow new brain tissue.[10, 11]

Suffice it to say here that exercise is one of the most effective "natural cures" on earth, and it is particularly effective against the vast majority of the diseases of aging. We'll discuss it more throughout the book, but especially in the section on bones and muscles.

SLEEP: LISTEN TO YOUR INTERNAL RHYTHM AND LIVE LONGER

Sleep is a big part of a longevity lifestyle. It's no secret that most of us don't get enough of it. Sleep affects how we work, how we relate to other people, how we make decisions, and how we feel in general. Not getting enough sleep can depress our immune system, raise our stress hormones, and contribute to weight gain.

This is a good time to take a brief moment to discuss a philosophic concept that underlies a lot of the thinking about longevity in general, and certainly underlies a lot of my personal beliefs reflected in this book. Although society has changed drastically in the past few hundred years, our genetics have not. Geneticists and anthropologists tell us that our specific human genome has only changed 0.01 percent in the past ten thousand years. Therefore, whenever possible, I think it makes sense to look to what our human genus was programmed for when it comes to basic things such as food, activity, and sleep.

For instance, our caveman ancestors ate from what I call the *Jonny Bowden Four Food Groups*: food you could hunt, fish, gather, or pluck. I've always maintained that this is the blueprint from which we should shape and choose our diet. The human genus has been on the planet for some 2.5 million years, homo sapiens about 100,000 years. Does it not make sense that when designing a diet for longevity, we keep in mind what I call *factory-specified fuel*—fuel that humans have run on for millennia, rather than the food that has come to dominate the modern landscape in the past half century?

Well, it's the same thing with sleep. Prior to electricity, we listened to our biological rhythms, which were in sync with the rhythms of the earth. We slept when it was dark out and awoke when it was light. We spent plenty of time in the sun. We moved around a lot. And when it was dark, we sat around the campfire and went to bed and slept like babies. When the sun rose, we started the day. This, if you will, was the natural order of things. This is the *factory-specified* sleep pattern for healthy humans. It's been wildly disrupted—and we've paid a great price in health and longevity.

Let me explain.

Circadian rhythms are roughly twenty-four-hour cycles in the biological and physiological processes of all living beings. The term comes from the Latin *circa* ("around") and *diem* ("day"). Our circadian rhythms are part of our makeup, but they are generated by external cues, the most important of which are light and dark. Because in the "olden" days there was no such thing as artificial light, our circadian rhythms were in sync with the natural rhythms of the universe. This cycle is incredibly important to human longevity; patterns of brain wave activity, hormone production, and all sorts of other regulatory metabolic functions are connected to this circadian rhythm and intimately connected with the quality and length of our sleep. When our sleep patterns deviate wildly from what we were genetically "programmed" for, countless systems (hormonal, metabolic) inexorably break down and systemic aging accelerates.

Sleep is the ultimate anti-aging strategy.

Anyone remember from the old movies how people who were stressed out and experiencing what was then quaintly called a "nervous breakdown" were sent away for the "rest cure"? Makes sense when you think about it—after all, when your dog gets sick what does he do? He usually curls up in a corner, won't eat, and sleeps a lot. He's basically taking a "rest cure." This is the animal's natural way of healing. No extra energy is spent on external things such as digestion, and all the body's resources are mobilized for the task at hand. Sleep and rest minimize the "output" and allow the body to replenish, renourish, and repair. We were programmed to get those eight hours at the end of every day to accomplish much of the same thing your dog accomplishes when he curls up and naps until he feels better.

Except that we're not doing it. Not even close.

Scientists don't even fully understand exactly *why* our bodies need sleep, but they know that we *do*. Sleep generates hormones, such as *human growth hormone*, the ultimate anti-aging hormone (released only in the deep stages of sleep), and *melatonin*, which appears to have anticancer properties. Biochemicals get replaced. And let's not forget that lack of sleep is a huge stressor, causing our bodies to secrete *cortisol*, whose aging effects we've already discussed. In short, not getting enough sleeping can shorten our life and diminish its quality in multiple ways.

And, to continue the parallel to food, it's not just the *quantity* of sleep that we get that's important; it's also the *quality*.

To understand the full anti-aging benefits of proper sleep we need to understand something about what's known as *sleep architecture*.

Sleep can be divided into two gross categories—REM sleep and non-REM sleep. Non-REM sleep has four stages. Stage one is when you move from wakefulness to drowsiness to falling asleep. (Stage one sleep is what you see when guys get dragged to the opera and start nodding off.) In stage two, eye movements stop, brain waves slow down, muscles relax, heart rate slows down, and body temperature decreases. Stages three and four, together called *slow wave sleep*, are characterized by brain waves

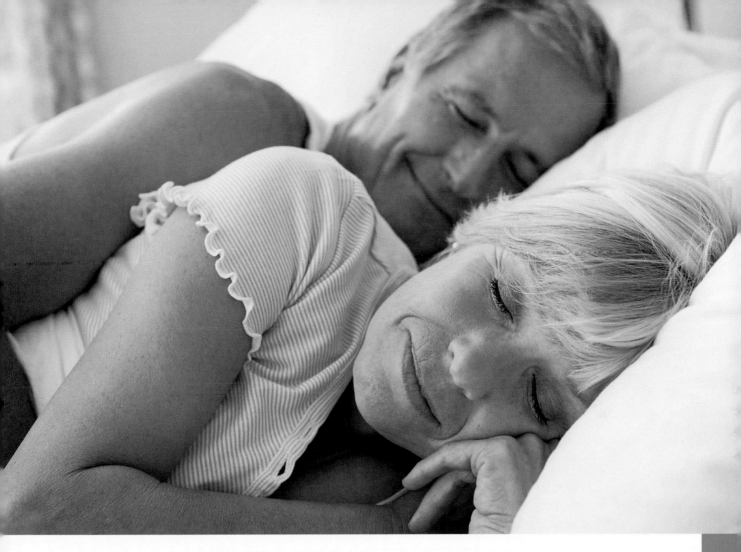

ANTI-AGING ACTION PLAN:

Reduce Stress with Sleep

Get seven to nine hours of sleep every night. Nature intended it to be that way for a reason.

Take the electronics out of the bedroom, remove the lights, and create a dark, warm, and inviting sanctuary where you can actually sleep undisturbed for the full length of time you were programmed to do.

called delta waves. Body temperature and blood pressure drop just a little more, breathing slows, and the body becomes immobile—the well-known "dead to the world" phase.

And finally, the pièce de resistance, REM sleep happens. This is when everyone in dreamland gets up to dance! REM (rapid eye movement) sleep is the stage where you dream. One complete sleep cycle consists of the four stages plus a period of REM sleep, and together they form a kind of "sleep symphony." One complete cycle is repeated anywhere from four to six times a night, and each cycle takes about 90 to 110 minutes.

Now as we age, sleep changes. It takes longer to fall asleep. The percentage of time in each stage changes (stages one and two increase and stages three and four and REM sleep decrease). The percentage of time spent in deep sleep

falls. But healthy, normal adults should still spend about 20 to 25 percent of their sleep in REM sleep, and when that's disrupted, all kinds of stuff happens, none of it good from a longevity point of view.

Sleep is essential to memory, mood, and cognitive performance, all markers for the youngevity lifestyle. All diminish as you get older unless you take good care of your sleep. Inadequate sleep is linked to increased anger, anxiety, and sadness, all diminishers of the quality (and potentially length) of your life. One study at the University of Pennsylvania showed that when subjects were only allowed to sleep 4.5 hours per night they exhibited significantly more stress, anger, and mental exhaustion.[12]

Then there's obesity and diabetes and all the life-shortening syndromes and conditions that come with being overweight and having an impaired metabolism. A 1999 study at the University of Chicago showed that under-sleeping for even a few days impairs sugar metabolism and disrupts hormone levels, in some cases to a prediabetic state![13] Under-sleeping also lowers levels of the appetite-regulating hormone *leptin* and increases levels of the hunger-increasing hormone *ghrelin*, both of which increase the likelihood of obesity.[14] All of this makes a pretty strong case for the connection between adequate and proper sleep and a longer and healthier life.

Sleep also affects immunity, in ways we'll discuss in chapter 10 on the immune system. In one study, flu shots were administered to men who had been restricted to just four hours of sleep per night for four straight nights and to another group that was allowed to sleep normally. Ten days after receiving the vaccination, the sleep-deprived group had a significantly lower immune response than the other group. The under-sleepers actually produced less than half as many flu-fighting antibodies![15]

The bottom line: Sleep matters. More than, perhaps, you realize. The old saying "I can sleep when I'm dead" used to be a badge of honor among Masters of the Universe types, but the irony is that those who live that way—ignoring the importance of sleep, with all its metabolic and hormonal anti-aging benefits—may find themselves dead sooner rather than later!

STRESS MANAGEMENT IS NOT A LUXURY

In August 2008, there were widespread warnings about Hurricane Gustav, which was about to hit New Orleans. No one wanted a replay of Hurricane Katrina, no one knew just how bad Gustav was going to be, and residents of the area were under a mandatory evacuation order "just in case."

One man who ignored the order was Russell Gore.

Gore told Gary Tuchman of CNN that he couldn't imagine leaving his home, which he rebuilt with his own hands after Katrina. He told CNN that his wife Cindy would have wanted him to stay.

When Katrina hit, Russell's home was flooded with nine feet of water. He and Cindy climbed to the attic, where they waited for the rescue helicopters. Russell kept his arms around Cindy the whole time, reassuring her that they would be okay. He told her not to panic.

"Next thing I knew, she leaned over towards me while I was talking to her—and she was dead," he told Tuchman, his voice breaking.

Cindy Gore—a healthy woman in her early fifties—had died of stress.

Although this story is heartbreaking, it illustrates something that few people understand: Stress kills. Granted, it usually doesn't kill as quickly and dramatically as it did in the case of Cindy Gore, but kill it does—slowly, insidiously, and deliberately. Stress exacerbates virtually every disease of aging and many others as well (herpes, asthma, allergies, and acne being just some of the more "minor" conditions that stress hormones can aggravate). Stress slows down recovery from serious illness. Stress shrinks areas of the brain that are intimately involved with memory and thinking. It increases the risk of heart disease. It decreases the effectiveness of the immune system. It deeply deserves its designation as one of the Four Horsemen of Aging, and many might reasonably argue that it is the most deadly horseman of all.

I tell you this so that you fully appreciate what I'm about to say: Without a way of dealing with stress, there simply *is* no "living longer."

Throughout this book we'll be talking about stress and it's effects, but make no mistake—managing stress is not a luxury. It's an important part of your longevity program (arguably the most important part of all). Stress reduction, or stress *management*, doesn't have to be done in expensive spas or yoga retreats. It can be as simple as walking in the woods, having dinner with friends, taking warm baths in candlelight, listening to relaxing music, or reading by the fireplace. Or it can be a more structured activity like doing deep breathing exercises (see page 128) or meditating.

My purpose here isn't to write a book on how to reduce stress; rather, it's to let you know how important it is that you do it. Once you're convinced how important stress reduction and management are to achieving the goal of a long, happy, and healthy life, I'm hoping you'll find the best ways to do it on your own. Chances are that without even thinking about it too much, you could easily name a dozen things that you personally would find relaxing, enjoyable, and soothing. These dozen things would automatically lower your heart rate, blood pressure, and stress hormones naturally.

Take my advice: Do them.

The longest-lived people in the world may not go to day spas or yoga retreats. But they have constructed their lives in such a way that their stress is naturally manageable. To the extent that you do the same—however that "looks" for you—you will be taking a huge step toward increasing the odds that you wind up living longer, better, and healthier.

EMOTIONAL INTELLIGENCE EXPLAINED

I've saved this section for last—in fact, it gets its very own section in the book—for a reason. And that reason can best be illustrated by using the analogy of a computer.

How well your computer works depends on a number of things: memory, speed of processor, and so on—all of which can be adjusted right on your desktop with a good repair person. You can upgrade the memory, defragment the disc, and do all sorts of other things I don't pretend to understand to make your computer run better. The stuff that lives on your own personal computer—the hard drive, the programs—are all things that are analogous to the systems we're going to discuss later on: the heart, the brain, the hormones, and so on. I'm going to talk about things you can do for those systems that are the human equivalent of making your own personal computer run better. By delving into how systems like the heart and the brain break down and age—and by determining what we can do to prevent such a breakdown—we will take some substantial steps toward extending our lives.

But there's a problem with this approach: It's incomplete.

See, whenever researchers have investigated long-lived people, they've looked at their diets, their activity levels, their genes, all sorts of things that pertain to the *individual*. We know, for example, that those long-lived Russians up there in the Bulgarian mountains eat lots of yogurt (but no fish). We know that the folks in Okinawa eat tons of fish (but no yogurt). Ultimately, there are very few elements related to diet or nutrients or detoxification or even sleep that are absolutely universal among all long-lived people.

Except one.

There is *one category* of human activity that is *absolutely universal* among every culture everywhere in which people live long and are healthy into their ninth decade and beyond. It's the closest thing we have to a "universal truth" about anti-aging. And it doesn't have very much to do with what we eat, how we sleep, or how we exercise, except indirectly.

See, to continue the computer analogy, computers don't live in a vacuum. My beautiful iMac may live in my house, but how it ultimately performs has a lot to do with a little thing called the Internet. You can't optimize your computer's performance (and extend its working life) unless it has clean connections to servers outside itself, has good browsers, doesn't crash, doesn't have viruses, and all the rest of the performance parameters that have to do with its *connections to the outside*.

It's exactly the same with us humans.

The absolute universal truth about anti-aging is that *there is no anti-aging without a strong social fabric*. Not one single long-lived society anywhere in the world is absent a set of strong social connections, including family, community, place of worship, and all the rest of the structures that go with living together as a cohesive group. That is our personal, human Internet, and without it, we are isolated PCs that might as well be sitting on a deserted island where we will quietly burn out in a matter of years.

In looking for a category for this kind of anti-aging behavior, I found there really wasn't one specific label that captured all the "nonphysical" things we can do to extend life (and improve its quality in the bargain). So I borrowed a term from psychology—it's called *emotional intelligence.*

I'm going to loosely define emotional intelligence as the sum total of everything in our lives that relates to our relationships with others, our relationship with ourselves (how we manage our emotions, for example), and our ability to communicate. If we can harness the power of emotions, we can use them to facilitate thinking, problem solving, communication, and connection to other people. All of these have profound implications for anti aging.

Our thoughts and emotions have powerful effects on our physiology. What we think about can literally affect our blood pressure, our heart rate, and the amount of hormones we release in our bodies, all powerful modulators of aging. Our emotional intelligence is intimately connected to our ability to manage stress, which, as we've already seen, is one of the most insidious of the Four Horsemen of Aging. And a big part of our emotional intelligence—its manifestation, if you will—is how we relate to and interact with others.

In fact, if there is one category of behavior that is most associated in the research with anti-aging, more perhaps than even food, supplements, hormone replacement therapy, exercise, detoxification, sleep, or any other individual behavior, it's our relationship with others. It's no accident that married men live longer than single men do. And it's no accident that there isn't a single long-lived society anywhere on earth where people live in isolation, unconnected and unattached to others.

Hence, the third section of this book. I'll be going into the details a lot more, but the important part to remember now is that anti-aging is a two-part affair. Yes, there are things you can do as an individual that dramatically improve your health, organs (the heart and the brain and the liver), muscles, hormones, and immune system. We'll discuss all of them in detail in the next section.

But all of these things pale in comparison to the life-extending effects of being connected to other people, being part of a community, and learning to know and accept yourself.

That's emotional intelligence, and it's the most powerful anti-aging tool of all.

Now let's get started!

7

Keep Your Heart in Shape

June 27, 2008, was a day like any other for the people who worked at NBC News. Writers were preparing copy, anchormen were broadcasting, television cameras were whirling away, BlackBerries were buzzing. The United States was in the middle of one of the most exciting presidential campaigns in memory, and the news was coming, as always, fast and furiously.

NBC News' Washington bureau chief Tim Russert, one of the most beloved and trusted on-air personalities in America, an energetic and almost daily presence in living rooms across the country, was recording a voiceover for *Meet the Press*.

And then, without warning, Russert suffered a massive heart attack. He collapsed in the studio and was dead within hours.

He was fifty-eight years old.

Although Russert's untimely death left thousands of people saddened and shocked, he was hardly the only person that day to succumb to heart disease. Nor was he the youngest. At present, heart disease is shortening the lives of millions of people and diminishing the quality of life for millions more. It's currently the leading cause of death in the world, accounting for 12.2 percent of all deaths worldwide, and an even higher percentage, 16.3 percent, in high-income countries.[1] In the United States alone, more than 652,000 people died from heart disease in the last year for which figures are available, more than four times the number of people who died from diabetes and Alzheimer's disease combined, and more than five times the number of people who died from accidents.[2]

That's more than 1,786 Tim Russerts a day, just in the United States alone. Many of these deaths are just as unexpected as Russert's was. In fact, for many people, the first and only symptom of heart disease will be death.

And it's not just men who are dying. Although most women are much more frightened of breast cancer than of heart disease, the sad truth is that heart disease is far more likely to kill them. One out of every two women's deaths in the United States is because of cardiovascular disease.

Heart disease is scary. And at the risk of stating the obvious, if you want to live long and live well, it's best to avoid it.

The thing is, a great deal of the risk for shortening your life from heart disease is actually under your control. Few diseases are as preventable, or at least modifiable, by lifestyle choices as heart disease is. Although there are certainly factors that you *can't* control, such as genes, they pale in comparison to the ones that you *can* control.

In fact, a massive amount of data suggests that five simple behaviors can reduce the risk for heart disease by a number greater than the effect of any drug on the planet.

The famous Nurses' Health Study, which followed more than 100,000 women for more than thirty years, found that a healthy diet and body weight, moderate physical exercise, no smoking, and limited alcohol consumption can lower the risk of heart disease by a staggering 83 percent.

"We're not asking people to run marathons," said Walter Willett, M.D., chairman of the nutrition department at Harvard School of Public Health and a coauthor of the Nurses Health Study ll. "Everyone could achieve these goals."

Indeed.

Another study, the Lyon Diet Heart Study,[3] looked at patients who were at serious risk for a heart attack. These were all patients who had survived a first heart attack. Most of them had all kinds of risk factors—these were not people for whom the insurance companies would have given reduced rates! The researchers divided the approximately six hundred participants into two groups and matched them according to blood pressure, weight, smoking status, and so on. For all intents and research purposes, the groups were identical.

A massive amount of data suggests that five simple behaviors can reduce the risk for heart disease by a number greater than the effect of any drug on the planet.

The first group didn't receive any specific dietary advice. Their doctors merely told them to "eat a prudent diet," which is code for the same old tired advice the American Dietetic Association has dished out for years—low fat, low cholesterol, all the usual things. This group ate a diet that was closest to the National Cholesterol Education Program's recommendations, which is pretty much what you've been told to eat by a conventional doctor if you are at risk for heart disease.

The second group was put on the Mediterranean diet.

Now there's some confusion about what a "Mediterranean diet" really is, because at least fifteen countries border the Mediterranean Sea and not all of the people in them eat the exact same food. But there are some shared characteristics. In this case, the folks in the second group consumed more vegetables, nuts, unsaturated fats such as olive oil, omega-3 fats, moderate amounts of fish and poultry, whole grains, not much red meat, and moderate amounts of wine.

Want to know what happened?

They stopped the study.

The group eating the Mediterranean diet got such outstanding results that the researchers felt ethically compelled to stop the study after a year and put everyone on the Mediterranean plan.

After a four-year follow-up, those still following the Mediterranean-style diet had a 50 to 70 percent lower risk of heart disease. Let that sink in for a minute. The absolute best result a cholesterol-lowering drug has been able to produce—and in my opinion, even this number is highly misleading—is a 33 percent lowered risk, and that's only in a tiny fragment of the population (middle-aged men who have already had a heart attack). These guys got a 50 to 70

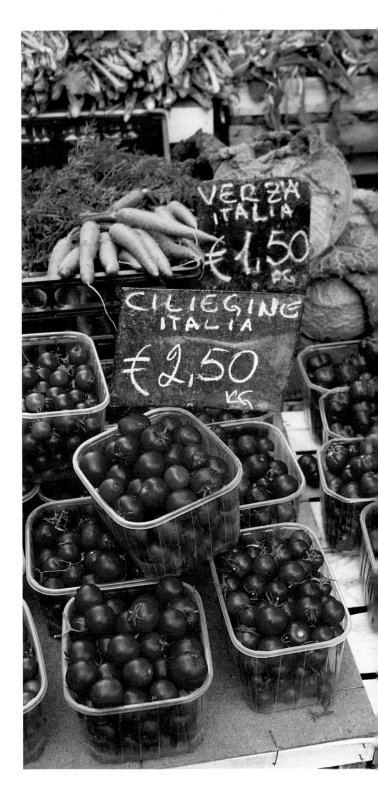

The Heart: A View From the Outside

Left Main
Coronary Artery

Circumflex Artery

Left Anterior
Descending Artery

Right Coronary
Artery

Directional Flow of Blood
Through the Heart

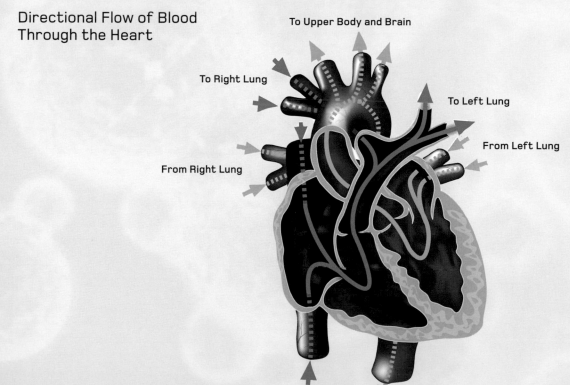

To Upper Body and Brain

To Right Lung

To Left Lung

From Left Lung

From Right Lung

From Lower Body

To Lower Body

percent reduction without a drug! (And needless to say, without the side effects or expense of a drug.)

And by the way, their cholesterol levels *didn't much budge*. (But that's a whole different discussion.) What matters here is that by changing their diet they were able to reduce their risk of cardiac death and nonfatal heart attacks by double digits.

Let me also venture to say that those folks did not know all of what you are learning in this book. They changed their diet—a huge deal, no question about it. But when you think about the results you might get when you *combine* diet changes with nutritional supplementation, stress reduction, exercise, and emotional intelligence, the possibilities are staggering.

A PRIMER ON THE TICKER

To understand what you can do to protect your heart, so you can live long and well and keep the old baby ticking away into your ninth decade and beyond, it helps to understand how it works. And to understand what can, and frequently does, go wrong.

Cardiovascular disease includes any arterial disease that affects the blood supply to the heart or the brain (or to the peripheral regions of the body). When the arteries supplying blood to the heart are affected, it's called *coronary heart disease*; when the blood supply to the brain is affected, it's called *cerebrovascular disease* (and the result is usually a stroke).

Sharp-eyed readers will note that in both cases the problem starts in the circulatory system. The health of those pipes carrying blood around the system is absolutely critical to the health of their destinations (heart, brain, and so forth). We'll come back to that in a moment.

Although there are two structures in the cardiovascular system that transport blood—the veins and the arteries—they are significantly different from one another. The vein is basically a tube through which blood flows. The arteries, on the other hand, are throbbing, pulsating, living structures that contract, dilate, and have their own version of a muscular system. "The arteries have thicker, elastic, and muscular walls that relax and open wide as the blood courses through them," explains my friend Mark Houston, M.D., M.S. Although arteries and veins have a similar construction, the arteries have an extra layer of smooth muscle tissue that allows for their contraction and expansion. It's invariably the arteries that are damaged or blocked in heart disease.

So even before we go any further, one thing should be extremely clear: The health of your arteries is of prime importance, especially as you get older.

ANOTHER CORONARY DISEASE MARKER

This is a really good time to introduce a new term, one that you may not have heard before but one which, I promise you, you will hear many times in the future. I'm talking about *endothelial dysfunction*.

Whoa, big words! Indeed. But here's the thing: They describe a condition that underlies virtually every circulatory problem, and certainly every problem that relates to the aging heart. You've got heart disease? You've got endothelial dysfunction. Not *some* of the time, but *all* the time. In fact, you've got endothelial dysfunction well *in advance* of the hard-core symptoms and traditional signs of heart disease, and if you can do something about it early, you may never progress to heart disease at all. Interested? Read on.

The Circulatory System

Superior
Vena Cava

Pulmonary
Veins

Interior
Vena Cava

Femoral
Veins

Aorta

Pulmonary
Arteries

Descending
Aorta

Femoral
Artery

Cross Section of A Blood Vessel

Endothelium

It's worth pointing out that the initials doctors use as a shorthand for endothelial dysfunction also stand for another well-known problem of aging, erectile dysfunction. And they are more than a little related. "I've never seen a case of ED (erectile dysfunction) that didn't also go with a case of ED (endothelial dysfunction)," quips Houston. (If you are a guy, you suddenly just became interested, even if you somehow weren't before!)

So here's the deal. The endothelium is a thin layer of cells that lines the interior surface of blood vessels (such as the arteries and veins). It is like an interface between the blood circulating in the inner tube of the vessel and the walls of the vessel itself. Endothelial cells line the entire circulatory system. But they're anything but passive—they don't just lie there like a rug. Far from it. They secrete substances, including the all-important *nitric oxide*, which helps the arteries dilate. They protect the smooth muscles of the artery from toxic substances in the blood, acting as a kind of protective barrier. They secrete chemicals that protect the artery after an injury, chemicals that send messages to both white blood cells and smooth muscle cells to mobilize quickly and get over to the injury site.

When the endothelium is not functioning well, all hell breaks loose. Absolutely every patient with atherosclerosis (i.e., hardening of the arteries) has endothelial dysfunction. Atherosclerosis begins with one of the Four Horsemen of Aging, inflammation. Endothelial cells respond to that inflammation by activating immune cells. These processes eventually damage the arterial wall and lead to plaque.

With aging, the endothelium starts to be leaky, like an old roof, offering less protection than before. It starts to be less vigilant about letting toxins through. These toxins enter the smooth muscle cells, which then gather at the site of an injury, causing the artery to lose more flexibility.

White blood cells start to congregate, and they release pro-inflammatory substances and damaging free radicals (another horseman of aging), which in turn attack the poor aging endothelium even more. The toxins soon penetrate the arterial wall, substances such as cholesterol and triglycerides accumulate and become oxidized by free radicals, and the cycle of damage and aging continues.

When the walls of the arteries that supply blood to the heart thicken, it's the beginning of trouble. That thickening is caused by small lesions in the wall, injuries (minor and not so minor) that get patched over with material that forms into plaque. The plaque itself can restrict blood to the heart muscle, much like a boulder in the middle of the highway can restrict traffic. Worse, if the cap covering the plaque ruptures, the blood may clot and completely obstruct the flow. The result is what doctors call a *myocardial infarction* and what the rest of us know as a heart attack.

The term *atherosclerosis* actually comes from the Greek word *athere*, meaning "porridge," and refers to the soft core of the plaque, which has an oatmeal-like consistency. *Sclerosis* means "hardening." Although there is indeed cholesterol in the plaque, that's hardly the only component, and researchers are beginning to discover that the cholesterol particles have to be oxidized (i.e., damaged by free radicals) before they become a problem.

Oxidated, or damaged, LDL ("bad") cholesterol is taken up by little PacMan-type structures called *macrophages*, which then become known as *foam cells*. Accumulation of these foam cells in the arterial wall leads to the first sign of atherosclerosis, or at least the first sign that's visible, a yellowish spot in the wall that merges into streaks (known as *fatty streaks*). As atherosclerosis progresses, the streaks become larger and more complex, eventually turning into lesions, and finally evolving into fibrous plaque.

The good news is that you can do something about it, and probably extend your life in the process. Because endothelial dysfunction *always* involves a measure of inflammation and oxidation, a diet that fights these two horsemen is synonymous with a diet that protects the heart and helps fight the kind of aging none of us wants.

IT'S WHAT YOU EAT

Okay, full disclosure. I'm *not* one of the people who believes that cholesterol is the most important thing you need to pay attention to when it comes to protecting the aging heart. I realize that conventional wisdom says otherwise, but I believe when it comes to the heart, emerging research is pointing in the direction of oxidation and inflammation as far more serious concerns. Cholesterol may accumulate at the site of injury, but if we want to slow aging and prevent damage, we need to better understand (and prevent) the injuries in the first place. Blaming cholesterol for heart disease is like blaming the St. Bernard for the avalanche.

That's why the true heart-healthy diet is not necessarily low in cholesterol. But it *is* high in anti-inflammatories and antioxidants.

Starting to make sense?

We've already seen (above) that cholesterol doesn't become a problem until it's oxidized. And that most of what happens when it comes to the development of plaque is, in fact, the body's attempt to repair injuries, usually caused by inflammation. Once again, these two important processes, *oxidative damage* and *inflammation*, are at the core of the problem, and addressing them seems to me to be

Now you have a real problem. The plaque itself can narrow the arteries, but that's only half of it. If a fibrous plaque becomes unstable, if it breaks or tears, blood clots called *thrombi* can form, further increasing the likelihood of a blockage that can result in a heart attack.

The interesting part of all this is that researchers now understand that atherosclerosis may actually be part of the body's attempt to mount a healing response to injury, an attempt that is initiated by the endothelium. And that injury may come in the form of *inflammation.* This is part of the reason that inflammation has gotten so much attention in recent years; it's clearly a big part of the problem in heart disease. Inflammation may well turn out to be much more important in determining your risk for heart disease than cholesterol.[*] At the very least, it's a factor you need to pay attention to.

---

[*] I'm being oh-so-politically correct here. The truth is, inflammation is much more important than cholesterol in determining your risk for heart disease, and the sooner conventional medicine accepts that, the better for all of us.

number one when it comes to keeping your heart young and vibrant.

And it starts with the diet.

More than a low-fat diet, and *much* more than a low-cholesterol diet, an anti-inflammatory diet is of paramount importance in keeping you young. And, as we've seen before and will see again, the very foods that are loaded with anti-inflammatories also tend to be loaded with antioxidants. When you eat these heart-healthy foods, you get a double dose of protection and a nice boost to your anti-aging strategy.

The importance of diet in preventing heart disease can't really be overstated, and even conservative doctors are beginning to realize this. Just as I was writing this chapter, the results of a new study from Greece appeared on my desktop. The study, published in the journal *Risk Analysis*,[4] concluded that knowing what a person eats significantly improves the ability to predict his or her risk for heart disease. In the past, doctors mainly used traditional measures of risk (such as cholesterol), which don't necessarily do a great job of predicting outcomes.[†]

These researchers found that by evaluating diet-related factors they could make much better predictions about who's at risk than they could by using just the traditional measures alone.

THE FIVE PRINCIPLES OF A HEART-HEALTHY DIET

So what exactly is a heart-healthy diet?

Let's cut to the chase. In 2002, two distinguished professors at Harvard Medical School, Frank Wu, M.D.,

and Walter Willett, M.D., examined a massive amount of research in the area of diet and heart disease.[5] They reviewed 147 studies to try to determine the basic principles of a heart-healthy diet. Here are the five principles they came up with. If you read no further and just follow these five mandates, you'll be in better shape from an anti-aging point of view than most of the world.

1. Increase your consumption of omega-3 fats from fish and fish oil supplements and even plant sources (such as flaxseed).
2. Substitute nonhydrogenated, unsaturated fats for saturated and trans fats.
3. Eat a diet that is high in vegetables, nuts, fruits, and whole grains and low in sugar and refined grain products.
4. Avoid processed foods.
5. Choose foods, food combinations, and food preparation methods that are low on the glycemic index.

This isn't just theoretical. Several years ago, explorer Dan Buettner visited four of the regions in the world where the inhabitants consistently lived longer and healthier than anywhere else. These areas also had some of the highest numbers of healthy centenarians in the world: Sardinia, off the coast of Italy; Okinawa, Japan; Loma Linda, California; and the Nicoya Peninsula, off of Costa Rica. Although there were differences in the diets of these four regions, what was remarkable were the similarities. The Sardinians' diet consists of whole-grain bread, beans, garden vegetables, fruit, and cheese

[†] Full disclosure: Political correctness once again. Cholesterol levels are a lousy predictor for heart disease. Fully half the people who have heart attacks have perfectly normal cholesterol, and half the people with elevated cholesterol do not. Using cholesterol levels to predict heart disease will give you slightly better results than using tea leaves to predict the weather.

high in omega-3 fats that's made from grass-fed sheep. The Okinawans eat a plant-based diet, including stir-fried vegetables and tofu, plus a high-antioxidant food called goyam which also contains compounds that lower blood sugar. Many of the Seventh Day Adventists in Loma Linda consume nuts at least five times a week (and have about half the risk of heart disease as those who don't). They also eat two or more servings of fruit a day and beans (or peas) about three times a week. And the Nicoyans in Costa Rica eat a nutrient-rich diet based around fortified maize and beans.

All of these societies eat meat, but in very small amounts. Plus, probably most important of all, the meat they *do* eat comes from healthy, locally raised, grass- or pasture-fed animals and is never filled with the hormones, steroids, and antibiotics that come with virtually every serving of feedlot-farmed meat in the United States.

And all eat a lower-calorie diet than the typical American.

They don't worry about the saturated fat or cholesterol in their diet, but by eating high-fiber foods like beans and consuming the tons of antioxidants and anti-inflammatories that come with a whole foods, plant-based diet rich in vegetables, they don't have to.

One thing to understand is that there is no single magic food that makes a diet heart healthy. It's the combination of low sugar, high antioxidants, high anti-inflammatories, high-quality protein, and omega-3 fats, and the absence of trans fats, that does the trick. And the exact details matter less than the way the parts fit together. That said, there are some superstars among the heart-healthy foods, and you should consider including them on a regular basis if you want to protect your heart and live long and strong.

GO WILD FOR SALMON

The ultimate brain food is also the ultimate heart food— salmon. (But not the farm-raised kind, the wild kind. More on that in a moment.)

Farmed salmon has more fat than wild salmon, but a much smaller percentage of that fat is from heart-healthy omega-3s and a much larger percentage is from pro-inflammatory omega-6s. Because, as we've seen earlier, the ratio of anti-inflammatory omega-3s to pro-inflammatory omega-6s is a big issue in the field of anti-aging (and human health in general), this is a disturbing piece of news.

Farmed salmon are fed pellets of grain and their meat is colored with artificial colors chosen from a device called a SalmoFan, which looks like one of those paint sample charts you see at Home Depot, and no, I am not making this up. Wild salmon get their red color naturally by consuming krill and other sources of the powerful antioxidant *astaxanthin*.

In addition, farmed salmon tends to have much higher levels of chemical contaminants that are known to cause cancer, memory impairment, and neurobehavioral changes in children.[6] A disquieting report from the Environmental Working Group indicates that farmed salmon are likely the most PCB (*polychlorinated biphenyls*)-contaminated protein source in the U.S. food supply.[7] Seven of ten farmed salmon purchased at grocery stores were found to be contaminated with this carcinogenic chemical at levels high enough to raise health concerns. Farmed salmon have about sixteen times the dioxin-like PCBs found in wild salmon, according to the group, a nonprofit advocacy agency based in Washington, D.C. And the group's research supports previous studies of farmed salmon contamination by scientists from Canada, Ireland, and the United Kingdom.

ANTI-AGING ACTION PLAN:

Eat Wild Salmon at Least Twice a Week to Protect Your Heart

Salmon grills up very nicely. You can also marinate it in olive oil and spices, wrap it in foil, and bake for just a few minutes (until flaky). I frequently make mine on a George Forman grill. Just remember not to overcook it—it only takes a few minutes to cook. (Check out the recipe on p. 31.)

Remember to eat wild salmon. Yes, farmed salmon has more fat than wild salmon, but a much smaller percentage of that fat is from heart-healthy omega-3s and a much larger percentage is from pro-inflammatory omega-6s. Because, as we've seen earlier, the ratio of anti-inflammatory omega-3s to pro-inflammatory omega-6s is a big issue in the field of anti-aging (and human health in general), this is a disturbing piece of news.

Another difference: Farmed salmon are fed pellets of grain while wild salmon get their red color naturally by consuming krill and other sources of the powerful antioxidant *astaxanthin*.

Okay, I don't want to scare you off eating salmon. There's no doubt that if there's a choice between eating farmed salmon and not eating salmon at all, you should choose to eat the fish. Two Cornell University professors, Barbara Knuth and Steven Schwager, studied the risks and benefits of the two types of fish and concluded that, in general, the net benefits of eating wild salmon outweigh those of eating the farmed kind. But they also noted that there were some substantial differences in the contaminant levels depending on where the farmed salmon came from. Chilean farmed salmon, for example, had the lowest levels of contaminants, while European (particularly Scottish) farmed salmon had the highest.

"Careful consumers with a history of heart disease could choose farmed salmon from Chile for their high omega-3 content and relatively lower level of contaminants," said Knuth. She also noted that farmed salmon from North America would be a better second choice than European farmed salmon.[8]

But if you have a choice, go for the wild variety. Although there's always some concern about mercury and other toxins that might be in wild fish, the overall benefits for your aging heart far outweigh any possible concerns for the vast majority of people. I personally eat salmon from Vital Choice, a company of Alaskan fishermen with the highest concern for purity and quality; they ship deep-frozen fillets directly to my door, as well as canned products (including tuna) that will make you wonder where they've been all your life. Their salmon comes from pristine Alaskan waters and tastes amazing. (You can find Vital Choice through a link on my website, www.jonnybowden.com. I've been a fan for years, and I'm in good company— Dr. Andrew Weil, Dr. Christiane Northrup, and Dr. Nicholas Perricone are also converts!)

And in case I haven't convinced you yet of how important cold-water (high omega-3) fish is to your anti-aging program, here's what the doctors at the Mayo Clinic are saying: "If you're worried about heart disease, whether you want to avoid it, or you already have it and want to get healthier, eating one to two servings of fish a week could reduce your risk of dying of a heart attack by a third or more."[9] Even the American Heart Association, a group far more conservative than I am, now recommends eating fish twice a week.

A postscript to the whole diet/fish/heart/anti-aging conversation: Readers of my book, *The Healthiest Meals on Earth*, may remember that the recipes in that book were based on a concept called *the polymeal*. If you didn't happen to read that book (which I hope you will), let me tell you the part that's relevant for our purposes here.

In 2004, a researcher named Oscar Franco published a paper in the *British Medical Journal* in which he suggested that dining regularly on a meal composed of specific ingredients (which he called "the polymeal") could boost the health of the heart and the blood vessels and cut the risk of cardiovascular disease by more than 75 percent. Franco projected that a diet rich in meals like the ones he described in his research would delay the average onset of a heart attack by nine years for men and eight years for women, increasing the average lifespan by between 4.8 and 6.6 years. Men could expect to live free from cardiovascular disease and its associated aging for at least nine extra years, and women could expect to do so for more than eight.

The main dish in the polymeal? Cold-water fish. In my book, that makes eating wild salmon on a regular basis a powerful anti-aging strategy. And for variety, herring, mackerel, sardines, and, to a lesser extent, tuna, are rich in the same omega-3s found in salmon!

Eat Broccoli as Often as Possible to Keep Your Heart Young

Include broccoli in as many meals as possible—an omelet for breakfast, a salad for lunch, and a side dish for dinner are just a few ideas. The anti-aging benefits are enormous.

Here's a quick and easy recipe from my book, *The Healthiest Meals on Earth*, on steaming broccoli (or another healthy green) with nuts.

STEAMED GREEN VEGGIES AND NUTS

Prep Time: 5 to 10 minutes

Cook Time: 3 to 10 minutes

Ingredients

4 cups asparagus, young green beans, or broccoli florets, washed and trimmed

4 tablespoons dry roasted nuts, chopped, such as almonds, walnuts, or pecans

Fit a large pot with a steamer basket, pour water in the pot to just under the basket line (so it doesn't come into direct contact with the veggies), and bring the water to a boil. Add the vegetables and steam until bright green and tender-crisp, for 3 to 10 minutes. Sprinkle the nuts over top and serve.

Yield: Makes 4 servings

PROTECT YOUR HEART WITH BROCCOLI

The cancer defense properties of broccoli (and the entire brassica group of vegetables, including cabbage and brussels sprouts) are well known and extensively documented. But broccoli is also a food you want to consume regularly if you want to keep your heart young!

Many studies have demonstrated that a diet rich in vegetables, especially the brassica group, is linked to a significantly decreased risk of stroke and heart attack.

ANTI-AGING ACTION PLAN:
Eat More Beans to Protect Your Heart

Try to include at least four servings of heart-healthy legumes (beans and peas) every week in your diet. Legumes help fight heart disease, contain a lot of fiber, don't raise blood sugar, and are a source of vitamin B. Plus, they're an inexpensive and versatile staple.

Eat them in the morning as many cultures do, sprinkle some on your salad for a protein boost, or create a main-meal soup out of them, such as minestrone. There are many legumes to choose from. Try one or more of these:

Beans (black, red, kidney, pinto, and garbanzo, for example)

→ Lentils

→ Peas

→ Soybeans

In my book *The 150 Healthiest Foods on Earth*, I wrote about a powerful plant compound in broccoli called *sulfuraphane*, which is known to activate detoxifying enzymes in the liver that may help the body get rid of cancer-causing chemicals.

When you want to study the protective effects of foods on blood vessels, diabetics are a good population to study, largely because they frequently have damage done to their blood vessels by uncontrolled levels of blood sugar. High blood sugar can cause free radical production to increase a great deal and damage human cells. Professor Paul Thornalley and his research team from the University of Warwick in the United Kingdom wanted to see what effect sulforaphane might have on blood vessels damaged by high blood sugar, so he studied a group of diabetics.

The results showed a significant reduction in free radicals. The presence of sulfuraphane actually reversed the increase in free radicals by 73 percent and doubled the activation of substances that protect cells and tissue from the aging effects of those free radicals. The researchers concluded that compounds such as sulfuraphane from broccoli may help counter processes linked to the development of vascular disease.[10]

Although this study was done on diabetics, there's every reason to believe that the same mechanism would protect the vascular system of those who are not diabetic. The benefits to the vascular system, together with the other demonstrated health benefits of broccoli, make an excellent case for including broccoli in as many meals as possible as part of an overall anti-aging strategy.

BEANS: MAKE THIS INFLAMMATION FIGHTER A PART OF YOUR DIET

There's an old saying that goes, "Beans, beans, good for the heart." And if you look at the research, it's clear that the old saying contains more than a little truth. One study, for example, followed more than 16,000 middle-aged men in seven countries for twenty-five years, looking for correlations between eating habits and risk of death from heart disease. After crunching the numbers, researchers found that those who ate the most legumes had—are you sitting down?—an 82 percent reduction in risk![11]

Almost 10,000 people participated in another ongoing study in the United States, called the National Health and Nutrition Examination Survey. Researchers followed these folks for nineteen years. One pattern that emerged clearly was that people eating the most fiber had significantly less risk for heart disease. People who consumed legumes merely four times a week saw a 22 percent reduction in risk for heart disease compared to people who ate them only once a week or less. "Our study indicates a significant inverse relationship between legume intake and the risk of coronary heart disease and suggests that increasing legume intake may be an important part of a dietary approach to the prevention of coronary heart disease in the general population," concluded the authors.[12]

If you look at what beans provide you can see immediately why they'd be a great weapon in your fight against aging. Take kidney beans: They're loaded with both folate and magnesium. Folate (folic acid) is one of the weapons against homocysteine, that nasty toxic compound that is a stand-in for systemic inflammation in your system. And magnesium is the great relaxer, helping the arteries contract and expand as needed and generally supporting heart health in all sorts of ways.

BLUEBERRIES: GO WILD, PART II

If any food on earth qualifies for the overused moniker *superfood*, blueberries certainly do. I've already talked about their memory-increasing capacity and how healthy they are for the aging brain in general. But blueberries are also a great food for the heart. The plant compounds that make blueberries that rich shade of blue are called anthocyanins, and they are powerful antioxidants that help protect the structures of the entire vascular system. "Blueberries and blueberry leaves represent some of the most powerful, naturally occurring antioxidants and anti-inflammatory agents found in vegetation," writes nutrition and training consultant Christine Lydon, M.D.[13]

Research at the University of Maine, Orono, concluded that a diet containing wild blueberries may reduce the risk from cardiovascular disease. Animal research suggests that blueberries have the potential to decrease the vulnerability of blood vessels to both oxidative stress and inflammation. Previous work by the same researcher, Dorothy Klimis-Zacas, Ph.D., demonstrated the positive effect of a wild blueberry-based diet on blood vessel function in animals.[14, 15]

EATING NUTS ISN'T CRAZY— IT'S HEART HEALTHY

Nuts are another food that suffered in the aftermath of the ridiculous low-fat dogma of the 1980s (and beyond). Hopefully, they're making a much-deserved comeback as a health food for many reasons, not the least of which is their powerful effect on the heart. Nuts contain fiber, plant sterols, antioxidants, minerals, and healthy fat, and they are a secret weapon in the fight against aging.

In one comprehensive review[16] of all the available epidemiological and clinical evidence, distinguished

ANTI-AGING ACTION PLAN:

Make Nuts a Regular Part of Your Diet to Lower Your Risk of Heart Disease

Consume 2 ounces of nuts at least three times a week. The health benefits are numerous: they contain fiber, plant sterols, minerals, and healthy fat, and are a staple in at least one of the longest lived societies on the planet in Loma Linda, California.

The nuts that contain the highest amount of monounsaturated, or "good," fat are almonds, Brazil nuts, hazelnuts, macadamia nuts, pecans, pistachios, and walnuts. So munch on them as a snack, top salads or soups with them, or mix them with fruit and yogurt.

professor of nutrition at Penn State Penny Kris-Etherton concluded: "To date, five large epidemiologic studies and 11 clinical studies have demonstrated that frequent nut consumption decreases the risk of coronary heart disease."[17] And in another study, published in the *American Journal of Clinical Nutrition*, researchers stated that "emerging evidence indicates that there are ... bioactive molecules in nuts that elicit (heart-protecting) effects. These include plant protein, dietary fiber, micronutrients such as copper and magnesium, plant sterols and phytochemicals."[18]

Kris-Etherton also did a study at Penn State where she asked a group of young men, whose reaction to stress suggested that they were likely candidates for developing high blood pressure, to consume pistachios every day. One group consumed 1.5 ounces of the nuts, a second group consumed 3 ounces, and a third group, for comparison, consumed none. After a month, the researchers checked the young men's blood pressure and did an assessment of the elasticity of their blood vessels. They also gave them two stress tests.

The results? Those eating 1.5 ounces of pistachios a day lowered their systolic blood pressure by 4.8 mm of mercury (so a reading of 130/80 would go down to 125/80) and also lowered their cholesterol levels.* The group eating the 3 ounces daily lowered their blood pressure by a little less but showed relaxed arteries and a slightly greater reduction in cholesterol levels. (Okay, I've said a million times that I don't think cholesterol is the most important thing to be paying attention to, but still, this is one more study to show the positive effects of nuts.) Pistachios also contain an

---

* This may not seem like an enormous amount, but with blood pressure, every little bit helps!

antioxidant called *lutein*, which is normally found in leafy green vegetables such as spinach.

And it's not just men who benefit from nuts. The famous Nurses' Health Study at Brigham and Women's Hospital in Boston and the Harvard School of Public Health, a study that monitors more than 80,000 women, found that women who eat more than 5 ounces of nuts per week—a tiny amount, about as much as you'd get in one of those silly airplane packets—had a whopping one-third fewer heart attacks than those who hardly ever ate nuts.

Note: The takeaway from this should not be that you should run out and buy family-sized bags of almonds and eat them all day. Nuts, with all their amazing health-promoting qualities, are still very high in calories. If you're trying to manage your weight, stick to a 1-ounce portion; if you choose to eat more, at least cut back on some other high-calorie items to make up the difference!

POMEGRANATE JUICE: IT GIVES MORE THAN JUST YOUR HEART A BOOST

A natural Viagra?

That's what volunteers called the substance they consumed in a study published in the *Journal of Impotence Research*. The substance? Pomegranate juice! Lead researcher Christopher Forest, M.D., summed it up this way: "Pomegranate juice has great potential in the management of erectile dysfunction."

Or, as the British paper, *The Sun*, quipped, "Nearly half the men who drank it for a month said they found it easier to rise to the occasion."

In the study, published in 2007, sixty-four volunteers aged twenty-one to seventy with mild to moderate erectile dysfunction drank about 8 ounces of pomegranate juice a day with their evening meal. Forty-seven percent of

the men reported that their erections improved with pomegranate juice.

So why am I bringing this up now?

You'll recall that earlier I told you that *erectile* dysfunction is almost always associated with *endothelial* dysfunction. The same antioxidants that help improve levels of nitric oxide (which relaxes blood vessel walls and makes erections easier) also improve endothelial function. It's no coincidence that pomegranate juice is one of the most heart-healthy drinks on the planet.

Researchers at Technion-Israel Institute of Technology in Haifa suggest that long-term consumption of pomegranate juice may help slow aging and protect

ANTI-AGING ACTION PLAN:

Drink 6 Ounces of Pomegranate Juice Daily to Help Your Heart—and Your Love Life!

Antioxidant-rich pomegranate juice has always been shown to help with erectile dysfunction and may help slow aging and protect against heart disease and cancer.

Pomegranates are also rich in potassium and contain vitamin C. They're grown all over the world and tend to be more available in October and November in the United States.

Less labor-intensive than eating pomegranates is drinking pomegranate juice. One brand that's commonly available is Pom Wonderful, but any brand that is primarily juice is fine. Just watch out for added sugars and for the infamous "juice drinks" that can contain as little as 10 percent actual juice!

against heart disease and cancer. According to the results of a study published in the August 2006 issue of *Atherosclerosis*, subjects reduced their risk of atherosclerosis significantly just by drinking 6 ounces of pomegranate juice a day. "Pomegranate juice contains the highest antioxidant capacity compared to other juices, red wine, and green tea," said professor Michael Aviram, who has been doing pioneering work in this field.

And wait, there's more. A study published in the *Journal of the American College of Cardiologists* had forty-five patients with ischemic heart disease drink either 8 ounces of pomegranate juice or a placebo for three months. Compared to those drinking the placebo, the patients drinking the pomegranate juice had significantly less oxygen deficiency to the heart during exercise, suggesting

increased blood flow to the heart. Pomegranate juice also inhibits the oxidation of LDL ("bad") cholesterol. And at least five studies have demonstrated a beneficial effect of pomegranate juice on cardiovascular health, including a study that showed a 30 percent reduction in arterial plaque.

"In most juices," Aviram explained, "sugars are present in free—and harmful—forms.* In pomegranate juice, however, the sugars are attached to unique antioxidants, which actually make these sugars protective against atherosclerosis."[19]

Now that's a heart-healthy beverage!

HEART DISEASE PREVENTION: IT'S NOT ALL ABOUT CHOLESTEROL

By now you're probably sick of hearing me say that cholesterol is probably not the most important thing to

---

* "Free" meaning the way they occur naturally in the food or juice, "harmful" meaning added stuff, such as high-fructose corn syrup.

worry about when it comes to aging well and avoiding heart disease, so I won't say it again. But I *will* tell you that two other risk factors are emerging that are turning out to be very important. Both are measures of inflammation, and both are things you can do something about immediately.

We've seen how damage to the arteries, and how endothelial dysfunction in general, are both caused in large measure by inflammation, one of our Four Horsemen of Aging. We've also seen in chapter 2 how inflammation—especially the chronic kind that causes long-term damage and aging—flies beneath the radar, often producing no symptoms and creating damage and destruction silently from within.

However, there's a problem here. *How do you know you have chronic inflammation?* (Remember, chronic inflammation doesn't hurt like acute inflammation does.)

Although you can assume that if you're breathing you have *some* inflammation, you might want to know the extent of the damage. Wouldn't it be a good thing if you could measure it, much like you can measure your blood levels of cholesterol or triglycerides?

Well, we don't have a *perfect* measure of systemic inflammation, but there are a couple of measures that, as the song says, "will do until the real thing comes along." Scientists have identified substances in the bloodstream that are excellent markers for systemic inflammation and may turn out to be highly valuable in assessing your risk for heart disease. And though I'd be the last person to say that by bringing these two measures down you're guaranteed to live to one hundred, I'd be foolish not to recommend that you get them down as low as possible. If you have high levels of either of these two

ANTI-AGING ACTION PLAN:

Take These Three B Vitamins to Lower Your Risk of Heart Disease

The toxic compound Homocysteine is a risk factor in heart disease and stroke. In addition to being tested for homocysteine levels in your blood, take these vitamins daily to lower your levels:

→ Folic Acid: 1 gram (up to 4 grams)

→ B_{12}: 1,000 mcg

→ B_6: 100 mg

If your homocysteine levels remain elevated, your doctor may suggest higher doses and may also add the supplement TMG (trimethylglycine), which usually does the trick.

compounds, well, as my grandmother used to say, "That can't be good."

The discovery of the first substance has an interesting story, and one you might want to pay attention to. It shows exactly how much resistance the medical establishment has to new ideas that fly in the face of conventional wisdom (and how hard it may be to correct the idea that living long and living healthy is about lowering cholesterol). But it's a feel-good story because it shows how persistence and a willingness to stand up for what you believe in can sometimes result in complete vindication.

Our story begins with an eight-year old boy who died of arteriosclerosis. The exact diagnosis was arteriosclerosis of the carotid artery with cerebral infarct (in other words, hardening of the artery leading to the brain with the death of brain tissue). This rather obscure and unusual case was reported in the November 23, 1933, issue of the *New England Journal of Medicine* (where it was referred to as Case 91471) and was promptly forgotten about for the next thirty years or so.

Fast forward to 1968.

A brilliant young doctor had just completed his education, including a residency and fellowship in chemistry, medicine, biochemistry, molecular biology, genetics, and pathology. His name was Kilmer McCully, and shortly after completing his studies at Harvard University (where he graduated cum laude) he was given an appointment and a research lab at the prestigious Massachusetts General Hospital in Boston.

McCully wanted to study diseases of genetic origin, so he began looking at weird genetic diseases and somehow came across Case 91471. Because McCully had an incredibly diverse background, he was able to do some medical detective work and, very (*very*) long story short,

he discovered that what killed the eight-year old boy was a little-known and recently discovered disease called *homocystinuria*, which produces an excess of a nasty little toxic compound in the blood called *homocysteine*.

More detective work and the beginnings of a theory followed. Homocysteine, in McCully's view, was linked to heart disease and might, just *might*, be more important than cholesterol. He published a paper stating this view in the *American Journal of Pathology* in 1969.

The conventional medical establishment was not amused. Here's McCully in his own words:

> For about six or seven years I continued work on this project. I made a number of observations and discoveries in homocysteine metabolism. Every experiment I conducted showed something new. It was an exciting time. In the early and mid-1970s I published quite a number of papers presenting evidence that supported the observation that homocysteine had something to do with vascular disease.
>
> Then in 1976, the chairman of my department at Harvard retired and the new chairman told me the elders at Harvard felt I had not proved my theory, and unless I could support my salary from grant money I would be cut off and have no position. They moved my lab into the basement where I had no contact with other people. They made the situation so unpleasant I decided I couldn't work there.
>
> I left in January 1979 and tried to find another position. For the next twenty-seven months I was unable to find a position in North America that would allow me to continue this work.

When asked why he thought he was given the heave-ho, McCully said the following:

> They told me later they didn't want to have Harvard or Massachusetts General Hospital associated with my theory because it appeared to contradict the conventional wisdom that cholesterol and fats were the causes of heart disease."[20]

Well, yes, we mustn't upset that $20 billion-a-year applecart, mustn't we?

But don't get me started.

This isn't a book about the idiocy and stubbornness of the conventional medical establishment, so I won't bore you with the details of what happened over the next thirty years. The bottom line is that McCully was reinstated at Harvard Medical School, homocysteine is now an accepted risk factor for heart disease and stroke, and the homocysteine test is widely available everywhere. As Michelle Stacy wrote in the *New York Times*, "Where once McCully's was almost a lone voice in homocysteine research, now dozens of articles have appeared in scientific journals, including one a few weeks ago in the *New England Journal of Medicine*. Where once the theory was shunned by the grant-giving powers that be, the National Institutes of Health recently put out a request for applications for further research, and at least one large-scale study of homocysteine in humans is already under way."[21]

John Rowe, M.D., and Robert Kahn, Ph.D., the lead researchers for one of the most comprehensive and significant studies ever done on aging in America (the MacArthur Foundation Study of Successful Aging), concluded that elevated homocysteine carries as much risk as hypertension. "The higher one's blood level of homocysteine, the greater one's risk of vascular disease," they wrote.[22]

There have since been a ton of studies on homocysteine and the risk for cardiovascular disease and stroke. Although virtually every one of them has shown a relationship, the exact size of the relationship has been hard to determine, and the results have varied from study to study, largely because people with elevated homocysteine also have *other* risk factors for heart disease. (Smoking, for example, drives homocysteine off the charts.) But when all is said and done, after adjusting for the effects of smoking, blood pressure, and cholesterol, merely lowering homocysteine by 25 percent is associated with an 11 percent reduction in coronary heart disease risk and a 19 percent reduction in the risk for stroke.[23] Considering how easy it is to bring down your homocysteine levels, I'd say those figures make it something worth doing.

Oh, and just for good measure, you might be interested to know that in addition to heart disease and stroke, excess homocysteine has also been correlated with Alzheimer's disease, osteoporosis, depression, and cognitive impairment.

Most anti-aging doctors that I respect like to see homocysteine levels no higher than 10, and the Life Extension Foundation recommends 7 to 8 as an optimal range. "My primary goal is below 7, but sometimes I have to settle for 8 because 7 may not be achievable," says my good friend David Leonardi, M.D., an anti-aging specialist and the medical director of the Leonardi Executive Health Institute in Denver. In most Western populations, the average concentration of blood homocysteine is about 12 umol/L, a full 33.33 percent higher than the best docs think is optimal.

So what can you do about this?

Three simple B vitamins will lower your homocysteine levels, documented by a ton of peer-reviewed published research. These vitamins are folic acid, B_{12}, and B_6. Normally, the body makes homocysteine as a by-product of the metabolism of an amino acid called *methionine*, and under ideal circumstances, "detoxifies" and remetabolizes it back into methionine and other beneficial or harmless compounds. It's only when that doesn't happen effectively and homocysteine builds up that you have a problem. Folic acid, B_{12}, and B_6 all play a role in turning homocysteine back into compounds that aren't a health concern.

Now in the interest of fairness, I want to point out that lowering homocysteine is not a magic bullet when it comes to reducing heart disease, nor when it comes to improving your odds of living longer and healthier.

In fact, at least one study, the SEARCH trial,[24] found no reduction in vascular events as a result of lowering homocysteine. So did the initial results of the Vitamin Intervention for Stroke Prevention, or VISP, study.

But when researchers reanalyzed the VISP study data, eliminating patients who had significant kidney problems at the start of the study, as well as patients who had uncommonly high or low B_{12} levels, high-dose vitamin supplements did indeed reduce stroke, death, and heart disease by a very nice 21 percent. Those findings were published in the journal *Stroke*.[25] And a large epidemiological study demonstrated that homocysteine levels above 10 µmol/L are associated with an up to threefold increase in heart attack risk.[26] A study published in the *New England Journal of Medicine* followed 587 people with coronary disease, a lot of whom had already undergone bypass surgery or angioplasty. Over the five years of follow-up, the mortality rate of those with homocysteine levels below 9 umol/L was 3.8 percent. The mortality rate for those with homocysteine levels of 15 or greater was a whopping 24.7 percent, more than six times higher than those with the lower, healthier levels of this toxic compound![27]

So let's review what we've got. Evidence shows this toxic by-product contributes to atherosclerosis, reduces the flexibility of blood vessels, and contributes to making platelets stickier, thus slowing blood flow. Net result: There's a direct correlation between high homocysteine levels and an increased risk of heart disease and stroke. And we now know that even small increases in homocysteine levels can significantly increase the risk of heart disease.

Still, this strategy is not a universal remedy. As I've pointed out before, anti-aging is a holistic endeavor, much greater than the sum of individual strategies and parts. There are more than a few good reasons to believe that lowering measures of inflammation, including homocysteine, throughout the body will have benefits down the road, particularly when combined with other life-extending strategies such as lowering insulin (see page 133), boosting immune system functioning, and lowering systemic stress. And the individual B vitamins needed to lower homocysteine, particularly folic acid, have so many other benefits (and virtually no downsides for the vast majority of people) that it doesn't seem like much of a stretch to recommend that you take them on a regular basis.

ASK YOUR DOCTOR TO MEASURE THIS INFLAMMATION MARKER

C-reactive protein (CRP), a compound first identified in the 1930s, is a component of the immune system and a substance produced in the liver in response to inflammation. The standard test for CRP has long been used to detect infections and as an assessment tool for such inflammatory conditions as arthritis and autoimmune diseases. The standard CRP test doesn't pick up the low levels of inflammation that can slowly age your body and contribute to heart disease. But the new, high-sensitivity CRP test does.

I think this is a test that should be part of every major blood workup.

C-reactive protein is a great marker for systemic inflammation and is beginning to emerge as a powerful predictor for coronary heart disease as well as for other diseases of the cardiovascular system.[28] Because the high-sensitivity CRP test (hs-CRP) is capable of picking up levels of CRP in the blood at the very earliest stages of vascular disease, you have a much better shot at treating inflammation early before it ages your body beyond repair.

Research has found that high-sensitivity cardiac CRP is able to predict the risk of myocardial infarction (heart attack), stroke, peripheral arterial disease, and even sudden cardiac death among healthy individuals with no history of cardiovascular disease! It can even predict recurrent events and death in patients with coronary syndromes. Researchers have concluded that higher levels of cardiac CRP are associated with higher risk for cardiovascular disease.[29] And here's what researchers writing in the prestigious journal *Circulation* said:

"In older men and women, elevated C-reactive protein was associated with an increased 10-year risk of coronary heart disease, regardless of the presence or absence of cardiac risk factors. A single CRP measurement provided information beyond conventional risk assessment, especially in (men and women at intermediate levels of risk)."[30]

And, in another perfect example of how lowering the risk factor for aging in one organ (the heart) can also lower the risk of aging in other systems, consider this: Increased C-reactive protein is also linked with a greater risk for developing type ll diabetes, age-related macular degeneration, and even the loss of cognitive ability in seemingly healthy people. It's also strongly related to major depression in men.

The simple message: Get your levels tested. And if they're high, get them down.

You may remember from earlier discussions that fish oil is one of the most anti-inflammatory substances on the planet. It may well turn out that fish oil (and even the omega-3s from plant foods such as flaxseed) may help keep CRP levels in check. In any case, the best protection we have right now, because there are no drugs that specifically lower CRP levels, is to eat an anti-inflammatory diet. The foods recommended in this chapter are a great beginning.

THE POTASSIUM CONNECTION

A lot of research, going all the way back to 1928, suggests that high potassium intake can reduce high blood pressure.[31] Large groups of people with a high intake of potassium have lower blood pressure than large groups of people who don't consume a lot of potassium. And there's research showing that this is true for individuals as well.

To understand why, it helps to understand the relationship of sodium and potassium. These two minerals operate in a kind of seesaw relationship in the body, performing all sorts of metabolic functions, including the regulation of blood pressure. Although we've heard a ton of warnings about too much sodium in our diet, the truth is a bit more nuanced and has to do with the *balance* between the two. Our Paleolithic ancestors consumed a hearty 5:1 ratio of potassium to sodium in their diet—the average American has that upside down, consuming about a 2:1 ratio of sodium to potassium.

"Too much sodium compared to potassium can tip the scales in favor of hypertension, while too little sodium compared to potassium can leave you with low blood pressure," says Houston.

So here's yet another reason why high fruit and vegetable consumption is associated with health and longevity and are a feature of the diet of every long-lived society ever studied: Fruits and vegetables are the best dietary sources of potassium on the planet.

"I recommend a potassium intake of 4,000 milligrams or more per day, with the bulk of it in food form," says Houston. Yams, beans, potato skins, Swiss chard, portobello mushrooms, winter squash, and kale are all great sources of potassium, as are apricots, dates, figs, apples, avocados, raisins, prunes, and bananas.

Magnificent Magnesium

In addition to potassium, magnesium may be one of the most helpful nutrients for maintaining healthy blood pressure. One reason: It helps the arteries squeeze and relax as necessary. Plus, it's an essential component of several hundred metabolic processes, including the creation of important hormonelike substances called *eicosanoids* (or *prostaglandins*) that help the arteries dilate (as opposed to constrict). In fact, you can think of magnesium as the "relaxing" mineral; think Epson salts, which are basically high-magnesium baths!

Once again, not surprisingly, magnesium is found everywhere in the plant kingdom. Shiitake mushrooms, navy beans, soybeans, leeks, kale, peppers, spinach, and chard are all great vegetable sources of this wonderful mineral, as are figs, prunes, peaches, apricots, and dates. And nuts and seeds are absolutely loaded with the stuff—pumpkin seeds, flaxseeds, almonds and almond butter, raw cashews, walnuts—if it's a nut or a seed, chances are it's a good source of magnesium.

Mineral Synergy

Nothing in nature works in a vacuum, and this is especially true with minerals in the diet. Although studies on calcium supplements and blood pressure have yielded mixed results, Houston believes that the relationship among the minerals calcium, magnesium, and potassium (and sodium) may be the key. And some people respond more to certain minerals (and nutrients in general) than others because of a wide range of individual factors.

"Each (of these minerals) influences the action of the others," says Houston. "For example, low magnesium will cause low potassium, so until the missing magnesium is replaced, taking potassium alone will not increase blood potassium levels. If you want to reduce blood pressure, taking more calcium, potassium, and magnesium together, coupled with a low sodium intake, will be more effective than doing any of these things by itself.

Research shows that, through the use of hs-CRP tests, we are now better able to predict the risks of heart attacks, stroke, arterial diseases, and even sudden cardiac death. Those with elevated CRP levels have up to three times greater risk than those with normal levels.

TAKING THE (BLOOD) PRESSURE OFF

Picture this: You're a primitive caveman on the African savannah enjoying a much-deserved snooze after a hard day of hunting and gathering. All of a sudden you spot a lion eyeing you with a look that says, "Hmm. Human. Tasty lunch."

We've already talked about how the stress response kicks in, getting you in gear and preparing you to either run like heck or (more stupidly, in this case) stay and fight. Now let's talk about a specific aspect of that response, one that has a lot to do with whether you actually *become* lunch or eat one. That aspect of the stress response is blood pressure.

See, if you're going to have the energy to flee or fight, you're going to need all the fresh, oxygenated, nutrient-rich blood your heart can pump, and you're going to need it rushed special delivery to all the tissues that require it posthaste. That increase in blood pressure is normal and important for survival. Whether you're running from a lion or running a 5K in New York's Central Park, your blood pressure and heart rate are going to increase, but once things return to normal they should go back down.

"With hypertension (high blood pressure)," says Houston, "your heart is often or *always* working harder than normal and your arteries are *always* narrow and constricted."

So why is this not a good thing from the point of view of aging? Let me count the ways.

Remember the endothelium we discussed earlier? That one-cell-thick lining between the blood itself and the blood vessel walls? Well, when blood comes pounding through the arteries like killer hurricane waves against the Santa Monica Pier, that lining gets damaged. This is way more of a problem than it sounds like. Remember that the endothelium secretes all kinds of substances that affect cardiovascular health.

"Damage to the endothelium speeds up what's called hardening of the arteries (atherosclerosis), a process that affects all of us as we age," says Houston. "These stiffened, narrowed arteries have a hard time supplying the body with enough oxygen and nutrients, which means the tissues and organs that they serve can be damaged." This is one way that high blood pressure will age you.

Endothelial damage, or endothelial dysfunction, is at the center of the problem of high blood pressure, but it hardly stops there. High blood pressure damages the heart, the brain, the kidneys, and the eyes. "It causes stroke by weakening and wearing away at the lining of the brain arteries, and choking these arteries with plaque," says Houston. "The damaged linings provide a perfect site for plaque deposition and the formation of blood clots."

And if you think high blood pressure doesn't affect aging, think again. "The higher your blood pressure, the shorter your life expectancy," says Houston. Here's a chart that shows the relationship between life expectancy and blood pressure for a thirty-five-year-old man.[32]

Blood Pressure (mm/Hg)	Life Expectancy
120/80	76
130/90	67 1/2
140/95	62 1/2
150/100	55

There are risk factors for high blood pressure that you can't change (such as genetics and race), but these are far outweighed by the ones you *can* change. The top of the list is smoking, but right up there with it is poor diet and lack of exercise. Regular exercise lowers blood pressure and the risk of cardiovascular disease. Merely losing weight will bring your blood pressure down. And do I really have to tell you about the ten million ways throwing out your cigarettes will extend your life? I thought not.

USE THE DASH DIET TO LOWER BLOOD PRESSURE NATURALLY

In 1997, the National Heart, Lung, and Blood Institute funded a classic study on the effect of diet on hypertension (high blood pressure). The name of the study was the DASH study, an acronym for Dietary Approaches to Stop Hypertension. The study compared three diets: (1) the standard (horrible) American diet (appropriate acronym SAD), (2) a diet similar to the SAD (standard American diet) but with more vegetables and fruits, and (3) the DASH diet, which was high in vegetables, fruits, and low-fat dairy, but low in saturated fat, total fat, and cholesterol.

At the end of the study, both groups 2 and 3 had much lower blood pressure, showing that fruits and vegetables really made a difference. But the people in group 3—the ones on the DASH diet—got the best results. And the most striking results happened for those who had high blood pressure to begin with. In fact, their results were just as good as those that had been obtained with medication!

Okay, fast-forward to a second study, called, guess what, the DASH-ll. This study divided folks into two groups. One ate the SAD diet and the other ate the DASH-ll diet, which was basically the same as DASH-l only with a reduction in sodium. (The first DASH diet didn't make any specific changes to sodium intake.) In DASH-ll, each person consumed a specific amount of sodium for a month at a time. They consumed 4,300 milligrams per day for the first month, followed by 2,400 milligrams per day for the second, and finally, 1,500 milligrams per day for the last month.

Regardless of whether people were on the standard American diet (group 1) or the DASH-ll diet (group 2), lowering sodium produced a reduction in blood pressure. But the reduction was greatest in group 2, those on the DASH-ll program, showing that combining sodium reduction with a high fruit and vegetable intake was the most productive approach to lowering blood pressure. Again, those that got the most stunning results were the ones in the most "trouble" (blood pressure–wise) to begin with.

Not long ago, the Hypertension Institute of St. Thomas Hospital in Nashville pioneered a program that went the DASH-ll diet one better. Under the direction of my old friend Houston, patients were given a specially modified version of the DASH diet that Houston believes is the best diet possible for people with hypertension. (You'll notice that this diet has a lot of overlap with the general dietary strategies recommended for anti-aging throughout this book; it's not a coincidence.) Check out the Hypertension Institute version of the Modified DASH Diet for reducing blood pressure (and for reducing its aging effects on your cardiovascular system) on page 112.

THE MODIFIED DASH DIET FOR REDUCING BLOOD PRESSURE

Food Group	Number of Servings	Serving Size	Suggestions
Cereals, grains, pasta	3–4 per day	1 oz dry flax or whole-grain cereal, ½ cup cooked cereal, 1 slice bread, ½ cup cooked whole wheat pasta	Eat whole-grain breads, cereals, and pastas with no added sugar or salt.
Vegetables	8–10 per day!!	1 medium vegetable, 1 cup raw (chopped) ½ cup cooked, 6 oz unprocessed vegetable juice	Eat your vegetables raw, or cook them lightly without adding salt or fats. You can substitute vegetable juice for one serving per day, but make sure it contains no salt.
Fruits	2–3 per day	1 medium fruit, 1 cup raw (chopped), ½ cup cooked	Eat your fruits raw whenever possible. If chopped, cut just before serving to preserve all the vitamins.
Meat, poultry, fish	2–4 per day	3–5 oz cooked	Eat lean cuts only; trim fat; skin poultry; cold-water fish is preferred.
Dried beans, seeds, nuts	1–2 per day	½ cup cooked beans, 2 tbsp seeds, ⅓ cup nuts, 3 oz tofu	Choose unsalted nuts or seeds. Avoid canned beans because of high sodium/sugar content.
Dairy	1–2 per day	1 cup nonfat or low-fat milk, buttermilk, or yogurt 1½ oz nonfat or low-fat cheese (low-sodium kind)	Dairy products are great sources of calcium, but also provide moderate amounts of sodium. Get the nonfat or low-fat and low-sodium varieties whenever possible.
Fats and oils	4–5 per day	1 tsp canola mayonnaise, 1 tsp virgin olive oil, 1 tsp spread made from omega-3 fatty acids (e.g., flaxseed oil mixed with butter)	Reduce saturated fat. Replace with monounsaturated oils, such as olive oil.
Sweets	None!		Avoid candy, pastries, sugar, honey, syrup, and jelly.

Adapted from *What Your Doctor May Not Tell You about Hypertension* by Mark Houston, M.D., with Barry Fox, Ph.D., and Nadine Taylor, M.S., R.D. Used with permission.

ANTI-AGING ACTION PLAN:

Lower Your Blood Pressure with Vasculosirt

My good friend, Mark Houston, M.D., recommends taking Vasculosirt as part of your program to lower blood pressure. Houston designed this supplement, which incorporates everything that current state-of-the-art research shows is important in reducing the risk of hypertension.

Vasculosirt is a blend of antioxidants, minerals, and anti-inflammatories like quercetin. It is available through its manufacturer, Biotics Research by calling 800.231.5777 or you can find it at vitamin and health food stores.

DR. HOUSTON RECOMMENDS

The list of supplements recommended at the Hypertension Institute as part of a program to lower blood pressure is naturally pretty long. Many of them, including omega-3s and resveratrol, overlap with supplement recommendations I've made elsewhere in this book. But if hypertension is an issue that concerns you—and if you have it, it should concern you very much—Houston has designed a supplement that incorporates everything that current state-of-the-art research shows is important in reducing the risk of hypertension.

The supplement is a potent blend of antioxidants like vitamin C and olive leaf extract, minerals like magnesium, and anti-inflammatories like quercetin. It's called VasculoSirt and is available through the manufacturer, Biotics Research, at 800.231.5777. Houston, who is not known for either hyperbole or unsubstantiated claims, told me, "VasculoSirt slows vascular aging and reduces vascular disease." Highly recommended.

EXERCISE: EVEN MORE IMPORTANT THAN YOU MIGHT THINK!

There probably isn't a person on the planet—certainly no one reading this book—who doesn't know by now that exercise is good for the heart. But the connection is actually more profound and interesting than you might have thought. To understand the way exercise actually influences things like blood pressure, it helps to understand how exercise affects the brain and the nervous system.

"The nervous system can be compared to the wiring in a house," says my friend, holistic chiropractor Ann Knight, D.C. (www.drannknight.com). "When the nerves and neurons are firing correctly, the system works as it should, just as when the wiring in the house is intact, the TV and other appliances work just fine."

In a house, it doesn't much matter whether the TV is on all the time, or the lights are switched off. When you need those lights, you just flip the switch and presto, there they are. And if you turn off the TV for a month and then decide you just can't live without those *Friends* reruns, you can be pretty sure that at the flick of a switch, Monica, Chandler, and the gang will be right back in your living room where they belong.

Unfortunately, the body doesn't quite work that way.

In the body, and the brain, it's "use it or lose it" time. The "circuits" (or wiring) that you use the most get stronger, and the ones that you don't use get weaker. (Much like in the gym, if you exercise your biceps, they get bigger, and if you don't, they eventually turn into pancakes.) Similarly, if you turn off your body's "television wiring" for a few months and then decide to turn it back on, you're likely to get a lot of static and snow instead of Rachel and Phoebe.

Now the nervous system has "wiring" that is permanently connected, like the electricity to the clocks in your house, and there is wiring that is voluntarily turned on and off (like the power to the TV). "The nervous system has some of these circuits that are always running," explains Knight. "These are very primitive circuits that are related to basic survival. These circuits control breathing, blood pressure, heart rate, digestion, and most other organ functions. They're the 'clocks' of the body. You don't have to think about them consciously to get them to function."

The part of the nervous system that controls these circuits is called the autonomic nervous system. The *autonomic nervous system* has two divisions—*sympathetic* and *parasympathetic*—one of which speeds things up and the other of which slows things down. The accelerator part is called the *sympathetic* nervous system. When you're resting comfortably on that African savannah we talked about and suddenly a lion eyes you hungrily, it's the sympathetic nervous system that makes your heart rate and blood pressure go through the roof. And when you're relaxed and about to sit down for a nice meal, it's the *parasympathetic* nervous system that slows your heart rate, lowers your blood pressure, and concentrates your energy on digestion and other tasks that are superfluous if you're trying to run away from a lion. (If you're trying to avoid becoming lunch, it doesn't make much sense to waste valuable metabolic energy on things like immunity or digestion.)

In the best of all possible worlds, these two systems work nicely together, like the accelerator and the brakes in a car.

To understand how exercise influences this equation, it's helpful to think about what happens when you break your arm. When you put a joint in a cast, Knight says, "you change the feedback that the joint sends to the brain. The brain will actually remodel itself to reflect that lack of movement of that particular joint. The area in the brain that represents that joint will actually become smaller. And the brain will also expand in other areas to compensate for that change. That remodeling happens very quickly, which is why it's so important to do proper rehabilitation after an injury where any body part is immobilized or put in a cast for any length of time."

But putting your arm in a cast is not the only way to stop movement. You can limit movement voluntarily or unconsciously, just by sitting at your desk all day or lying on the couch all night and eating bonbons. The brain doesn't really know the difference; it treats this inactivity the same way it would treat inactivity caused by a cast.

ANTI–AGING ACTION PLAN:

Get Moving to Keep Your Heart Healthy

Exercise doesn't have to be intense to benefit the brain systems that keep the heart healthy. Ping-Pong, tai chi, and ballroom dancing are just a few of the many ways to strengthen the parasympathetic nervous system's ability to keep your heart healthy and your body young.

Although you can get cardio benefits from as little as three half-hour sessions a week, the optimal number seems to be the equivalent of thirty to sixty minutes five days a week.

Now, because the circuits that run the accelerator are on all the time, this inactivity doesn't affect them much. As long as you're breathing, they keep your heart beating and your blood pressure pressuring whether you move around a lot or not. But the circuits that *calm things down* can use all the help they can get. And when you officially become a couch potato, those "braking" circuits begin to lose their power to get the job done. Without the brakes to balance things out, the accelerator has a field day.

This is one of the reasons blood pressure rises as you age. It's like a teenager without supervision or an id without a superego—absent any adult supervision to tone things down, the brain continues to send signals to speed things up without enough complementary balancing activity to slow them down. Those circuits are like your neglected biceps in the gym. "Remember, when the brain is activated it provides brakes to the system," Knight says. "It slows down the heart rate, decreases the blood pressure, and allows for the digestive organs to digest food and provide the brain with nutrients."

All operations that tend to "deteriorate" with age.

But they don't have to.

"The whole process of brain aging occurs subtly, and often the symptoms don't appear until this process has been underway for many years," Knight told me. "When the process is detected, often heroic efforts such as pharmaceuticals must be used to lower blood pressure and heart rate in an attempt to prevent the damaging, aging effects of a sustained high heart rate or hypertension."

Enter exercise.

Exercise will increase blood pressure and heart rate, too, as Houston reminds us, but exercise *also* activates brain areas that allow the brakes to be put on. This is the real gift of exercise to the person who wants to age optimally and healthily. And it's why exercise has a positive effect on blood pressure and on the heart in general.

So when you're going for a walk, stretching your muscles, learning the mambo, or doing tai chi, you're actually helping circuits fire in the brain that have the effects of strengthening the "brakes" and protecting your heart from aging.

This is why brain experts such as Daniel Amen, M.D., and Larry McCleary, M.D., recommend activities like Ping-Pong and ballroom dancing. It's not all about the aerobics and the pumping heart; it's also about messages to the brain to keep it flexible and active. "With exercise, you get so much firing from the joints and muscles that it actually increases brain activity," explains Knight. By "uncasting" those joints, you are flooding the brain with signals that allow it to keep your heart healthy and your blood pressure down.

SUPPLEMENT YOUR DIET WITH THESE ITEMS

These are some of the nutritional supplements I think are most important for protecting the heart.

Fish oil: Fish oil helps prevent heart disease. There, I've said it, no disclaimers, no "these statements haven't been evaluated by the FDA," no "results aren't typical" in the small print, just a clear, measured opinion statement based on a reading of literally hundreds of studies showing the overwhelming benefit of omega-3 fatty acids for just about every organ and system in the human body.

Of course, this is not just my opinion. In a study in the *Journal of the American Medical Association*, researchers from the Harvard School of Public Health reported that women who consumed fish two to four times per week reduced their risk of heart disease by 30 percent.[33] Another study in the same publication found that men who had no evidence of prior heart disease but consumed omega-3 fatty acids had a significantly reduced risk of sudden death.[34] And finally, Italian researchers reported in the journal *Circulation* that consuming 1 gram a day of omega-3 fatty acid supplements translated to a significantly reduced risk of sudden death among heart attack survivors.[35]

Omega-3s also seem to reduce the risk of stroke, lower triglycerides (an independent risk factor for heart disease), reduce blood pressure, and improve blood-clotting mechanisms.

CoQ10: Coenzyme Q10 is a powerful antioxidant that is normally made in the body, but we make less of it as we age. In Japan it was approved as a drug for congestive heart failure in 1973. Researchers have long known that there's a deficiency of CoQ10 in people suffering from heart disease.[36] "If a surgeon would like his heart patients to recover better and have a stronger heart muscle, CoQ10 supplementation should be a real option to use," says Franklin Rosenfeldt, M.D., head of the research unit at Alfred Hospital Cardiac Surgical Research Unit in Melbourne, Australia. Both statin drugs (cholesterol-lowering medications) and beta-blockers can inhibit CoQ10 activity in the body. If you are on a statin drug, for goodness's sake, supplement with CoQ10. Health professionals recommend 100 to 300 milligrams a day for those on statin medications. I recommend 100 milligrams a day for people who want to protect and nourish their heart.

L-carnitine: L-carnitine is an amino acid–like substance that helps with cellular energy. It acts as a little transport shuttle, moving fatty acids out of the bloodstream and into the power centers of the cells (mitochondria), where they can be burned for fuel. Because the heart is a hugely important muscle in the body, it uses a lot of energy. "The normal heart derives 60 to 70 percent of its fuel from fat, so for anyone with heart disease, efficient fat delivery to the mitochondria is a must," says my friend cardiologist Steven Sinatra, M.D. [37]

He also points out that L-carnitine is burned up in the heart under strain. So although healthy people might not need supplementation, those with any level of heart disease definitely could benefit. "The more advanced the heart disease, the lower the L-carnitine concentration present and the greater the need for it," says Sinatra.

The highest levels of L-carnitine (the word comes from the Latin *carnis*, meaning "meat") come from mutton, lamb, beef, and red meat. Most vegetarians don't get enough, and we make less of it as we age. "Having enough L-carnitine available to metabolize fatty acids efficiently lets the heart do more with less oxygen," says Sinatra. I've found the combination of CoQ10 and L-carnitine to be an excellent "energy cocktail" and wrote about it in my book, *The 150 Most Effective Ways to Boost Your Energy*.

For general prevention, and especially for vegetarians, Sinatra recommends 250 to 750 milligrams daily of L-carnitine. "Our heart patients take 1 to 2 grams once or twice a day," he says. There's been much written, and much controversy, about whether it's better to use plain old L-carnitine or a kind of "super" carnitine known as acetyl-L-carnitine (which appears to benefit the brain, but is more expensive). Opinion is divided as to which is best. My friend Mark Houston, M.D., recommends the acetyl-L-carnitine form, 500 milligrams twice a day. Either way, you can't go wrong.

Sip Green Tea to Protect Your Heart

Five cups a day seems to be the magic number for maximum benefits and heart protection. Alternatively (or in addition), take an EGCG supplement of 250 milligrams per day.

Garlic: Garlic has a number of properties that make it worth including in any program for heart protection. Yes, the conservatives will tell you that the studies are mixed, which they are, but the effects of garlic depend a lot on the kind of garlic used and on the method of preparation. Varying amounts of studies show that garlic lowers blood pressure, "bad" cholesterol, and triglycerides. One study showed that regular garlic consumption made the arteries of elderly people more elastic.[38]

The bottom line on garlic, which is one of the oldest medicinal foods on the planet and one on which more than 1,200 pharmacological studies have been done, is that it may influence the genesis and progression of cardiovascular disease through a number of different biological effects, including lowering LDL cholesterol, triglycerides, and blood pressure. And because it has other demonstrated medicinal properties, and may help knock out pathogens that contribute to inflammation, it makes sense to make it part of your diet. (If you take supplements, be sure to use a high-quality brand such as Kyolic Aged Garlic Extract or Allicidin by Designs for Health.)

"Studies show that garlic reduces multiple cardiovascular risk factors, including blood pressure, cholesterol, homocysteine, and platelet aggregation and adhesion, while stimulating nitric oxide generation in endothelial cells and raising HDL," says Sinatra. He has his patients with heart disease supplement with a minimum of 1,000 milligrams a day. The protocols at the Hypertension Institute at St. Thomas Hospital include a high-quality stable form of garlic called Allicidin by Designs for Health as part of their dietary and supplement regime for both hypertension and high triglycerides.

GREEN TEA: THE LONGEVITY DRINK

Japanese people live longer than people in any other country. One reason just might be the tea.

Japanese researchers[39] analyzed data from a National Cohort Study that began in 1994 and included more than 40,000 participants, aged 40 to 79. Everyone who started the study was free of stroke, heart disease, and cancer. For the next eleven years, researchers watched what happened. They found that people who drank five or more cups of tea a day had a significantly lower risk of death compared to the folks who drank only one cup or less a day. The five-cup drinkers had an especially lower risk of dying from cardiovascular disease and stroke.

The more green tea people consume, the less likely they are to have coronary artery disease. Underlying mechanisms for the heart-beneficial effects of tea include vasculoprotective, antioxidative, antithrombogenic, anti-inflammatory, and cholesterol-lowering properties of tea flavonoids.

And if you do, God forbid, have a heart attack, you probably have a better chance of recovering well if you're a green tea drinker. During a heart attack, a ton of inflammation and inflammation-related compounds are released. They promote even more (oxidative) damage, which in turn kills more

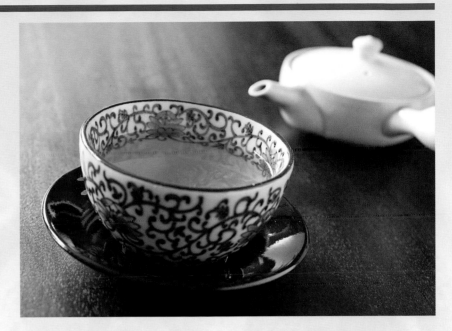

heart cells. The primary catechin in green tea, EGCG, prevents heart muscle damage by blocking the activation of some of these inflammation-related compounds. EGCG also appears to speed the recovery of heart cells.

Another way green tea helps protect the heart is by lowering blood pressure and helping prevent hypertension. Tea increases the body's production of nitric oxide, which dilates arteries and thereby reduces blood pressure.[40, 41] A study[42] published in the July 2004 *Archives of Internal Medicine* found that among persons consuming tea regularly for at least one year, the risk of developing high blood pressure was 46 percent lower among those who drank ½ cup to 2½ cups per day, and 65 percent lower among those consuming more than 2½ cups per day.

Green tea also shows promise in the prevention of stroke.[43] Furthermore, the green tea polyphenols, particularly EGCG, have been shown to protect brain cells from destructive processes following a stroke.[44, 45, 46]

How to Keep Your Brain Sharp

There may be a baby boomer or two who doesn't worry about losing their memory, but if there is, I've yet to meet them.

In fact, in talking to baby boomers around the country, the single fear I hear repeated most often is not the fear of dying, but the fear of losing one's faculties. Of not being able to remember the names of loved ones. Of being infirm and incapacitated and not even knowing what's going on. Of being kept alive, a virtual empty shell of the person you once were.

To many of us, that's a fate way worse than death. No wonder Nancy Reagan famously described life with her husband during the Alzheimer's years as "the long goodbye."

"Because people tend to forget that their brains are flesh and blood," says Dharma Singh Khalsa, M.D., author of *Brain Longevity*, "they often overlook the physical care and maintenance of their brains." There's an enormous disconnect between the amount of time we spend trying to build and protect our muscles and our skin and even our hearts all the while virtually ignoring what we can do to protect and nourish our brain, arguably the most important organ in the body.

The brain is responsible for cognitive tasks including attention, thinking, and memory, all of which decline when we age. But hundreds of other unconscious processes, such as the release of hormones, are mediated through signals that originate in the brain, and these processes have profound implications for our health and longevity. The aging brain affects us not only mentally, but also physically. If you think about the brain as an airport traffic control system, imagine what happens to all the planes if, all of a sudden, the phone lines get jammed up. Because

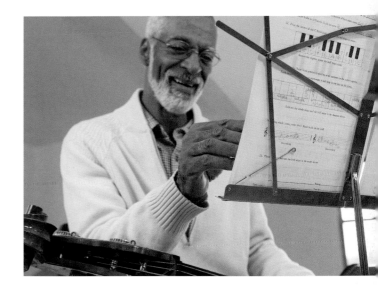

your brain is air traffic control central for your body, it's easy to see why an aging brain can also affect your sex drive, muscles, immune system, hormones, bones, heart, and every other destination that requires, directly or indirectly, signals from the brain to perform optimally. So anything we can do to keep the brain nourished and fully functioning is going to be a powerful strategy in the anti-aging arsenal. First, let's get the bad news out of the way: Starting in your early twenties, your brain begins to shrink. It does so at the rate of about 0.2 percent a year, and by your seventh decade or so it will be about 10 percent smaller than it was in your twenties. Sorry.

But here's the good news: *It may not matter.*

What *really* matters is the ability of the remaining neurons—and don't worry, there are billions of them—to make connections. In fact, making connections, or reorganizing your brain networks, is the single most important anti-aging strategy for keeping your brain young. (Don't worry if you don't yet know what I'm talking about because it will all become clear in this chapter.)

ANTI-AGING ACTION PLAN:
Revitalize Your Brain with Fish Oil

Taking fish oil is good for the cell membranes in the brain. The fatty acids it contains (EPA and DHA) get incorporated into the membranes, making them fluid enough for information to get in and out easily and facilitating cellular communication and, ultimately, a sharp mind! Take a minimum of 1 gram daily.

BRAIN BASICS

The average adult has somewhere around 100 billion neurons in his or her brain. (For comparison purposes, you have trillions, that's thousands of billions, of cells in your entire body.) Cells of the nervous system, known as *nerve cells* or *neurons*, are specialists with a particular job description. They have the ability to carry messages to other cells, much like a giant email system. (And the chemical messengers whose job it is to transmit those messages are called *neurotransmitters*—"neuro" for brain and "transmitters" for, well, transmitting!)

Neurons share certain characteristics with other cells in the body. They're surrounded by a cell membrane, they have a nucleus (which contains genes), and they have cytoplasm, the jellylike fluid encased inside the membrane where most of the cellular activities occur. Within this cytoplasm are little *organelles*, which are specialized subunits with specific functions. (One of the most important is the *mitochondria*, little structures that are ground zero for energy production.)

Because the membrane is like the casing for the cell, its health is very important. It acts like a spam detector on your computer's email system—tough enough to keep out the request for your bank account number from that Nigerian prince who wants to smuggle $20 million out of the United States, but not so tough that it rejects your wife's reminder to pick up the milk on the way home. If the cell membrane is too stiff, nothing, including valuable signaling information, can get in and out easily, but if it's not stiff enough, the boundaries aren't protected.

THE REAL INFORMATION SUPERHIGHWAY

That brain of yours is the server network for the biggest information superhighway in the world: your body. And the ability of your brain cells to form connections with other brain cells is of paramount importance in living long and living well, maybe even more important than the number of brain cells you actually have.

Here's a rough example. Suppose your goal is to reach up on the top shelf of your kitchen cabinet for your favorite coffee cup, which is hidden back there somewhere. But you hurt your right shoulder during golf yesterday, so stretching up there with your right hand is painful and difficult. What do you do?

You reach up with the *left* hand. Result: You still get to drink your coffee in your favorite mug.

Now suppose instead of reaching for a physical object (e.g., the coffee cup) you reach for a memory. Or a word that's on the tip of your tongue. Or a name you can't quite recall. When certain pathways or neurons have deteriorated, making it difficult to "reach" that memory (e.g., remember a name), the adaptable brain can "reroute" (e.g., use the "left hand"). It learns new sequences and develops new networks. That's why the actual physical shrinking, and concomitant loss of neurons, doesn't matter nearly as much as your ability to create these new *networks*, these alternative ways of "reaching" for what you want. And that's why a mnemonic device, such as remembering that a colleague's name is Peter because his nose looks like a pretzel, is so effective. It's an alternative way to access the memory.

Making new connections is a vital part of anti-aging, both literally (in the brain) and metaphorically (in life) and something that's much more under your control than you might think.

You see this all the time when someone relearns to walk or speak after a stroke. When certain pathways or neurons are damaged, the brain simply improvises, using new pathways to accomplish the same activity. It would be as if a tree fell on a hiking trail, cutting off the usual path to the mountaintop. Then, slowly and surely, hikers begin to take an alternate route until a new pathway develops, a trail is laid down, and eventually there's a whole new way to

get to the same end point. (Think: a right-handed person learning to write with the left hand.)

The ability to form these new neural networks is one of the most adaptive things our brain can do, and it is one of the keys to protecting the aging brain and keeping it young and active.

Remember the old riddle, "How do you get to Carnegie Hall? Practice, practice!" It's the same thing with your brain. You can practice network formation. You can strengthen the ability to form new connections, just as you strengthen your biceps by doing dumbbell curls. You can practice network formation and strengthen your brain's ability to do it by living what I call a *life of learning*. Brain expert Randy Buckner, Ph.D., of Harvard University, suggests that adults take university courses as a strategy to stave off brain aging. And why not? The key is to engage the brain in new activities and new challenging tasks.

Personally, I'm addicted to the Teaching Company courses (www.teach12.com). You may know them from their ubiquitous magazine ads. In the past few years I've taken "A Brief History of the World," "Fundamentals of Western Civilization," "The American Presidency," and an eighty-lecture series on the history of the United States. Just for fun, I memorized every U.S. president and can recite them in order, including the years they served. (I'm now a favorite party guest wherever friends play Trivial Pursuit. Want to know how many U.S. presidents were assassinated or died in office? Just ask me!)

Sounds silly, but it isn't. The important thing here is *learning new information.* Think about it: The average person slows down mentally when the kids leave the house. They're less engaged. They watch television and spend most of their leisure time being entertained rather than being actively involved. If they've worked at the same job for decades, the tasks they do, no matter how complicated, start to be performed by rote.

Learning new skills, such as studying new subjects (learning a language or the order of the U.S. presidents or a hundred breeds of dogs, or anything that might strike your fancy), engages the very networks whose health your youngevity depends on. It almost doesn't matter *what* you learn; rather, it matters *that* you learn. Anecdotally speaking, I'm sure it's no accident that some of the longest-lived folks on earth are musical conductors, who are constantly learning new scores or reinterpreting old ones. (And it doesn't hurt that they send a lot of oxygen into their brain by waving their hands around for two hours a night. Talk about "neuroaerobics"!)

"No matter how badly damaged your brain is, it can grow new cells and get more 'thinking power' out of old cells," says Khalsa.

THE LESSON FROM THE CANARY SCAM

Back in the 1930s, one of the most popular pets was the common yellow canary. People loved them because they could sing. But nature wasn't just—it only gave the ability to sing to the male of the species, rendering the females a lot less valuable to the bird-buying population. (Hey listen, there have to be *some* species where the males have an advantage, don't there? It's only fair!) So what to do about these tone-deaf female canaries? Well, unscrupulous pet store owners improvised. They somehow discovered that injecting the female birds with testosterone, the potent male hormone, temporarily turned the previously undesirable females into a bunch of operatic divas.

Over the past few decades, researchers have investigated this phenomenon more scientifically and discovered that injecting testosterone into female canaries produced an interesting side effect: It caused them to grow new brain cells.

Now before you throw this into the "so what?" file, consider that the prevailing wisdom at the time was that it was *impossible* to grow new brain cells, that you're born with as many nerve cells (neurons) as you will ever have, and that within the first year of life you start to lose them! The human brain contains about 100 billion nerve cells and a staggering 100 trillion connections, but by late adulthood those cells are dropping like flies; just in the course of normal use you'll lose about 100,000 brain cells a day (more if you play around with alcohol and drugs). So the notion that you could actually *grow new cells in the brain* was revolutionary.

"The philosophical implications of this discovery are profound," says Khalsa. "It means that people are not limited to just the brain cells they were born with."

WALK A DAY AND GAIN A SIZE

The work of Arthur Kramer, Ph.D., at the University of Illinois[1] has shown that a simple activity can actually increase the size of the brain. The activity? Walking.

Kramer and his colleagues put a group of sixty volunteers in an MRI machine, which pinpoints changes and abnormalities in body tissues. "These folks were basically couch potatoes," Kramer told me, "healthy but sedentary, and ranging in age from sixty to eighty." Then the researchers divided them into two groups. One group went into an aerobics program, the other into a "toning and stretching" program.

"We started the aerobics group at fifteen minutes a day at a pretty slow pace," Kramer said, "but after two months they were up to forty-five to sixty minutes, three days a week." And they kept it up for six months. "The other group did some very basic stretching exercises with exercise bands," he said. Good stuff, but not enough to get their heart rates up. Then after six months, the subjects went back into the MRI machine and the experimenters examined their gray and white matter.

The gray matter of the brain is composed of neurons or *computational units*, while the white matter is the axons, or interconnections, kind of like telephone wires between the neurons. The researchers specifically wanted to see whether any changes in either type of tissue had taken place over the course of the study.

ANTI-AGING ACTION PLAN:
Walk to Build Your Brain Power

Walking is one of the easiest ways to get exercise, so I recommend walking at a moderate pace for thirty minutes every day. All you need is a good pair of shoes. Once you start walking regularly, you can increase the pace and duration of your walks.

Starting in our early twenties, our brains begin to shrink, at a rate of 0.2 percent a year. So by your seventh decade, it will be about 10 percent smaller than it was in your twenties. However, studies show that exercise, such as walking, can actually increase the size of the brain. So get moving!

This was a novel approach to looking at the changes in the brain that exercise produces. Although plenty of studies have shown that exercise produces changes in the brain's *functional* abilities (e.g., improved memory, the ability to count backwards, etc.), no one had investigated *structural* changes. Kramer's work was unusual precisely because it focused on the *size* of the brain, not how it functioned. "This was pure anatomy," he told me.

I know you're on the edge of your seat wondering whether the brain actually got bigger, so I won't keep you in suspense: "Both the gray matter *and* the white matter showed increased volume," said Kramer.

In other words, exercise actually *increases* the size of the brain. And, at least when it comes to the brain, size does matter. More good news: It doesn't take much exercise to accomplish this minor miracle. Forty-five to sixty minutes, three times a week, seems to do the trick.

As we'll see countless times in this book, strategies that affect one organ or system in the body often influence others. The body is truly a "global economy" in which benefits spread from system to system without regard for parochial boundaries. In this case, exercise, one of the strongest anti-aging strategies on the planet for the heart (not to mention the bones and the lungs), affects the brain in the same way. "What's good for the heart is good for the brain" has been said by more experts than I can possibly count, largely because it is 100 percent true. Even Kramer's eight-year-old daughter was able to grasp the relationship when she summarized it thusly: "Exercise your heart and get really smart!"

PROTECT THE BRAIN: THE CORTISOL CONNECTION

In the first section, we discussed stress as one of the most important factors in the aging of every body organ and system. And there's no better way to show you how stress causes the brain to age than to tell you a story about fish.

It is a story passed down by one of the great neurological researchers of our time, Robert Sapolsky, Ph.D., and has been repeated in many classrooms and books ever since. Khalsa nicknamed it "the fish story." It goes like this:

One of the greatest feats of energy in the animal kingdom is performed by salmon, which literally swim upstream over long distances to spawn. After that, however, it's pretty much curtains for the salmon. They don't live to spawn another season. The journey exhausts them.

The fish need a ton of energy for that journey, which is an amazing feat of strength and endurance. Where do they get it? From our old friend cortisol, the stress hormone produced by the adrenal glands, the one I introduced in section I. Now when the fish start this journey, their normal cortisol-regulating mechanism is working just fine. But the journey requires the cortisol factory to work overtime.

So the adrenals just pump the stuff out, working tirelessly until the goal of spawning is achieved.

See, high cortisol, destructive though it is in the long run, can be energizing. A good example of this is the well-known phenomena of the "adrenaline junkie." The biochemical effect of cortisol can actually feel *good*, almost like a high, to some people, and it clearly acts as an "upper" to the fish. It's this rush of cortisol through the salmon's system that gets them, against all odds, up the river.

But this overproduction of cortisol during the exhausting journey has a price: The salmon die.

After they spawn, the salmon have hugely swollen adrenal glands, peptic ulcers, lesions on their kidneys, and a depleted immune system (making them far more likely to succumb to opportunistic infections and parasites). Their entire hormonal system is a complete mess. They die—very quickly.

But, Sapolsky tells us, a miraculous thing happens when researchers remove their adrenal glands right after they spawn. Cortisol production stops, obviously, and the salmon return to their previously healthy state and actually live another entire year. "The moral of the fish story," says Khalsa, "is that cortisol overproduction, which also happens to stressed-out people, wreaks havoc upon the body, the brain, and the nervous system."

THE THREE WAYS THAT STRESS AGES YOU

Stress, in the form of the stress hormone cortisol, ages your brain in three primary ways. The first is by decreasing glucose metabolism. See, the brain needs a certain amount of glucose (blood sugar) to function properly. But cortisol interferes with the hippocampus's ability to use blood sugar. When you don't have enough blood sugar, you

Reduce Stress Every Day by Doing Deep Breathing Exercises in a Quiet Place

Here's a great way to get started, and you can actually do it in fewer than ten minutes:

1. Lie down in a comfortable position (but try not to fall asleep!). In yoga, this is called Savasana (corpse pose), which should give you some idea of how relaxed you should be. The pose is used in yoga to practice stilling a hyperactive brain by gaining control over breathing.

2. Your arms should be by your sides, rolled out so your palms are facing up.

3. Your legs should be relaxed. Put support (like a rolled towel) under your knees and allow them to naturally roll outward.

4. Close your eyes.

5. Breathe normally for about a minute. Pay attention to your breath.

6. On each exhalation, imagine that all the points of contact between your body and the floor are softening.

7. After one or two minutes of normal breathing, gradually begin to extend the length of your exhalation. Exhale deeply and slowly.

8. The goal is to inhale fully on a count of four and then exhale fully on a count of eight. In other words, your exhalation should be twice as long as your inhalation.

9. Continue this 1:2 ratio for four to five minutes.

10. Go back to regular breathing for one to two minutes.

Don't get too hung up on the specifics, the counts, or the number of minutes. The idea is to simply breathe in slowly and breathe out even slower and to do it consistently. There are dozens of variations on this theme, including several I've written about in *The 150 Most Effective Ways to Boost Your Energy*. I also wrote about one method called "The Relaxation Response," which I wrote about in *The Most Effective Natural Cures on Earth*. Whatever technique you feel most comfortable with is just fine.

(Thanks to my dear friend, holistic health counselor Jeanette Bessinger of Balance for Life, LLC, for contributing this particular exercise. Visit Jeanette at www.balanceforlifellc.com.)

basically don't have enough fuel to lay down a memory. You may experience putting down the car keys or saying hello to your daughter, but you may not remember doing so. This is probably why short-term memory problems are so common under stress. The second way cortisol ages your brain is by interfering with its neurotransmitter circuits. You may recall that neurotransmitters are those chemical messengers that send information to the brain cells and are necessary for the creation of memories. Under high levels of stress, those memories are, in Khalsa's words, "like downed telephone lines in a storm." They exist, but they can't be accessed. The third and possibly most insidious way that cortisol ages your brain is by killing brain cells. Cortisol somehow allows too much calcium to get into the brain cells, and the calcium eventually produces free radicals (remember them?), causing oxidative damage and destruction. And just when you thought it couldn't get any worse, consider this: Cortisol literally shrinks the hippocampus, an important brain structure deeply involved in memory and one of the first regions of the brain to suffer damage in Alzheimer's disease. Cortisol does this through what Khalsa calls "the terrible feedback loop," or the destructive cascade. Here's how it works:

When you're under a lot of stress, what happens in your brain is like an army going into action. Your hypothalamus is like the general as it releases something called *corticotropin-releasing factor*, whose job it is to send a signal to the field commander (the pituitary), which puts out a second hormone called *ACTH* (also called *corticotropin*). ACTH then rushes down to the adrenals (the troops) and puts in the order for more cortisol. All this happens in less time than it takes to read one word of this sentence.

So far so good. Efficiency, clear chain of command, no problem. But whose job is it to turn off the cortisol

production once it's no longer needed? Who calls the troops back home after the battle is over?

Turns out the main responsibility for doing that falls to the hippocampus. But the hippocampus is the *very area of the brain most damaged by cortisol*! So now you have this terrible "degenerative cascade" in which the structure responsible for moderating the whole shebang is being damaged by the hormone it's trying to shut off. As a result, you may have more cortisol than you need running around your body even when you're not under stress!

There's a ton of research going back to the late 1960s demonstrating the link between high levels of cortisol and the major symptom of brain aging, memory loss.[2] Researcher Sonja Lupien, M.D., a neuropsychologist and assistant professor of psychiatry at McGill University, has published a number of papers linking stress and memory impairment. In one of her studies, she found that approximately one-third of fifty-one healthy subjects in

TRAIN YOUR BRAIN TO REMEMBER!

One thing aging can do to brain function is slow down the speed at which you process information. Mayo Clinic researchers investigated whether a computer program might improve the speed and accuracy of brain processing and discovered a fascinating side benefit of the program—it improved memory!

For five days a week for two months, men and women over age sixty-five, all of whom were healthy and none of whom had a diagnosis of cognitive impairment, worked on computer-based activities in their homes. The experimental computer program used six auditory exercises that were specially designed to improve both the speed and the accuracy of processing (such as distinguishing between low- and high-pitched sounds presented at an increasing speed). At the end of the eight weeks, researchers used standardized tools to measure changes in memory (such as the ability to repeat words or numbers after hearing them once).

Those in the experimental group improved twice as much over the course of eight weeks as the group that didn't play with the computer program. What's especially intriguing about this study is that the program really didn't "train" memory. Instead, it trained processing speed, but it improved memory nonetheless. Best of all, the participants in the experimental group reported that their memory had improved in day-to-day tasks as well.

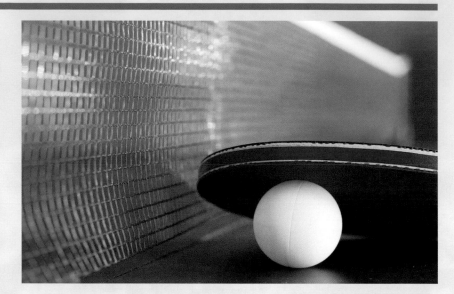

"The study indicates that choosing a memory-enhancing approach that focuses on improving brain processing speed and accuracy, rather than memory retention, may be helpful," said study author Glenn Smith, Ph.D., of the Mayo Clinic.[3]

It's way too early to know which of the many "brain training" programs sprouting up all over the place will actually work. But this study indicates that there may be some promising choices on the horizon when it comes to computer programs for the brain. Keep your eyes open!

And you don't need to wait for technology to come up with the perfect "brain training" program to start doing some work on keeping your mind sharp (not to mention hand-eye coordination). Why not take my friend Dr. Daniel Amen's advice: Pick up a Ping-Pong racket.

Ping-Pong is an activity tailor made to train your brain's ability to process information quicker. Who knows? That increasingly popular little sport— easily done into your nineties or even beyond—just might be the ticket to keeping your brain young and vibrant for a long time.

a study had sustained high levels of cortisol over a five-year period. This group was consistently terrible at remembering images they had been shown only twenty-four hours earlier. They also took much longer to find their way through a maze that was specially designed to measure spatial memory.[4] Research has shown that even people taking cortisone pills (which turns into cortisol in the body) don't remember word lists as well as people taking placebo (sugar) pills.[5]

Further, in a paper published in 2002, researchers from Beth Israel Medical Center and Harvard Medical School concluded that "stress has a major impact upon neurodegenerative and mental disorders." They also pointed out that the amount of stress you're under on a daily basis plays a significant role in how susceptible you are to the degenerative diseases associated with brain aging, not to mention the progression of those diseases and their eventual outcome.[6]

And now, just when you are close to being thoroughly depressed about the effect your overstressed life is having on your brain and your ability to age, well, it's time for the good news.

Much of this is reversible.

When the salmon's cortisol factory was shut off, the damage reversed and they lived for another year. We know from research that the hippocampus of a rat that's been stressed will return to normal size once the rat is left alone and cortisol production returns to normal. All this, and other research, indicates that if you can "down-regulate" the cortisol production factory, you may be able to reverse much of the aging damage that's been done.

Good news, especially if there is something we can actually *do* to return the cortisol manufacturing plant to its normal hours of operation. And there is.

It's called meditation.

More effective than any other anti-aging technique for reducing cortisol (and stress) and arresting any further aging of the brain that's caused by stress is simple meditation. And if that's too esoteric for you, deep breathing works just as well. Basic deep breathing exercises pioneered by Herbert Bensen, M.D., of Harvard University have been found to positively affect a host of syndromes related to aging, including stress.

THE SUGAR–INSULIN CONNECTION

The link between diabetes and Alzheimer's is both well documented and troubling. Several large studies show that people with type II diabetes have double the risk of developing Alzheimer's when compared with nondiabetics of the same sex and age. One study even found that those with borderline diabetes were an incredible 70 percent more likely to develop Alzheimer's than those with normal blood sugar.[7]

Although it's long been suspected that the connection might be due to cardiovascular problems caused by diabetes (resulting in blocked blood flow to the brain and contributing to dementia), other theories are emerging that center around the hormone *insulin*.

Here's how it works: When you eat sugar—or food that converts into sugar easily and quickly (such as white bread and pasta)—your blood sugar rises and your body (specifically your pancreas) responds with a squirt of insulin, a hormone whose many jobs includes escorting that excess blood sugar into the muscle cells, where it can be used for energy. But diabetics usually develop a condition called *insulin resistance* in which this system of regulating blood sugar doesn't work very well. Blood sugar goes up (especially when you eat high-carbohydrate brain. Every (metabolic) cloud has its silver lining, and all that, right?

Well, it *would indeed* be a good thing if there *were* more insulin in the brain. And that is exactly what you would reasonably expect to be the case if there was a lot of insulin hanging around in the bloodstream. What *actually* happens is the exact *opposite*.

With high levels of insulin in the bloodstream, the whole insulin signaling system gets screwed up. The transporters—those little structures responsible for getting insulin from the bloodstream into the brain—start to turn down the volume and become less active, with the result that *less* insulin actually gets into the brain, not more. And this *low* level of insulin in the brain, the direct result of having too *much* in the bloodstream, isn't good for either the brain or memory.

One of the many good things insulin does in the brain is break down a nasty, toxic little protein called *amyloid*. So one major effect of this whole sugar-insulin "deregulation" (and of the resulting lowered brain insulin) is that less amyloid gets broken down. Amyloid builds up, leading to plaques and causing more inflammation and injury to the brain. It also increases the amyloid plaques that are prominent in the brains of those with Alzheimer's. In the absence of insulin, the amyloid structures bind more readily to nerve cells, which results in—here we go again—*inflammation*! Neurons wind up disconnecting from one another, destroying the very connections that are the basis for all thought. "It's the first step in the degenerative process that eventually results in Alzheimer's disease," says McCleary.

Another feature of Alzheimer's and dementia, indeed of brain aging in general, is the loss of an important neurotransmitter called *acetylcholine* (more on that later).

foods), the body tries to protect itself by squirting even higher levels of insulin into the bloodstream, but the cells become resistant to its actions. This requires the pancreas to release even *more* insulin in a futile attempt to get your blood sugar back down where it belongs.

So now you have high insulin in the bloodstream. Which is not a good thing at all.

What does that have to do with the brain?

Well, a lot actually, and here is where it gets tricky, so pay close attention! Insulin performs a lot of important functions in the brain, most of them *good*. "Insulin in the brain acts on nerve cells to form new connections between brain cells and to resist the dents and dings of aging. It even increases neurogenesis (the formation of new neurons)," explains my friend, renowned brain surgeon Larry McCleary, M.D., author of *The Brain Trust Program*.

But wait, you might think. It sounds like this excess insulin that's carousing around the bloodstream as a result of insulin resistance is actually a *good* thing, right? Insulin resistance means more beneficial insulin for the

Acetylcholine deficiency has long been seen as an early abnormality in those who develop Alzheimer's, and it is linked to dementia as well. We need acetylcholine to think and remember. Researcher Suzanne de la Monte, M.D., at Brown University, shows that the enzyme that actually *makes* acetylcholine is regulated by—drum roll, please—*insulin*!

"Insulin is the controlling factor in (many features) of Alzheimer's disease," she says. "If you don't have enough insulin or the ability to respond to insulin is impaired, then neurons will not function well and they will probably die." De la Monte has actually coined the term *type III diabetes* to refer to the form of insulin deficiency in the brain that is increasingly linked to brain deterioration (and with the insulin resistance found in type ll diabetics, made worse by high-sugar diets).

To recap:

THE HORSEMAN RETURNS

So our old friend inflammation has shown its face again, this time as a major player in the aging and deteriorating brain. What about oxidation?

Researchers at Salk Institute and University of California, San Diego Department of Pathology wanted to investigate why diabetes seems to predispose people to Alzheimer's disease, so they induced diabetes in mice. The mice suffered damage to the blood vessels, largely due to the overproduction of free radicals. These free radicals caused oxidative damage to the cells that line the brain's blood vessels.[8]

If you think you know where all this is leading, you're probably right. Sugar, long known to be a major culprit in obesity, diabetes, heart disease, and even some cancers, is your worst enemy when it comes to protecting your aging brain.

And you don't have to have diabetes to benefit from getting off sugar (or at least decreasing its presence in your diet substantially). Just as this book was being written (spring 2009), new research from Columbia University Medical Center found that having high blood sugar levels may be to blame for memory lapses, the well-known "senior moment." This research indicated that *even in people who were perfectly healthy*, with not a hint of diabetes, keeping blood sugar under control might just be the key to preserving memory!

Spikes in blood sugar, typical of eating high-carb foods, seems to damage a particular area of the hippocampus called the *dendrate gyrus*, an area that actually helps us form memories. In one study, conducted by Scott Small, M.D., and his colleagues, the researchers did some interesting detective work. They scanned the brains of 240 elderly folks to try to find something that could be related to

Be a Sugar Detective to Guard Against Premature Aging

Read the label of every food you eat for sugar content. Remember that 4 grams equals 1 teaspoon. A high sugar diet can prematurely age you, resulting in sending high levels of insulin to the blood stream and low levels to the brain. When it comes to sugar, the less you consume, the better.

the damage in their aging brains, specifically to the dendrate gyrus.

They found it: sugar.

The researchers reported that the effect on the dendrate gyrus could be seen even with *moderately* elevated blood sugar (or glucose). Because physical activity helps regulate blood sugar, Small told the *New York Times*, "We have a behavioral recommendation—physical exercise."

I have another one: Dump the sugar.

Eliminating sugar may just be one of the best anti-aging strategies I know. To the extent that you can eliminate or reduce sugar in your diet, including sugar in the form of high-carb, processed foods, which have the same effects on your brain, you will be doing your brain the greatest possible favor, and possibly extending its useful shelf life by many years. What better result could you ask for from an anti-aging strategy?

FEED YOUR BRAIN, EXTEND YOUR LIFE

Let's cut to the chase: Want to start protecting your aging brain big time? Eat fish. At least twice a week, preferably more. Your grandmother was right about fish being brain food.

Cold-water fish (such as salmon) contains two critically important fatty acids that have significant effects on brain function and go by the unwieldy names of *docosahexaenoic acid* and *eicosapentanoic acid*, but we can call them by their nicknames, *DHA* and *EPA*. People have written entire books extolling the virtues of these omega-3 fats for the heart, brain, and overall human health, but the critical thing to remember for our purposes is that these essential fatty acids are highly concentrated in the brain and are your secret weapon in the fight against aging. (A new baby's brain is about 60 percent fat by weight and most of it is DHA!)

Omega-3s are particularly important for cognitive function (like memory). You may recall that these omega-3s are incorporated into cell membranes, making them fluid and thus making it easier for information from neurotransmitters to get in and out. Research has shown that including omega-3 fatty acids in the diet protects against such brain injuries as stroke caused by plaque buildup and blood clots in the arteries leading to the brain. In fact, eating at least two servings of fish per week can reduce the risk of stroke by as much as 50 percent, according to the University of Maryland Medical Center.[9]

> "Old neurons are like old married couples that don't talk to each other much anymore," says Joseph. The blueberries opened the lines of communication.

THE HIGH-ORAC EATING STRATEGY

You may remember from section I that antioxidants are powerful protection against damaging free radicals. You may also remember our discussion of high-ORAC foods, those that have been tested for antioxidant power and found to be outstanding performers. (As a reminder, ORAC stands for *Oxygen Radical Absorbance Capacity*—now you know why we like to simply call it ORAC!)

Well, there was a reason we spent so much time on that! High-ORAC foods may slow aging, and they seem to have a *particularly* powerful effect on the brain. In studies on middle-aged rats, high-ORAC foods helped protect the loss of function in brain cells, protected blood vessels against oxygen damage, and prevented the loss of long-term memory and learning ability. "If these findings are borne out," said Agricultural Research

ANTI-AGING ACTION PLAN:
Eat One Cup of Blueberries Three Times a Week for a Memory Boost

Eat more if you like! Blueberries are the ultimate "memory food." They are loaded with compounds that fight both oxidation and inflammation: two of the four horsemen of aging.

Blueberries can be added to cereal, eaten with yogurt, even sprinkled on green salads. They go great in smoothies. And best of all, you don't need to be limited by their seasonal availability—they're absolutely fabulous frozen. I actually eat them direct from the freezer (mixed with frozen cherries, yogurt or raw milk, and sprinkled with coconut flakes and almonds). Feel free to defrost if you don't like the "faux ice cream" effect!

Eat Cold-Water Fish Two to Three Times a Week for More Omega-3s

Best sources: wild salmon (like the Vital Choice brand linked on my website, www.jonnybowden.com), as well as mackerel, halibut, sardines, tuna, and herring.

A DEPRESSED BRAIN IS AN AGING BRAIN

With the relationship between depression and unhealthy aging becoming increasingly clear, consider anything that may help mood and optimism a strong asset in an anti-aging program. Omega-3s fit the bill.

At least one clinical study of patients hospitalized for depression has shown measurably low levels of omega-3 fatty acids (and the ratio of inflammatory omega-6s to anti-inflammatory omega-3s as especially high). Those who incorporated fatty fish two to three times a week into a healthy diet for five years experienced significant reduction in feelings of depression. Omega-3s are clearly mood enhancers, and by reducing depression they just may extend your life.

Service administrator Floyd P. Horn, "young and middle-aged people may be able to reduce the risk of diseases of aging—including senility—simply by adding high-ORAC foods to their diet."

One of the best researched foods for protecting the aging brain is blueberries. Just ask Jim Joseph, Ph.D., a researcher at the U.S. Department of Agriculture Human Nutrition Research Center on Aging at Tufts University. Specifically, ask him about the dancing rodents.

Joseph rigged up something he calls the "rat Olympics" in his research lab. Using various mazes and Rube Goldberg–type contraptions, he put his little rat subjects through various tests of memory, motor function, muscle strength, and coordination. Rats, like us, tend to slow down on all these measures during middle age.

Until you feed them blueberries.

Mental deterioration? Gone. Loss of coordination? Gone. Loss of balance? Ditto. The blueberry-eating rats performed like mambo-dancing youngsters. If you happen to be a rat, Joseph found you the Fountain of Youth.

So why blueberries? Well, as I've said before in this book (and as I talked about at length in *The 150 Healthiest*

Foods on Earth), blueberries are absolutely loaded with compounds that fight both oxidation and inflammation. They contain plant chemicals called *anthocyanins*, which protect the brain. And special compounds in the blueberries called *polyphenols* actually help neurons (brain cells) talk to each other. "Old neurons are like old married couples that don't talk to each other much anymore," says Joseph. The blueberries opened the lines of communication. Connections could be formed more easily, memories laid down and accessed, and a youthful vitality restored.

LOWER YOUR RISK OF COGNITIVE DECLINE

Can a diet actually protect your brain against one of the most devastating diseases of aging, Alzheimer's? Well, to quote an infamous American politician, "You betcha!"

Researchers looked at the eating habits of more than 1,300 people who had no particular cognitive problems as well as almost 500 folks who had what's called *mild cognitive impairment*, a condition that affects about 20 percent of

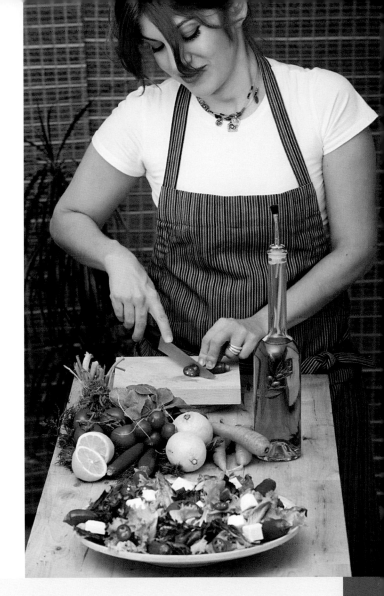

ANTI-AGING ACTION PLAN:
Follow the Mediterranean Diet to Slow Cognitive Decline

The Mediterranean diet emphasizes the consumption of vegetables, fruit, legumes, fish, and olive oil. (The diet is most decidedly not low fat, but the amount of junk food and processed carbs is somewhere between very little and zero.) There are many terrific books on the Mediterranean diet (although some tend to demonize saturated fat a bit more than I'm comfortable with). Nonetheless, you can find some excellent information and recipes in all three of the books listed in the resource section. Or Google "Mediterranean diet" and you'll be kept busy for days.

SPICE IT UP AND PROTECT YOUR MEMORY

Want a spice that can protect your brain? Look no further than the stuff that makes curry yellow—turmeric.

I've been a fan of this incredible spice ever since I wrote about it in *The 150 Healthiest Foods on Earth*. Turmeric contains active ingredients called *curcuminoids*, and these have been found to have potent anti-inflammatory and antioxidant properties. They have particular importance to the brain.

The general name for curcuminoids is *curcumin*, and it has been found to prevent the death of neurons (brain cells),[11] reduce oxidative damage, and decrease the formation of inflammatory factors in the brain.[12] And it reduces, or even, amazingly, reverses, the formation of amyloid plaques.[13, 14] Think of curcumin as a kind of natural NSAID (non-steroidal anti-inflammatory drug, such as ibuprofen). In that sense, it works much like omega-3 fatty acids from fish and flaxseed, and that may be part of the reason they are protective against Alzheimer's. Just for the record, the rate of Alzheimer's in the United States is nearly four times that of India, where turmeric is always on the menu.[15]

Research conducted in Singapore took a look at the role of curcumin (turmeric) in the prevention of basic cognitive decline, the kind that supposedly comes "naturally" with aging. The researchers measured decline by looking at scores on a test called the *MMSE* (Mini-Mental State Exam). The MMSE is a simple,

eleven-question test that's pretty standard for measuring cognitive decline. Questions include asking the person to name the date or follow simple instructions such as recalling three objects, counting by sevens, or repeating a simple phrase. The test is quite effective at identifying those with mild cognitive decline. Those who regularly consumed curry scored significantly higher on average compared to those who never, or rarely, did.

Turmeric, the whole spice, contains 2 to 6 percent curcumin. Although curcumin supplements are available, most experts recommend using the whole spice (turmeric) because it may contain a host of related compounds that work synergistically. Turmeric tastes delicious and you really can't overdo it. I sprinkle it on virtually everything, and it's my favorite seasoning for everything from scrambled eggs to soup.

the population over seventy. Mild cognitive impairment is a kind of middle stage between the "normal" cognitive decline of aging and the real serious stuff (e.g., Alzheimer's or dementia). The researchers put each patient into one of three groups, depending on how strictly they followed a Mediterranean-type diet (meaning large amounts of vegetables, fruits, fish, legumes, and olive oil, with relatively small amounts of meat and dairy).

What they found was that the patients who adhered most closely to a Mediterranean-type diet had an almost 30 percent lower risk of developing mild cognitive impairment (compared to those who followed it the least). They also noted that even in those who already had mild cognitive impairment, following a Mediterranean-type diet seemed to slow their decline.

It gets better. The most incredible finding of all was this: Those who followed the Mediterranean diet consistently had a 48 percent lower risk of developing Alzheimer's![10]

Although there is some variation in the Mediterranean diet depending on which part of the Mediterranean you live near, the foods mentioned above seem to hold across all regions.

Given that this kind of eating strategy has shown health benefits across a wide range of conditions, and that some of the healthiest and longest-lived people eat a diet not dissimilar from the one just described, it's reasonable to assume that this kind of eating style will protect your brain from aging badly as well as or better than any other dietary strategy on the planet.

PROTECT YOUR BRAIN WITH THESE SUPPLEMENTS

Inside most cells in the body there lives a tiny little structure called a *mitochondrion* (plural: *mitochondria*). The mitochondria are where all the action takes place for energy production in the cell, as well as burning fuel and supplying chemical energy to run the body. Some cells have only one mitochondrion and some have thousands. (Muscle cells, for example, are teeming with the little devils while fat cells—not so much.)

Brain cells have a lot of mitochondria.

The mitochondria play a huge role in aging. Not only are they responsible for energy, but they also put out a host of enzymes that are critical for the smooth operation of the brain. When the mitochondria are damaged—through oxidation and inflammation, for example—not only is their effectiveness as energy producers compromised, but so is their ability to manufacture these critical enzymes. Result: Your brain gets old, fast.

In a real sense, successful aging is all about avoiding damage to these critical energy-producing structures. When mitochondria are damaged, your energy drops, your heart doesn't function as well, memory declines, muscles start to ache, you don't feel as sharp, the whole nine yards. All of which makes perfect sense, because every function in the body requires energy. In general, diseases of aging all involve damage to the basic energy factories in the body.

The general term for this damage is *mitochondrial dysfunction.*

In the brain, damage to mitochondria can affect memory and thinking. Recently researchers have begun classifying nutrients that have a protective effect on these

Take Brain-Protecting Nutrients

To Keep Your Brain Firing on All Cylinders, Take These Supplements Daily:

→ Acetyl-L-carnitine: 1,000 mg (500 mg twice daily)

→ Alpha-lipoic acid: 100–300 mg

→ Phosphitadylserine: 150–300 mg

→ GPC (GlyceroPhosCholine): 600 mg

→ Gingko: 120-240 mg

Recommended: Take with 1,000–2,000 mg of omega-3 fatty acids

Note: These dosages are general-purpose recommendations. Individual requirements may vary.

functions as *mitochondrial nutrients*. Taken alone or, better yet, together, they can significantly reduce the risk of mitochondrial dysfunction, protecting your brain and its various functions well into your ninth decade or beyond.

The major way these mitochondrial nutrients help the brain is by protecting the energy centers of the cell against oxidative damage. Several research studies indicate that oxidative damage, the kind we talked about extensively in section I, is a major risk for the initiation and progression of both Parkinson's and Alzheimer's. One review, titled, "Can We Prevent Parkinson's and Alzheimer's Disease?" published in the *Journal of Postgraduate Medicine*, concluded that "reducing oxidative stress appears to be a rational choice for the prevention and reduction in the rate of progression of these neurological disorders."[16]

These nutrients act as PacMen toward free radicals and inhibit the damage to brain functioning they can cause. Chief among these mitochondrial nutrients are acetyl-L-carnitine and alpha-lipoic acid, both of which have been shown to protect the brain in significant ways. Other nutrients that work synergistically to keep your brain active and functioning include *phosphatidylserine*, *GPC* (GlyceroPhosCholine), and *ginkgo biloba*.

Let's take a look.

Acetyl-L-Carnitine: Teaching an Old Beagle New Tricks

As noted before in this book, L-carnitine is an amino acid–like compound that is derived from two other amino acids (lysine and methionine). We get it in the diet from red meats such as beef and lamb and we make it ourselves in the liver and kidneys. It's critical for energy production in the cells, including the cells in the brain.

Acetyl-L-carnitine is a form of L-carnitine that is kind of tailor made for the brain. In the acetyl-L-carnitine form, carnitine readily enters the brain, where it may help delay the progression of Alzheimer's, relieve the depression associated with senility and dementia, and improve memory in the elderly.

When researchers feed old rats acetyl-L-carnitine, both their memory and their physical activity levels improve. When they feed older beagles acetyl-L-carnitine in conjunction with alpha-lipoic acid (see below), the Snoopy dogs' ability to learn as evidenced by their performance on standard dog behavior tests improves markedly.[17] And a number of studies have shown positive effects of acetyl-L-carnitine supplementation in Alzheimer's patients, particularly on tasks that require attention and concentration.[18]

Acetyl-L-carnitine isn't just for those diagnosed with Alzheimer's. It's a powerful brain protector that you can begin taking right now. According to the prestigious (and conservative) *Physicians' Desk Reference for Nutritional Supplements*, preliminary evidence shows that acetyl-L-carnitine can slow mental decline in the elderly who are not afflicted with Alzheimer's.

Alpha-Lipoic Acid: A Triple Value for Your Supplement Dollar

Alpha-lipoic acid is a remarkable substance with myriad uses and a particular quality that makes it unique among antioxidants—it functions in both water and fat. This "all-access" pass allows it to do its magic act everywhere in

the body. Alpha-lipoic acid, an organic compound found in every cell in the body, is not only one of the most powerful antioxidants on the planet, but it's also able to revitalize and refurbish two *other* antioxidants, water-soluble vitamin C and fat-soluble vitamin E. When you take alpha-lipoic acid as a supplement, you're really getting triple value for your supplement dollar.

Alpha-lipoic acid as a brain nutrient first gained attention through the work of one of the most respected researchers in nutrition and biochemistry in the country, Bruce Ames, Ph.D. Ames performed a series of experiments in which he gave old rats a combination of acetyl-L-carnitine (see above) and alpha-lipoic acid. The results on aging were remarkable.

"With these two supplements together, these old rats got up and did the Macarena," said Ames. "The brain looks better, they are full of energy—everything we looked at looks more like a young animal." Not a bad endorsement from a professor of the graduate school division of biochemistry and molecular biology at the University of California!

When researchers analyzed the rats' brain tissue, they found substantially less damage to those little energy furnaces in the cells, the mitochondria. There was also substantially reduced oxidative damage to the hippocampus, the memory center of the brain.[19]

Alpha-lipoic acid's benefit to the brain (and aging) may well come because of its incredible power as an antioxidant. "If your brain is being devoured by free radicals," says David Perlmutter, M.D., author of *The Better Brain Book*, "you will not be able to think clearly, stay focused, or retrieve information when you need it." Perlmutter, a neurologist and nutrition expert, also points out that alpha-lipoic acid is one of the few antioxidants that can significantly boost *glutathione*, arguably the body's most important antioxidant and one that is nearly impossible to get from the diet or supplements because it is poorly absorbed. Alpha-lipoic acid, however, helps you "roll your own."

Phosphatidylserine: Finding Misplaced Keys

When it comes to protecting the brain, membranes matter.

You may recall that we discussed this earlier, and for good reason. The membranes are the outer casing for the cell, and when they're in disrepair, the free flow of information both into the cell and back out of it is severely compromised. Damaged cell membranes act like a virus in your email program, slowing down everything. The ultimate anti-aging strategy means protecting your cell membranes. "The first step in treating patients with Alzheimer's disease is to rebuild defective membranes," says neurologist Jay Lombard, M.D., author of *The Brain Wellness Plan*.

Enter phosphatidylserine.

Phosphatidylserine is a member of a class of chemicals called *phospholipids*, which is a critical component of cell membranes. And it's mostly concentrated in the brain. It's been available as a supplement for several decades and has been shown time and time again to help restore brain function. Phosphatidylserine can improve learning, name recall, concentration, face recognition, and even the ability to remember telephone numbers and find misplaced objects (like your keys).

One of the main jobs of phosphatidylserine is to help regulate the release of neurotransmitters, those chemical messengers that relay information into and out of the brain cells. Supplementing with phosphatidylserine may have "cognition enhancing activity," meaning it can sharpen your thinking and help slow brain aging, according to the *Physicians' Desk Reference*.

One of the ways it may do this is by acting in the body in a way similar to that of a major Alzheimer's drug called Aricept. See, one of the neurotransmitters most needed for sharp thinking, learning, and memory is called *acetylcholine*. When people have less acetylcholine in their brain, they start to experience the classic signs of the aging brain—cognitive impairment and memory loss being among the most common. Acetylcholine is broken down in the brain by an enzyme with a cumbersome name (*acetylcholinesterase*, if you really want to know). If we could somehow slow down the activity of that enzyme, we'd keep more acetylcholine in the brain and our memory and thinking would be sharper. It would be like the Fountain of Youth for the brain.

Aricept works precisely by slowing down the activity of the acetylcholine-destroying enzyme. And so does phosphatidylserine. Several double-blind studies suggest that phosphatidylserine can help maintain a youthful brain in older individuals and may improve memory and learning skill in some. Phosphatidylserine has also shown some ability to slow age-associated memory impairment and general mental deterioration even in non-Alzheimer's dementia.

My good friend, biochemist and nutritionist Parris Kidd, Ph.D., states (in his lilting Jamaican accent) that "dietary supplementation with phosphatidylserine can alleviate, ameliorate, and sometimes reverse age-related decline of memory, learning concentration, word skills, and mood."

For biochemical reasons far too esoteric to bore you with here, you need omega-3 fats to get the best results with phosphatidylserine. One product I like, PS/Omega-3 Synergy, by Crayhon Research (available on my website, www.jonnybowden.com), actually combines phosphatidylserine with omega-3s for you in one pill, so you don't have to worry. If you don't take this brand, include some omega-3s in your diet or supplement program along with your phosphatidylserine.

If you're trying to protect your brain against aging, you should be doing that anyway!

GPC—Not Your Car's Navigation System

Like its relative, phosphatidylserine, GPC (GlyceroPhosCholine) is a member of the class of biochemicals called *phospholipids*. As a supplement it has been researched extensively for its effect on mental performance, attention, memory formation, and concentration.

There's a great series of experiments that demonstrate what GPC can do. One of them is so ingenious you're going to love it (or at least love it as much as you can anything as generally boring as a scientific experiment). See, there's a substance called *scopolamine* that causes amnesia. Get yourself some scopolamine and take it by mouth or injection and presto, you've forgotten everything. All information skills, including memory, attention, and learning, just seem to evaporate into the ether. The effect is only temporary, wearing off in a few hours, but for those few hours you pretty much can't remember a thing.

Clever researchers used the scopolamine phenomena to test the hypothesis that GPC might have a protective effect on the brain. For ten days, they gave a bunch of healthy young volunteers a daily dose of either GPC or a placebo (an inert substance). After that, they gave the subjects a nice big dose of scopolamine and sat back to watch the fun begin.

The thing is, the subjects who received the GPC were *significantly protected* from the effects of the drug. Although the drug normally produces amnesia for a full six hours, in the GPC subjects it produced only three hours of forgetfulness and memory impairment. In one test, called the free recall test, the GPC subjects held off the amnesia the entire six hours! And remarkably, even before the administration of the drug, the subjects who took GPC scored higher on a baseline test of word recall. That means the GPC had a positive effect on their brains even before the administration of the drug!

"GPC has a proven track record against age-related decline and other brain damage," says Kidd. "Along with phosphatidylserine, these are the two most clinically proven brain nutrients and both are widely needed, especially since there are no pharmaceuticals available that provide lasting benefit against cognitive decline."

Ginkgo for the Prettiest Brains

I'm a huge fan of my friend Daniel Amen, M.D., who is always pushing the envelope when it comes to brain health (and how to preserve it!). Amen is famous for his SPECT scans, which are pictures of the brain that show where stuff is going on. Amen can read a SPECT scan like

HOW MUCH VITAMIN D IS ENOUGH?

Think you're getting enough vitamin D? Think again.

There is overwhelming evidence that we need far more vitamin D than previously believed. We now know that vitamin D is intimately tied to better physical performance, preservation of muscle strength and physical function, prevention of cancer and heart disease, improved immune function, and happier moods, not to mention being absolutely essential for strong bones (see page 150).

As of this writing, two major medical organizations—the American Academy of Pediatrics and the Canadian Pediatric Society—have updated their recommendations for vitamin D intake for children. Although the increase in recommended daily allowance is a step in the right direction, many nutritionists, myself included, feel they don't go far enough.

Michael Holick, M.D., professor of medicine at Boston University School of Medicine and an outstanding crusader for updating vitamin D intake recommendations, has found that 76 percent of the mothers coming into his hospital were severely vitamin D deficient and 81 percent of their infants were as well. Researchers have found that fully one-third of the toddlers in urban Canada have less than the recommended levels of vitamin D, as do 14 percent of toddlers in Boston.[20]

The Dearth of Vitamin D

Why are we so lacking in vitamin D?

One reason might be sun phobia. (Remember, one of the best sources of vitamin D is the sun, which is the fuel that allows our body to manufacture its own vitamin D.) We've been so conditioned to fear the sun that many of us slather on SPF 45 just to go out to the corner grocery store, effectively limiting the major source of "raw material" for vitamin D production.

Another reason might be the definition of adequate intake. When health professionals believed the main purpose for vitamin D was preventing rickets, they set the bar for adequate intake pretty darn low. So although we might get enough vitamin D by the "old" standards of adequate intake—meaning rickets prevention—we're not getting nearly enough to achieve the many documented health benefits that researchers are now discovering vitamin D has to offer.

And with the highly unpopular cod liver oil being the top source of vitamin D in the diet (followed by nine kinds of fish, none of which has the amount of vitamin D many health experts recommend for optimal intake), it's easy to see why we're so deficient.

Older adults should pay special attention. Research from Wake Forest University School of Medicine in North Carolina shows that older adults who don't get enough vitamin D are at higher risk for disability.

Dosage Dilemma

How much is enough? The way things are going, that number seems to be a moving target. What we do know is that up to 2,000 IUs daily for one year is safe in adolescents (and results in desirable vitamin D levels), according to a study in the *Journal of Clinical Endocrinology and Metabolism*.[21] The National Osteoporosis Foundation recommends that adults fifty and older get 800 to 1,000 IUs but claims "some people may need more." (I call that putting it mildly.) The Institute of Medicine has set the "safe upper limit" for vitamin D at 2,000 IUs per day, but many health professionals believe that vitamin D is safe at even higher levels.

"It is difficult to get too much vitamin D unless a person is taking a prescription dose of the vitamin," says the National Osteoporosis Foundation.[22]

Before determining an appropriate dosage, get tested. Although there are two tests for vitamin D, the one you want is called the *25(OH)D*, also known as the *25-hydroxyvitamin D* test. Some doctors will order an "activated vitamin D" test (also known as *calcitriol*). Calcitriol will tell you nothing about your vitamin D sufficiency. "If your doctor insists on ordering a calcitriol level to determine your vitamin D nutrition, find another doctor," writes John Cannell in the *Townsend Newsletter for Doctors and Patients.*[23]

Levels of vitamin D (25-hydroxy-vitamin D) below 30 ng/mL are considered deficient. Optimal levels are now considered between 30 and 65 ng/mL, with some arguing for an even higher upper limit of optimal. The Vitamin D Council states that the minimal acceptable level is 50 for children and adults all year-round.[24] (Levels over 100 indicate possible excess.)

If you don't want to wait to have your doctor test your levels, there is now a simple and accurate test for vitamin D recommended by the Vitamin D Council that you can do at home. It's called the Vitamin D Blood Spot Testing Kit and is available through ZRT Labs (www.zrtlab.com) or through a link on the Vitamin D Council's website (www.vitamindcouncil.org).

a geographer can read a complicated map—he can tell you where the damage is and what impact it's having on functioning.

Amen knows what a healthy brain looks like.

"The prettiest brains I've ever seen are those that are on ginkgo biloba," he told me.

Admittedly, that's not much of a hard science statement, but it contains a lot of truth nonetheless. Ginkgo is a terrific neuroprotector. In Germany, ginkgo biloba extract is registered as an herbal medicine to treat "cerebral insufficiency," a diagnosis that covers a wide range of conditions. According to the German Commission E monographs—the standard for therapeutic use of herbal medicines—the primary target groups for ginkgo are dementia syndromes. And it's also a powerful antioxidant.

Master herbalist Kerry Bone believes that taking ginkgo on a regular basis might actually help you live longer.[25] When researchers investigated whether ginkgo might help prevent dementia, according to Bone, they found that regular users of the extract had a significantly lower mortality rate from all causes!

Full disclosure: I'm a fan. I take ginkgo on a regular basis, generally about 240 milligrams a day. I like the idea that if Amen ever scanned my brain, he'd class it among the "prettiest" ones he'd ever seen!

VITAMIN B12: THE HOMOCYSTEINE FIGHTER

Okay, my vegan friends are going to hate me, but the truth is you can't get vitamin B_{12} from plant foods (at least not enough to make any difference at all). And you need vitamin B_{12} if your brain is going to perform well.

This presents a bit of a conundrum to those of us who wish to live long and keep our faculties. Why? Because to digest and assimilate vitamin B_{12} you need something in the stomach called *intrinsic factor*. And we make less of it as we get older. (This is why you may have heard of people who take B_{12} injections; this bypasses the stomach and gets the vitamin directly into the bloodstream.)

Even before B_{12} gets bound to intrinsic factor, the body has to extract it from food. And we do this with the help of hydrochloric acid, another secretion we make less of as we age. When we have inflammation in the stomach (a condition called *atrophic gastritis*), we produce fewer gastric juices (including hydrochloric acid), and that means less vitamin B_{12} in the system. Up to 30 percent of adults fifty and older have this condition and may be unable to normally absorb vitamin B_{12} in food.[26]

Researchers have been interested in the potential connection between vitamin B_{12} deficiency and dementia for a long time.[27] The connection is long and involved, but B_{12} deficiency may decrease levels of different substances needed for neurotransmitters—those chemicals that transmit information in the brain—to do their job properly. If your neurotransmitters aren't firing well, it may result in cognitive impairment. Vitamin B_{12}, you may remember, is also one of the three nutrients (folic acid and B_6 being the others) that brings down levels of that nasty inflammatory compound called homocysteine (see page 104), the same compound that increases the risk for Alzheimer's, stroke, and heart disease.

Vitamin B_{12} is so safe and nontoxic that the Institute of Medicine of the National Academies of Science did not establish a recommended upper limit for this vitamin. The Institute of Medicine did, however, recommend that adults over fifty get their B_{12} from supplements or fortified foods.

ANTI-AGING ACTION PLAN:

Take Vitamin D Supplements Daily to Protect Your Bones and Brain

Vitamin D is the latest superstar of supplements—and it should be. Research shows that people are becoming more and more deficient in vitamin D, which is needed to protect bones and may help protect the brain and prevent cognitive decline.

However, it's hard to get vitamin D from food, which is why supplementation is important. Take 1,000–2,000 IUs of vitamin D daily. Some people may benefit from more; doses of up to 2,400 IUs daily in healthy people rarely cause adverse reactions.

VITAMIN D: THE SUPPLEMENT SUPERSTAR

I don't want to leave this chapter without at least a mention of the latest superstar of supplements, vitamin D. "In recent years...no major nutrient has garnered as much research attention as vitamin D, nor produced as many significant positive results," says the *Physician's Desk Reference for Nutritional Supplements.*[28] We'll talk about vitamin D at length in the chapter on muscles and bones, but it's worth pointing out that vitamin D's resume extends well beyond protecting bones and may have important abilities to protect the brain and help inhibit cognitive decline.

A recent study looked at the relationship between blood levels of vitamin D and scores on the Mini-Mental State Examination or MMSE, mentioned earlier in this chapter. Patients with "sufficient" levels of vitamin D were found to have significantly higher MMSE scores.[29] The U.S. Census Bureau has estimated that nearly nineteen million Americans will be age eighty-five by 2050 and that more than half of these will have some form of dementia. Given that elderly populations worldwide are 40 to 100 percent (!) deficient in vitamin D and that the benefits of vitamin D supplements are broad and dramatic, it makes sense for every adult to supplement with this important vitamin. Few foods are natural sources of vitamin D, making supplementation even more crucial as an anti-aging strategy.

VINPOCETINE MAY BE RIGHT FOR YOU

Vinpocetine, an extract of the periwinkle plant, helps improve blood flow to the brain. "In my practice, I have seen vast improvement in patients using the supplement; practically overnight they become more lucid, sharper, and more on the ball," says Perlmutter. But vinpocetine is not for everyone; it's primarily useful if you have high levels of homocysteine and/or a history of heart disease or vascular dementia (senility caused by impaired blood flow within the brain).[30]

MORE BENEFITS OF RESTRICTING CALORIES: BETTER MEMORY!

Throughout this book I've alluded to the fact that cutting calories by 25 to 33 percent may be one of the most tested and effective anti-aging strategies of all. In the lab, it's virtually the only thing that's been shown to extend the life of every species tested, from yeast and fruit flies to monkeys.

It may also improve memory.

Researchers in Germany asked one group of elderly volunteers to eat the food they normally ate but to eat about one-third less, primarily by just eating smaller portions. After three months on the diet, they were given a memory test. Compared to two other groups that ate their regular number of calories, the group eating 30 percent fewer calories had significant improvement in memory.[32] "To our knowledge, the current results provide first experimental evidence in humans that caloric restriction improves memory in the elderly," said the researchers.

Why would calorie restriction improve memory? The answer may lay with two of the Four Horsemen of Aging. Scientists aren't sure of the exact mechanism by which calorie restriction helps the brain, but the two most prevalent theories are that calorie restriction reduces inflammation and oxidative damage, both of which are known brain agers.

Vinpocetine has been used in Europe and Japan for more than two decades to treat stroke victims and people suffering from dementia. A 1987 study in the *Journal of the American Geriatric Society* reported that 56 percent of patients treated with vinpocetine made "good to excellent improvement" and scored "consistently better on all evaluations of effectiveness of treatment."[31]

"More than fifty clinical studies have documented that vinpocetine can improve blood flow to the brain, promote better oxygen utilization, increase energy production in the brain, and help prevent blood clots," says Perlmutter. "It is also a potent antioxidant."

Note: Don't use vinpocetine with a blood thinner like Coumadin.

How to Protect and Maintain Strong Bones, Muscles, and Joints

Here's a riddle for you: What medical condition that almost no one has heard of yet will affect nearly every older person in the world?

The answer: sarcopenia.

Sarcopenia, from the Greek meaning "poverty of flesh," is just a fancy word for muscle loss. It's the gradual loss of strength and muscle tissue that every person experiences to some degree or another as he or she ages. And don't fool yourself because it's not some minor problem that has no effect on the quality of life, nor is it without significant social and economic costs. In 2000, the estimated health care costs directly attributable to sarcopenia in the United States alone were $18.5 billion.[1] (Just for comparison: U.S. Major League Baseball took in about one-third of that amount, $5.2 billion, in 2006.)[2]

One thing to know about sarcopenia is that it starts imperceptibly, when you're young, around the age of thirty, and progresses throughout your life. (It's no accident that the vast majority of athletic record holders are thirty or younger, a fact that I'm painfully aware of every time I hit the tennis courts.) A second thing to know about sarcopenia is that it can be pretty debilitating. It's not easy to live a robust, active life if you can't open a jar or lift the groceries out of the trunk of the car.

And a third thing to know about sarcopenia is that you can easily prevent it. Okay, maybe that's an exaggeration. Even trained athletes experience some muscle and strength loss, no matter how hard they work out. But you can slow it down so much that the amount of loss won't significantly impair your life or well-being. And—spoiler alert—the solution is simple: exercise. (More on that a little later on.)

When it comes to the skeletal system, muscle loss isn't the only thing we need to worry about—there's also bone loss and joint problems. Let's take those one by one.

OSTEOPOROSIS: ONE MAN'S CRUSADE

As far as I'm concerned, there's no one on the planet who can teach us more about aging bones than R. Keith McCormick, D.C., a certified chiropractic sports physician, a former varsity cross-country runner at Stanford University, the winner of the 1975 North American Pentathlon Championship, and a former member of the U.S. Olympic team (XXI Olympiad in Montreal).

One day, while running a track workout, he became suddenly lame with hip pain. Several MRIs and X-rays later, he was diagnosed with severe osteoporosis.

At the ripe old age of forty-five.

"Wow, you have worse bone density than a hundred-year-old woman," blurted the X-ray technician who evaluated his films.

"My first reaction was embarrassment," McCormick says in his book, *The Whole-Body Approach to Osteoporosis.* "How could I have this? I'd eaten well all my life, or at least I thought I had. I'd always drunk a lot of milk. I'd never smoked, drank alcohol, or used any type of drug or medication. I'd never done anything 'wrong.' I'd always done everything 'right' to be healthy. It just didn't make any sense. Osteoporosis, a disease associated with frailty, was the antithesis of who I thought I was."

Unlucky for McCormick (at least at the time—he continues to compete in triathlons in all distances, including, thank you very much, Ironmans), but very lucky for us.

Why, you ask?

Because McCormick's diagnosis led him to study the disease of osteoporosis with the passion of someone who has a horse in the race—which he does. What he discovered has a great deal to teach us, not only about osteoporosis, but also about aging, longevity, and the interconnectedness of everything in the body. (It's also helped *him* stay in the race.)

"Osteoporosis is not just the weakening of bones," McCormick told me. "It is a weakening of the body's entire physiology. When you have a chronic disease, you have to treat your whole body."

Indeed. And a quick explanation of what goes wrong when bones weaken will illustrate exactly what he means. (Stay with me now, it will be worth it!)

The large cast of characters in the drama of bone building makes the New York City phone book look like a grocery list, but these two characters deserve special attention:

The osteoblasts are the cells that form what's called the *bone matrix*, a honeycomb-like structure onto which minerals like calcium are deposited (or absorbed), resulting in nice, hard, mineralized bones. But this is not a one-way street. While minerals continue to be deposited on that honeycomb, other cells called

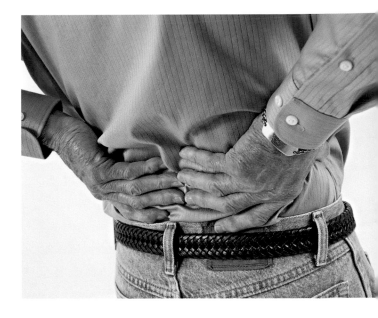

osteoclasts are busy removing minerals in a process called *resorption*. The delicate balance between adding and subtracting, between mineralization (building up) and demineralization (breaking down), between absorption and resorption is called, appropriately enough, *remodeling*.

"Osteoporosis is not just the weakening of bones. It is a weakening of the body's entire physiology. When you have a chronic disease, you have to treat your whole body."

—Keith McCormick, D.C.

It's actually very much like what happens if you remodel your bathroom. Workers remove debris (old, broken tiles) while other workers bring in fresh material (new tiles) and cement them down on the floor (the honeycomb, or bone matrix). The osteoclast workers remove debris, while their osteoblast partners begin the process of setting in new tile.

"The process ensures a continual replacement of old bone weakened by the microfractures caused by daily activity with new bone," explains McCormick. (A third type of cell, *osteocytes*, are like the supervisors or foremen on this whole construction project, orchestrating the complicated process.) "At any one moment, 2 to 5 percent of your skeleton is being remodeled," says McCormick. "Right now there are millions of these tiny areas of bone undergoing active repair in your body."

Now that you know the cast of characters, here's where it gets really interesting.

The way the two types of cells, osteoblasts and osteoclasts, communicate is through a molecule called *RANKL*. This molecule allows the workers bringing in the new stuff to coordinate with the workers removing the debris. When the osteoblasts release RANKL, it tells the osteoclasts to "take out" just the right amount of trash.

A perfect system, right? Well it is, until inflammation enters the picture.

REENTER THE HORSEMEN

As we've learned throughout this book, when you have chronic inflammation your immune system is working overtime. One of the first things the immune system does when it's activated is release T-cells, those sentries of immunity that are summoned whenever the body senses an injury (like inflammation).

Well guess what the T-cells do?

They produce RANKL.

Which tells the osteoclasts to keep on removing minerals, significantly weakening your bones. "When the immune system is constantly activated, you have too much RANKL," explains McCormick. "You can take all the calcium in the world and it would be like a person walking around with a little squirt gun trying to put out a fire in your house while there's a guy with a kerosene can throwing gas on it at the same time. When we reduce inflammation," he adds wisely, "we don't need as much calcium."

Inflammation is intimately connected to the loss of "quality" bone, but it's not the only horseman of aging that plays a role. Remember the stress hormone cortisol? "Cortisol activates receptors on the osteoblasts [bone builders] and shuts them down," McCormick explains. This leads to an imbalance between mineralization and demineralization; the cells "taking out the trash" are working just fine, but the ones replacing it with new minerals have been put to sleep by stress hormones.

Oxidation, another horseman of aging, plays a part as well. Free radicals, also known as *reactive oxygen species*, stimulate the osteoclasts (the cells that tear bone down). While not all free radicals are bad (some perform valuable functions in the cells), when there are too many of them the osteoclasts become overstimulated. The now turbo-charged osteoclasts go into overdrive and you get too much bone resorption. This is why antioxidants are a big part of McCormick's recommendation for keeping bones strong (see below).

McCormick is a particular fan of a powerful antioxidant known as *NAC (N-Acetyl-Cysteine)* because it specifically lowers reactive oxygen species within the osteoclasts themselves. "Every woman should be on 600 to 1,200 milligrams a day of NAC," he told me, "especially after menopause." (Estrogen helps reduce bone resorption; without it, you need even more help keeping the osteoclasts from getting too busy!) McCormick thinks NAC is a good idea for men as well. (N-Acetyl-Cysteine is widely available as a supplement; a particularly good brand can be found through a link on my website vitamin store, www.jonnybowden.com.)

And finally, there's our old friend glycation, another of the Four Horsemen of Aging. You may remember our discussion (back in chapter 3) about AGEs (advanced glycation end products), which form as a result of glycation in the body. (Briefly, when excess sugar in the bloodstream gloms on to proteins, the resultant molecules form nasty little compounds appropriately called AGEs that do exactly what they sound like—they "age" you in the ways discussed earlier.) Those AGEs damage your bones as well.

"The more AGEs, the more brittle bone collagen becomes, because AGEs stick like glue to the collagen fibers," McCormick says. He believes that is why diabetics have a higher fracture rate than nondiabetics, "even though," he adds, "they might have higher bone density."

IT'S NOT JUST BONE DENSITY, IT'S BONE QUALITY

Osteoporosis itself doesn't kill people, but fractures can.

Fractures are serious stuff. There are more than 300,000 hip fractures a year in America alone, estimated to go as high as 500,000 by 2040. Someone who sustains a hip fracture is more likely to die than a person of the same age who does not experience this injury. About 20 percent of people who have a hip fracture die within a year of their injury and only about one in four persons have a total recovery from a hip fracture.[3]

At the very least, fractures can significantly reduce quality of life, in some cases forever. "The real concern is breaking bones," writes Gillian Sanson in her excellent book, *The Myth of Osteoporosis*. "The preoccupation with measuring bone mineral density tends to eclipse this obvious and important indicator. You may have low bone density and never fracture; or you may have normal bone density and fracture."

Sanson goes on to point out that the bone mineral density definition of osteoporosis has contributed to the medicalization of aging women. The British Columbia Office of Health Technology Assessment review of the evidence for the effectiveness of bone mineral density testing echoes her concern: "BMD testing is unable to accurately distinguish women at low risk of fracture from those at high risk," the authors write.[4]

Bone mineral density tests may turn out to be very much like cholesterol—an interesting piece of information that has been enormously overrated in terms of its ability to tell us something important about what we really need to know—in this case, our risk of fracture. "Hip fractures that occur between the age of 80 and 90 are invariably linked to factors other than osteoporosis," writes Sanson. "Falling and breaking a hip is most often a marker of generally frail health. A man or woman who remains fit and well is less likely to fracture."

Bone quality—the strength or brittleness of the bone, and its tendency to fracture—is something we should all pay attention to. See page 154 for recommended tests that assess bone quality.

ANTI-AGING ACTION PLAN:
Eat These Foods For Strong Bones

Sardines, broccoli, almonds, prunes, oranges, and onions—these are Keith McCormick's favorite foods for building strong bones. Make them part of your regular diet by eating them every week.

"These are great foods for bone health," says McCormick, D.C. "They provide bioactive compounds that have been shown to increase bone density, and I recommend them to my patients all the time."

In his excellent book, *The Whole-Body Approach to Osteoporosis*, McCormick recommends tests for bone health that go well beyond the traditional evaluation of bone density and look at what's going on in the whole body. Although bone density is important, it's far from the whole picture. "It's a natural thing to lose bone, just not too much or too rapidly," he says. "That's why looking at bone density exam results alone isn't good enough. You want to look at bone quality."*

Among the various tests McCormick recommends to assess bone quality are the NTX or DPD urine tests,† both of which show you how much collagen is being lost in the urine. "That's a reflection of how much resorption is going on," he says. "If it's too much, that's an indication of poor bone quality."

He also looks at blood sugar levels. "The higher your blood sugar is, the more it's likely that you'll make AGEs in your body," he says.

Finally, he recommends a blood test for vitamin D, which makes total sense. Vitamin D is an essential component in bone health and helps ensure that the body absorbs calcium, which, of course, is critical for building strong, healthy bones, according to the *U.S. Surgeon General's Report on Bone Health and Osteoporosis* (2004). Without adequate vitamin D, you can take all the calcium

---

* The definition of bone quality is difficult and elusive and beyond the scope of this book, but it involves looking at markers for structural integrity, such as how well put together the collagen fibers are.

† These are standard tests available from any doctor.

in the world and it won't do you much good. Vitamin D deficiency has often been linked directly to osteoporosis. Research shows that more than 70 percent of women ages fifty-one to seventy and nearly 90 percent of women over seventy are not getting an adequate intake of vitamin D from food and supplements. Low levels of vitamin D are associated with reduced calcium absorption, bone loss, and increased risk of fracture.[5] (For more on vitamin D, see the sidebar on page 144.)

It's interesting that the guru of osteoporosis should reach many of the same conclusions as so many of my respected colleagues who question conventional wisdom when it comes to health ("wisdom" that includes an obsession with cholesterol scores, the demonization of saturated fat, and the advocacy of high-carb diets, to cite just a few examples). His dietary recommendations tellingly contain such bullet points as "go easy on the dairy products," "reduce the grains," "limit refined carbohydrates," and "eat protein" (you can see why I'm such a fan). And, of course, "Eat five to nine servings of fruits and vegetables each day." You can read more about McCormick's recommendations (and the reasons why he makes them) in his book.

ARREST THE ROBBERS

What you eat is critically important for the health of your bones, muscles, and joints, not to mention all the other body systems we've discussed in this book. But when it comes to bone health, it's particularly important to avoid what we call the "bone robbers."

"If you want good bones, you have to limit your alcohol intake, stop smoking, not salt your food excessively, go easy on the sugar, and not consume cola beverages," McCormick says. Sodas in particular are

loaded with phosphoric acid, a known robber of calcium. "By eliminating the unhealthy aspects of your lifestyle and diet, you will have better bones."

And what about supplements? Can they help? Absolutely. Here's McCormick's list of the top supplements for bone health:

- Daily multivitamin-mineral
- Calcium: 1,000 to 1,200 mg daily
- Magnesium: 500 to 600 mg daily
- Vitamin D3: 1,000 to 2,000 IUs daily
- Vitamin K: 1 milligram or more daily
- Daily antioxidant supplement:
  - Fish oil: 2 to 3 g
  - Flaxseed meal (like Barlean's Forti-Flax): 2–4 tablespoons
  - Probiotics: 3 to 20 million viable cells

But note well: "Calcium and vitamin D, although integral to your skeletal health, may do you little good if your body is . . . in a constant state of destruction," McCormick says. "Eliminating excess oxidative stress, systemic inflammation, and gastrointestinal dysfunction* are far more useful for healing purposes than overloading your body with calcium. Your major objective, instead of simply swallowing a few key nutrients, should be to build up your whole body."

Amen to that!

A PRIMER ON ARTHRITIS AND JOINT PAIN

"Oh, my aching back."

Heard that refrain lately? Said it yourself?

If so, you're hardly alone. One-half of all working Americans admit to having back pain symptoms, and back pain is the second most common reason for doctor visits and the first most common reason for missed work. It's estimated that as many as 80 percent of us will experience a back problem at some point in our lives.

And it's not just the back. All our joints are subject to wear and tear as we age. Once again, inflammation rears its ugly head. In fact, the very term *arthritis* comes from the Greek *athro* (meaning "joint") and *itis*, meaning "inflammation."

There are more than a hundred different types of arthritis and related conditions, but by far the most common type is *osteoarthritis* (OA), a chronic condition characterized by breakdown of cartilage (the part of the joint that acts as a cushion between the ends of the bones). When cartilage is intact, your joints can move easily

(which is good), but when the cartilage breaks down there's less of a cushion and your bones wind up rubbing against each other (which is not so good). The result is pain, stiffness, and loss of movement in the joint, typical symptoms of OA. It's not fun to live with.

And it's one of the most frequent causes of physical disability among older adults. Loss of joint function is also one of the major causes of reduced quality of life, potentially limiting people who suffer with it from walking a few blocks, climbing a flight of stairs, or engaging in all kinds of physical activities that they might otherwise enjoy, according to the Arthritis Foundation. It's also expensive. Arthritis and related conditions cost the U.S. economy nearly $128 billion each year in medical care and indirect expenses, including lost wages and productivity.[6] The total annual cost per person living with OA is approximately $5,700.[7]

By age sixty-five, more than half the population has X-ray evidence of OA in at least one joint, most frequently in the hips, knees, neck, low back, or fingers. (Interestingly, only about a third of these folks report actual pain or other symptoms.) And even X-rays don't tell the whole picture, because you can have pain without X-ray confirmation of damage. "X-rays are limited in their capacity to reveal how much joint damage may have occurred in osteoarthritis," says Ann Knight, D.C. "You may not see osteorthritic damage on X-rays until there's been a significant loss of cartilage."

What to do, what to do?

The different classes of arthritis medications tend to fall into five categories: NSAIDs (nonsteroidal anti-

---

* Gastrointestinal dysfunction is a huge source of inflammation in the body; when the gut isn't healthy, all sorts of problems can occur, including the overstimulation of the immune system.

inflammatory drugs, which include over-the-counter drugs like ibuprofen and prescription drugs like Celebrex); analgesics (painkillers); corticosteroids; DMARDs (disease-modifying antirheumatic drugs); and the newer biologics, which are primarily used in the treatment of a different type of arthritis (rheumatoid arthritis). Obviously, a discussion of all of these would take us way off course, but what's worth pointing out is that of the four classes of drugs most commonly used to treat OA conventionally, three of them (NSAIDs, corticosteroids, and DMARDs) are all about fighting inflammation! (The fourth class, analgesics, consists of painkillers.

So once again we have a major degenerative disease of aging in which the most common symptom is chronic inflammation.

Although the above-mentioned drugs fight inflammation, they are hardly without side effects. Some 10 to 50 percent of patients can't tolerate NSAID treatment because of side effects, including abdominal pain, diarrhea, bloating, heartburn, and upset stomach, and approximately 15 percent of patients on long-term NSAID treatment develop ulceration of the stomach and duodenum.[8] A type of NSAID known as a COX-2 inhibitor works by inhibiting an enzyme responsible for inflammation, but it, too, is not without problems. One of the most famous of the COX-2 inhibitors, Vioxx, was withdrawn from the market in September 2004 because of an increased risk of myocardial infarction (heart attack) and stroke.

GET RID OF INFLAMMATION—WITHOUT THE SIDE EFFECTS

So let's review. Arthritis is a condition in which inflammation is always present, usually with

accompanying pain. So whatever else we choose to do about it, reducing inflammation has to be the first order of business. We've talked about the most anti-inflammatory substance on the planet—fish oil—more times than I can count, but it's worth pointing out that it's one anti-inflammatory you can take with no danger of side effects.

Another nutritional strategy is to use turmeric—the spice that makes Indian food yellow—as often as possible. Turmeric has myriad health benefits, one of which is that it is highly anti-inflammatory, largely due to the active ingredients in the spice known as curcuminoids. (You can also take that active ingredient in supplement form. It's called curcumin and it's widely available. A particularly good brand is Vital Nutrients, available on my website, www.jonnybowden.com.)

Two other supplements are also useful for arthritis, and both of them are also without side effects.

Glucosamine is a nutritional supplement that can normalize cartilage metabolism, keeping it from breaking down. It's now widely accepted even by the conventional medical establishment as being very helpful for arthritis, particularly arthritis of the knee.

Two studies of the many that have been conducted on glucosamine are worth mentioning in particular. In one of them, 212 patients were put on 1,500 milligrams of glucosamine a day, followed for three years, and compared with a control group given a placebo. The researchers measured changes in the space between the joints and found that those taking glucosamine experienced no loss

of joint space (while those on the placebo continued to show progressive cartilage loss).[9] A second study followed 202 patients on the same 1,500 milligrams of glucosamine per day and compared their progress to a matched group of patients who received a placebo. Once again, researchers saw no joint space narrowing in the patients on glucosamine, and once again, those on the placebo continued to see their joints worsen.[10] In addition to these two studies, a systematic review of published randomized trials whose aim was to determine the effectiveness of glucosamine in OA found that each one of the included studies demonstrated a positive effect.[11]

But preventing cartilage loss wouldn't mean much to the average person if it didn't also decrease pain. "A seemingly overlooked, yet remarkable, finding in both of these trials was the improvement that was seen in joint pain over the years of study follow-up," write University of Utah School of Medicine professors Daniel O. Clegg, M.D., and Christopher Jackson, M.D., in the National Institute of Health's *Encyclopedia of Dietary Supplements*,[12] adding that "sustained lessening in pain of the degree and duration suggested by these trials has never been reported before for any agent in the management of osteoarthritis."

The Natural Standard, an international multidisciplinary collaboration of researchers and clinicians devoted to the rigorous evaluation of research on complementary and alternative therapies, gives glucosamine an "A" rating ("strong scientific evidence") for use in treating knee arthritis, and a very respectable "B" rating ("good scientific evidence") for use in treating OA in general.

On a personal note: I have been blessed to be the guardian of many animals over the past fifteen years, who have variously been attended by more than a dozen vets in three cities. I have yet to meet a single vet who does not routinely use glucosamine for animals with arthritic joints. You can't get "placebo effects" (the power of suggestion) with animals. And vets are remarkably free of the political in-fighting that frequently occurs between proponents of natural supplements and the pharmaceutical industry. Vets just use what works.

If you want to use glucosamine for arthritis, and I strongly recommend it, the usual dose is 1,500 milligrams per day,* usually in conjunction with chondroitin sulfate (see below). "The safety profile of glucosamine in the published studies . . . is uniformly favorable," write Clegg and Jackson.[13]

Chondroitin sulfate is a key component of normal cartilage, but arthritis sufferers have substantially less of it than normal. It draws in precious fluid to the cartilage, protects the cartilage, and stops it from breaking down.[14] Chondroitin sulfate also inhibits certain "cartilage chewing" enzymes, according to chemist and pharmacist Richard Stenlake.[15] A number of studies have reported statistically significant improvement in pain with the use of chondroitin sulfate. Most of these studies have reported important benefits in terms of symptoms (such as pain), function (such as mobility), and reduced medication requirements (such as anti-inflammatories).

"The published medical literature at present suggests that chondroitin sulfate is well tolerated and may be of benefit in alleviating the symptoms of osteoarthritis," write Jackson and Clegg.[16]

The Natural Standard gives chondroitin sulfate an "A" (for "strong scientific evidence") for use in OA. The recommended dose is between 800 and 1,200 milligrams per day, and it's generally used in conjunction with glucosamine (above).

Finally, there's one thing you can do that will most assuredly help you reduce the pain of arthritis and will have tremendous collateral benefits as well: Lose weight. For every 1 pound of weight lost, there is a 4-pound reduction in the load exerted on the knee for each step taken during daily activities.[17] Losing as few as 11 pounds can cut the risk of developing knee arthritis by 50 percent for many people.[18]

> For every 1 pound of weight lost, there is a 4-pound reduction in the load exerted on the knee for each step taken during daily activities.

---

* Some research indicates that higher doses, in the range of 2,000 to 2,500 milligrams, may be needed for people who weigh more than 200 pounds.

ANTI-AGING ACTION PLAN:

Lose Weight to Take Stress Off Your Joints

When you're carrying extra weight around, you're putting added stress on joints, wearing them down and exacerbating pain. Maintaining a healthy weight nearly always improves the pain of arthritis.

Dozens of research papers have demonstrated that losing even 10 percent of your body weight—a goal considered by most experts to be completely attainable by almost anyone—will significantly benefit your health. It will certainly benefit your joints!

THE SINGLE MOST IMPORTANT ANTI-AGING STRATEGY

So what do all these conditions—sarcopenia, osteoporosis, and arthritis—have in common?

Simple: They all respond favorably to exercise. "Studies have shown that even elderly adults over age eighty who have done active exercise and weight-bearing programs can significantly increase their bone density over a short period of time," says Michael Lam, M.D., M.P.H., a specialist in

nutritional and anti-aging medicine. Exercise is the go-to intervention for slowing the negative effects of aging on the entire musculoskeletal system. Exercise builds muscles, countering the effects of sarcopenia, strengthens bones, and is one of the best things you can do for arthritis.

I'll be honest with you—I generally don't like books that try to be all things to all people (a diet book plus cookbook plus exercise manual plus travelogue)! So I hesitated before including the following pages, but I decided to do it because I wanted to offer a simple, fairly painless manual for how to keep your muscles strong and supple. In no way do I think this is a comprehensive exercise manual, (of which there are plenty; see page 268 for a couple of my favorites). But performing these seven basic exercises will hit all your major body parts and keep your chest, shoulders, back, arms, legs, and abs perfectly strong and functional for a very long time.

Truth be told, you only need to do the series twice a week. That probably won't result in a body that will be featured on the cover of *Bodybuilding Monthly*, but it'll keep you mobile, strong, and fit, especially when you couple these exercises with the aerobics I've recommended throughout this book (e.g., walking at least thirty minutes a day) and the stretching exercises I've included afterward (more about those later on).

DR. JONNY'S BASIC PROGRAM FOR MAINTAINING MUSCLE STRENGTH AND BONE MASS

All you need for exercises below is hand weights (dumbbells), available everywhere. The exact weight will differ from person to person and from exercise to exercise—your legs, for example, are much stronger than your shoulders. Pick a weight with which you can do 8 to 12 repetitions. If you can easily do 12, the weight is too light, and if you can't complete 8, the weight is too heavy. As you get stronger, use heavier weights.

One space- and money-saving trick is to use two water bottles instead of dumbbells. Those plastic gallon-size bottles you get in the supermarket are perfect because they have handles. Fill the water bottle up just enough to make it difficult, but not impossible, to complete the 8 to 12 reps. You can even use a magic marker to indicate the right fill point for different exercises.

Crunches for the Abdominal Muscles

Lie on the floor with your legs bent, feet flat on the floor, and hands clasped behind your head with your elbows touching the ground. Your head should be in position with the body so that you could hold an apple between your chest and your chin.

Imagine Velcroing your lower back to the floor. You may feel like you're doing a small pelvic thrust slightly forward to accomplish this. Keep your lower back nice and stable in this position.

Curl your upper body forward and up, holding the highest position for a full second before lowering your upper body back down to the ground. Don't pull on your neck when you come up.

When you lower your upper torso back to the ground, don't return all the way to the "relaxed" position where your weight is supported by the ground, but instead just come down to the point where your upper body is just above the ground and your abs are still contracted. Go back up from this position, so the abs remain tense for the entire time.

Remember to keep your elbows all the way back while doing the movement.

Repeat for as many repetitions as you can manage in good form. The goal is to try for 10 to 20 repetitions.

Note: I constantly used to hear from people who say they're doing "hundreds of crunches" a day. The minute I hear this, I know they're doing them wrong. (I also know there's a good chance they're using momentum rather than strength, and are setting themselves up for a lower back injury!) If you do a crunch properly, it's hard! The good news is that when you do them correctly, you don't have to do nearly as many as you think to get good results.

Beginners: Remember that if you can only do one or two, that's fine. You'll work up to more. Don't dwell on what you can't do; concentrate on what you can do.

Squats for the Legs and Lower Body

Stand with your arms at your sides. (Do this exercise without weights, or hold a dumbbell in each hand.) Keep your feet shoulder-width apart and your head up. There can be a slight arch in your lower back.

Slowly bend your knees while pushing your rear out, until your thighs are about parallel to the ground. Squeeze your thighs and glutes for added contraction. At the same time as you bend, bring your arms up straight in front of you for balance until they're extended straight out at shoulder height, palms facing each other.

Now come up until you're standing again, dropping your arms back to your sides, and do 10 to 15 repetitions.

Don't lock your knees when returning to the standing position. Adjust your foot stance until it feels comfortable.

Chest Presses

Lie down on a bench, your feet resting comfortably on the floor. (If you don't have a bench, you can use a step or even the floor.) For an added challenge, try raising your feet as in the photos above. Grasp a dumbbell in each hand.

Extend your arms overhead, shoulder-width apart, palms facing out, so that the dumbbells are positioned directly over your shoulders.

Bend your elbows about 90 degrees, gradually lowering the weights until they are above and a little behind your shoulders.

Now push the dumbbells up with an arcing motion until they're back in the starting position.

One-Arm Rows for the Back

Bend over and rest your left hand on a bench or stool about 2½ feet high (this doesn't have to be the exact height). Extend your right leg behind you so that you're far enough away from the bench that your back is flat; make sure you don't round your back and instead keep it as flat as possible (you may actually have to arch it a little to keep it in this position). The right arm will be hanging down, straight. Your back should be like a tabletop in this position.

Take a dumbbell in your right hand and bring it straight up toward your hip by bending your elbow and bringing it up behind you toward the ceiling. It should be almost like starting a lawnmower in slow motion. When the weight is about hip level, lower it back down. That's one rep. Do 10 reps and repeat with the left arm.

Biceps Curls for the Arms

Stand with a pair of dumbbells in your hands, palms facing out and shoulder-width apart.

Keeping your elbows stable and next to your sides, raise the dumbbells toward your shoulders and then bring them slowly back down to the original position. Repeat for 8 to 12 repetitions.

Triceps Dips for the Arms

Sit on the edge of a bench or step, with your hands on the edge of the bench and your fingers facing forward.

Lift your butt off the bench and lower it toward the floor by bending your arms at the elbows. Make sure you stay perpendicular to the ground, back straight. Don't push the hips forward.

Lift yourself back up by straightening your arms, but don't rest your butt back on the bench until you're done. Repeat for 8 to 12 repetitions.

Lateral Raises for the Shoulders

Take a dumbbell in each hand and hold them at the sides of your body, palms facing inward. Stand with your feet shoulder-width apart, knees slightly bent. Don't lean backward.

Raise your arms up and out to the sides until they are parallel to the ground, or "cross" position, then lower back down. Repeat for 8 to 12 repetitions.

Although this routine won't make you into Mr. or Ms. Olympia, it will do wonders for keeping your muscles from atrophying, and the weight-bearing activity will strengthen your bones and joints. Best of all, a pared-down routine of one set per exercise takes less than half an hour (even with a five-minute warm-up and cool-down added in). And research by noted exercise physiologist and strength researcher Wayne Wescott, Ph.D , shows that merely two weight-training sessions per week is all you need. Just do them on nonconsecutive days so your muscles get a rest in between.

"Research with both older and younger people [produces] an increase in muscular strength of approximately 50 percent after just two months of twice-a-week (weight) training," Wescott writes.

DITCH THE PAIN WITH THESE SUPPLEMENTAL STRETCHING EXERCISES

Although strength-training exercises are great for keeping your muscles and bones young, they won't necessarily get you out of pain. But dozens of other exercises (and stretches) will. The following stretches, courtesy of my good friend Ann Knight, D.C., have specific therapeutic benefits for problem areas of the body. They are designed to strengthen the targeted areas as well as stretch them. Virtually all of them can be done with no equipment and are not very difficult. You can do all of them, or just choose the ones that are most appropriate for whatever area of your body feels tight and stiff. Many more rehab exercises are available on Knight's website (www.drannknight.com), along with terrific animated videos of how to perform them properly.

Pelvic Tilt for the Abs and Back

Purpose: To strengthen abdominal and back muscles

1. Begin by lying on your back with you knees bent and feet on the floor.
2. Push the lower part of your back into the floor by tightening your abdominal and buttock muscles. Rotate your pelvis upward without bringing your back off the floor.
3. Hold for 5 seconds and then return to the starting position.
4. Relax for 5 seconds.

Tip: Keep your lower back flat against the floor. You may use a folded towel to support your lower back.

Basic Abdominal Strengthener

Purpose: To strengthen abdominal muscles

1. Lie on your back with your knees bent. Place a towel underneath the small of your back. Keep your lower back pressed against the towel.
2. Tighten your abdominal muscles and hold.
3. In one continuous move, slowly straighten your left leg, pause, and then bring it back to the starting position. Do the same with your right leg. Let your heels slide across the floor.
4. Maintain the tightened abdominals as you alternate legs.

Tip: When you are unable to keep pressure on the towel with your lower back, stop.

Cat and Camel for the Back

Purpose: To stretch the lower back

1. Start on your hands and knees, with your shoulders vertically above your wrists and your hips above your knees.

2. On an inhalation: Arch your back upward and lower your head. Try to round your spine as much as is comfortably possible. Tuck your pelvis under using your abdominals and buttock muscles.

3. Hold for 5 seconds.

4. On an exhalation: Lift your head upward and push your chest and abdomen toward the floor.

5. Hold for 5 seconds and then repeat, starting with step 2.

Tip: Move slowly, feeling a gentle stretch in your lower back. On an inhalation, avoid compressing your lower back; instead, feel your chest expanding.

Kneeling Stretch for the Back

Purpose: To stretch the lower back, hips, and sides
(the *quadratus lumborum*)

1. Get down on your hands and knees, reach forward
   with your left hand, and grasp a secure object.
2. From this position sit back diagonally toward the left
   buttock, elongating the left side.
3. The left arm may be internally rotated to increase
   the stretch.

4. Work on elongation of the left side by dropping
   the pelvis further diagonally backward and toward
   the hip.
5. Hold for 5 seconds.
6. Repeat on the opposite side

Tip: Pull your head slowly.

Knee-to-Chest Raise for the Lower Back

Purpose: To loosen and warm up the lower back

1. Begin by lying on your back with you knees bent and your feet on the floor.
2. With both hands, pull (don't lift) your right knee as close to your chest as possible. Keep your left knee bent with your foot flat on the floor. Hold for up to 30 seconds.
3. Repeat using your left knee.

Tip: Don't "lift" your legs with your hands and arms; just pull until you feel a gentle stretch in the lower back. If you have bad knees, put your hands under the knee and pull. To intensify the stretch, straighten the supporting leg.

Prayer Stretch for the Back for the Lower Back

Purpose: To warm up and gently stretch the lower back

1. Start on your hands and knees, with your arms stretched out in front of you.
2. Extend your hips backward and move your face close to the floor. Try to touch your buttocks to your heels.
3. Hold for 10 seconds, and then return to the s tarting position.

Tip: Slide your hands while maintaining your arm position. Keep your back straight.

Mid-Back and Shoulder Stretch

Purpose: To strengthen the mid-back and shoulder girdle
(the lower *trapezius*)

1. Begin on your hands and knees, sit back on your heels, and
   bend forward, resting your forehead on the floor.
2. Pull your shoulder blades down and back. Do not squeeze
   your shoulder blades together.
3. Hold for 3 to 5 seconds. Repeat 5 times.

Tip: A variation can be performed by lying on your stomach.

Chest Stretch

Purpose: To stretch the shoulders and chest

1. Start by facing a wall. Reach your right hand straight out to the side, against the wall, just below shoulder height. Place your left hand firmly on the wall at chin height.
2. Bend the left elbow down to bring the right shoulder blade down and back. Maintain this position as the feet turn 90 degrees so they are parallel to the wall.
3. Press your right fingertips against the wall to help turn the chest to the right.
4. Slowly turn your chest further around to the right, opening both sides of the chest and feeling a stretch in the front of the right shoulder and chest.
5. It is important not to allow the right shoulder to elevate during the stretch.
6. Hold for 3 to 5 seconds.
7. Repeat on the left side.

Tip: Do not arch your back during this exercise.

Wall Press for the Back and Chest

Purpose: To stretch the upper back and chest

1. Start by standing at arm's length from the wall. Place both hands on the wall at shoulder height.
2. Squeeze your shoulder blades together and down.
3. Slowly bend your arms and touch your nose to the wall. Keep your spine straight.
4. From this position push your shoulder blades apart, tuck in your chin, and push your mid-back away from the wall.
5. Hold for 5 to 10 seconds, and then return to the starting position.

Tip: Keep your spine as straight as possible.

Outer Thigh Stretch

Purpose: To stretch the outer thigh muscle
(*tensor fascia latae*)

1. Start with your right knee on the ground and your left foot on the floor, keeping your knee bent. Rest your left arm on a chair for support. Your right arm should rest at your side.

2. Pull in your stomach and posterior. Tilt the pelvis forward by using the left leg, particularly the hamstrings. Then, shift the hips from left to right, maintaining a strong posterior pelvic tilt, and contract your buttocks. You should feel a stretch on the outside of your right hip.

3. Stretch for a total of 5 to 10 seconds.

4. Switch sides and repeat on the left side.

Hamstring Stretch

Purpose: To warm up and stretch the back of the legs (the hamstring muscles)

1. Begin by lying on your back with your arms at your sides. Keep your left leg straight on the floor.
2. Lift your right leg to approximately 90 degrees and place both hands behind your right leg.
3. Keep your elbows straight and slowly straighten your right knee to feel a stretch behind the right leg.
4. Hold for 1 to 5 seconds.
5. Slowly return your leg to the floor and relax.
6. Repeat with the left leg.

Tip: Use a belt or towel to elevate your leg. You should feel no pain in your lower back.

Standing Quad Stretch for the Legs

Purpose: To stretch the front of the thigh (the quadriceps)

1. Place your right foot behind you on a bench or chair with your knee flexed.
2. Keep your right buttock tight and tucked under by tightening your stomach muscles.
3. Bend your left knee and allow your right knee to flex or bend further until you feel a stretch in the front of the right thigh.

Tip: Do not allow your back to arch!

Upper Neck Head Nod for the Neck

Purpose: To stretch the upper neck at the base of the skull

1. Sit upright in a chair and place your fingertips on your chin.
2. Tuck in your chin and draw the back of your head forward and down. You should feel the stretch at the base of your skull.
3. Hold for 3 to 5 seconds.
4. Repeat 5 times.

Tip: Use your fingers to help guide your forward motion.

Neck Stretch

Purpose: To stretch the neck muscles (the *levator scapulae*)

1. Sit upright in a chair and turn your head to the right. Place your right hand on top of your head.

2. Slowly bend your neck toward your right shoulder. Do not pull your head; simply allow your hand to support the head and neck in this position.

3. With your left hand, grasp the chair and slowly lean your torso toward the right and slightly forward until you feel a stretch.

4. Hold for 3 to 5 seconds.

5. Repeat on the left side.

Tip: Move your head slowly.

10

Boost Your Immune System

Think for a minute about one of those prime time television police shows that we love to watch. Invariably, there's the discovery of a dead body in the woods somewhere. Inevitably, some *CSI*-type cop comes and takes a look and, with uncanny accuracy, provides the exact time of death. For visual effects they'll often show a sensitive cop turning away from the corpse in horror and they leave it to your imagination to figure out what decay and deterioration he's just witnessed.

Sorry for the horrible visual image, but it's a good way to segue into a discussion of immunity.

Think about it for a second: Why is it that all those bacteria, microbes, and parasites have a field day with the body once it's no longer alive? Clearly they didn't just jump out of the germ hotel and colonize a corpse out of the clear blue sky. It's reasonable to assume those little microbes run around all over the place *all the time*, not just when someone dies, and that you might even come into contact with some of them while you read this page.

But they don't cause you to look like corpses on television crime shows, do they?

Here's why: You've got an amazingly protective mechanism in the body called the immune system. And as long as it's up and running at full speed, most of those viruses, toxins, parasites, and bacteria don't have a chance.

The immune system is a perfect place to really get into the nuts and bolts of anti-aging. After all, if your immune system is working great, you are far less likely to succumb to the little things that sideline mere mortals, such as colds, fevers, flu, and the like, and also less likely to be felled by some of the big-picture degenerative diseases of aging. A healthy, robust immune system won't protect you for eternity, but by keeping it in tip-top shape, you can do an awful lot to "rectangularize the curve," keeping infirmity mercifully brief and limiting it to the very end of a (hopefully long and vigorous) life.

Which is, after all, what we want. And what this book is about.

LOOK TO THE HOST

Louis Pasteur is a name known to every high school student. A famous French chemist and microbiologist, he was best known for inventing a process to stop milk and wine from making people sick, a process that came to be called *pasteurization*. But what is less well known is that Pasteur spent most of his life engaged in research that supported the then-controversial "germ theory of disease," a theory that holds that nasty little microorganisms like the ones that show up on the television corpse are the causes of many diseases.

So what do you think this brilliant scientist, who dedicated his life to showing that germs cause diseases, said on his deathbed?

"Look to the host."

What Pasteur had realized was that when it came to explaining illness, it wasn't enough just to identify microbes, even though that's what he had spent all of his life doing. He realized that his life's work had focused on only half of the equation of illness.

And when you think about it, this is something you know intuitively from your own experience. Remember the last time "something was going around" your office and half the people were out sick? Then you also probably remember that half the people did *not* get sick. And some were probably sidelined for a day or so while others were still dragging around trying to "shake the bug" two weeks later.

In other words, there was a pretty big variance in the reaction, even though the same germs were involved. In fact, it's safe to assume that everyone in the office had probably been exposed. But not everyone reacted the same way. Why?

"Look to the host," said Pasteur. The "host" is the *person* who is exposed to the microbe. Pasteur's final words were a mandate to those who came after him to explore the secrets of immunity and discover just why some people get sick while others don't. This is where the action is.

After all, you can't do much about a hurricane. But you *can* build a stronger house.

If you want to strengthen the immune system, it helps to understand how it works. Then, as we have with the brain and heart, we can understand where it breaks down and how we might protect it from such breakdown. By doing so, we greatly increase the odds of living longer and in greater health.

Let's get started.

THE HALO EFFECT

As you've probably deduced from reading the above, I'm a big fan of Pasteur's final message to the world. How sick you get depends only *partially* on the germs you're exposed to. In my view, getting sick (and even the process of aging itself) is the product of two variables, the person and the environment. Under the heading of "person" is everything from the food we eat to the lifestyle choices we make, and under "environment" is everything else, from the toxins in the air to the germs we pick up in the office bathroom. These overlapping variables form hundreds of feedback loops, interacting with one another in countless ways, right down to the cellular level. Sickness—and aging—is the *product* of these interactions, not of any one single variable.

In fact, immunity can be *strengthened* by any one of these variables. Although it would be great to have strength and power in all areas of life, from your food to your exercise to your relationships and environment, in truth, excellence and strength in one area can be so powerful that it can often make up for a bit of a deficit in another.

I'll give you an example from my own personal experience, an admittedly highly unscientific observation, but worth telling nonetheless. Once, I was participating in a workshop given by the great motivational speaker Les Brown. In attendance was a remarkable guy whose energy and optimism just radiated out of his body. He dressed fashionably, had virtually no body fat, his skin glowed with good health, and his eyes sparkled. When you spoke to him, he exuded warmth, friendliness, and peace. Turns out he was a missionary and chaplain who periodically visited Africa on humanitarian missions and when he wasn't doing that he attended to his "flock" back in England. He had a spiritual "center" that was powerful and contagious and extremely attractive.

Here's the thing: For breakfast, he ate Pop-Tarts and drank a Coke.

Now this doesn't make any sense unless you take a theoretical leap and consider whether being highly evolved in one area of your life might have such a "halo" effect on other parts that it could act as a powerful counterbalance. Call me crazy, but I believe the reason this enormously healthy guy was able to survive on the worst diet in the world was because of how highly evolved he was in other areas of his life. I believe that the spiritual area of his life was so "elevated" that it boosted his immunity, enough so that

he was able to manage a "deficit" in the area of his life called "diet." I suspect that same diet would have decimated his immunity if everything else were equal.

If you're a sports fan, think of a baseball player. He might not be able to run very fast or catch as well as Willie Mays, but if every time he goes to bat he hits a home run, his *overall* value as a player is going to be high. In much the same way, a person who is deeply evolved spiritually—think the Dalai Lama or my friend from the Les Brown seminar—might bring a kind of "low blood pressure, low stress" sensibility to everything he or she encounters and as a result might be able to weather the horrible effects of a bad diet. I suspect that even if the Dalai Lama ate nothing but potato chips all day, he'd still be pretty healthy overall. But of course, that's just a guess.

And even if it's true, the fact remains that most of us aren't the Dalai Lama.

So we'd all benefit by boosting the quality of all the components that go into strengthening the immune system—our food, supplements, environment, and even spirituality. (We'll talk about how the mind influences immunity in a bit.)

THE IMMUNE SYSTEM: KEEPING OUT THE RIFFRAFF

If you had to write a job description for the immune system, it would probably boil down to this: "Keep the bad guys out." The number one task of the immune system is to be alert to substances that don't belong. In that sense, the entire immune system (with all its component parts) acts like a big burly doorman at an exclusive nightclub. The immune system's job is to decide who belongs and who doesn't, and to dispatch with the riffraff as quickly and efficiently as possible.

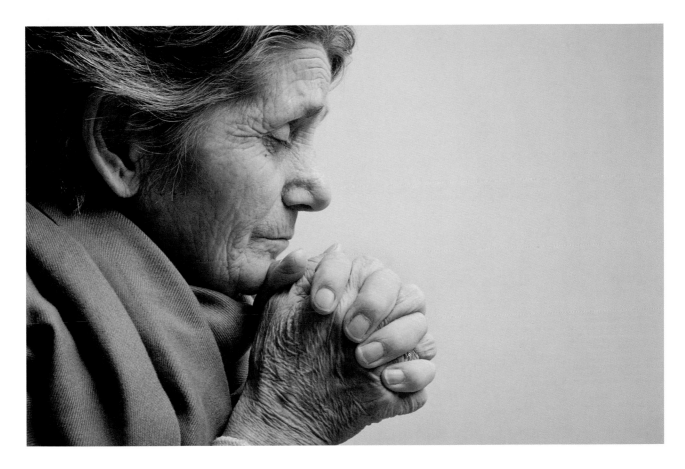

All the rest is details.

The best place to start our journey into those details is with a discussion of the lymphatic system. The lymphatic system consists of all kinds of organs, nodes, and ducts that transport a watery fluid called *lymph* throughout the body. Lymph also interacts with the circulatory system (blood) to drain fluid from tissues and cells. (The term *lymph* actually means "clear water"; it's the fluid and protein that's been drained out of the blood.) Lymph also distributes immune cells—it's kind of like a giant Amtrak train delivering the cellular defense army to all the places it needs to be.

The primary lymph organs include bone marrow and the thymus gland, while the secondary lymph organs include the lymph nodes, spleen, tonsils, appendix, and the all-important liver.

In the cellular army of the immune system, the main troops are white blood cells, the technical name for which is *leukocytes*. Their job is to defend against infectious disease and any other foreign invader (or what the body *perceives* as a foreign invader). This last caveat is important, because sometimes the body makes a mistake and thinks something (like pollen or ragweed) is more dangerous than it actually is, mounting a disproportionate attack against a relatively innocuous compound. Sometimes, too, the body gets confused and attacks its own tissues and cells (autoimmune disease). But for the most part, when things are working as they should, the leukocytes identify the bad guys accurately and then dispense with them in a variety of ways. It's in our interest to keep this system healthy and vibrant and fully functioning for as long as possible. In fact, a strong, healthy immunity is one of the foundations of healthy aging.

Just to get the cast of characters out of the way, it's helpful to understand that there are many different types of white blood cells (leukocytes). The chart below describes some of the major ones, which, if you've ever looked at your blood test results, will seem vaguely familiar. Now, when you see these names listed you'll know what your doctor is looking at. If, overall, the number of white blood cells (the types of which are listed below) is wildly off, it's valuable information about the behavior of your white blood cell army (and hence your immune system in general).

For science nerds, like me, only *neutrophils, eosinophils,* and *basophils* are collectively referred to as *granulocytes* because they all contain granules in their cytoplasm that stain under a light microscope. These granules in the granulocytes are actually enzymes that help digest bad-guy particles that the cells trap within the cell membrane. White blood cells that appear to have *no* granules in their cytoplasm are classed as *agranulocytes.* (Now you know.)

THE LYMPHATIC SYSTEM

TYPES OF LEUKOCYTES (WHITE BLOOD CELLS)

Type	Approximate Percentage in Adults	Main Target
Neutrophils	54–62 percent	Bacteria and fungi
Eosinophils	1–6 percent	Parasites/also involved in allergic reactions
Basophils	<1 percent	Involved in allergic reactions
Lymphocytes	25–33 percent	Varies according to type

The lymphocytes require special attention here. There are three main types, all are important in immunity, and all play an essential role in the body's defenses.

Most of the large lymphocytes are known as *NK cells*, or natural killer cells. (Remember these guys because they're really important!) We want our NK cells to be high performing. In fact, we want our whole NK army to be as well trained and elite performing as the Navy Seals. Why? Because NK cells are like poison dart guns for the bad guys. They "kill" by releasing nasty little granules that cause their target to die. NK cells work to contain viral infections and also play a major role in the rejection of tumors.

The smaller lymphocytes are T-cells and B-cells. You may have heard of T-cells because any discussion of AIDS invariably contains a reference to them. (One of the diagnostic criteria for determining whether HIV has progressed to AIDS is when a person's T-cell count has dropped below 200.) T-cells are an integral part of something called *cell-mediated immunity*, which means it is an immune response that *doesn't* involve antibodies. Cell-mediated immunity, with T-cells as one of its major weapons, is most effective in removing virus-infected cells but also plays a role in defending against fungi and cancers.

The third type of lymphocyte is the B-cell. These guys are the principle warriors for a type of immunity called *humoral immune response* (the balancing counterpart to the cell-mediated immune response mentioned above). The major job of the B-cells is to make antibodies! (Note to trivia buffs: The "B" in B-cells stands for—you'll never guess—*bursa of Fabricius*, a tissue found in a type of bird in which B-cell development was first described and which is remarkably similar to bone marrow, where B-cells develop in humans.)

In fact, *all* lymphocytes come from stem cells in the bone marrow; they just take different paths to their full development. Cells destined to become B-cells when they grow up, stay, and develop right there in the bone marrow, while cells destined to become T-cells migrate from the bone marrow up to the thymus gland, where they mature. (There is a bit of a scientific storm brewing over the exact origins of NK cells. Up until recently, scientists believed that NK cells also started out in the bone marrow just like B-cells and T-cells, but research at Ohio State University has questioned that belief.)

To simplify matters, think of the B-cells and T-cells as a kind of one-two punch against invaders. The B-cells are like a military intelligence system that seeks out targets and sends defenses (antibodies) to go after them, while the T-cells are like the soldiers trying to wipe out the invaders that the B-cells have identified.

The "invaders" are called *antigens*, foreign substances that trigger B-cells to produce antibodies. The antibodies lock on to specific antigens like a magnet to a refrigerator. But even though B-cells can recognize antigens and produce antibodies, they can't knock the little buggers out without help, which makes me think of crime in Los Angeles.

Why, you ask? Because in LA, whenever a crime is committed, you'll commonly see helicopters zooming and dipping and eventually hovering directly over the escaping criminal. But the helicopters, like the B-cells, rarely take the criminal out. That job is left for the on-the-ground troops (like the cops), who zero in on the identified perpetrator and make the actual arrest. This is pretty much how T-cells (the cops on the ground) and B-cells (the cops in the helicopters) work together.

Once the B-cells have produced antibodies they continue to exist in your body, so if that same antigen happens to sneak in again, you've already got your antibodies ready. That's why once you've had chicken pox, you're not likely to get it again. You already have the antibodies from the first time, and they're not about to allow the pox to take root a second time.

There's another classification of leukocytes (white blood cells) that's really cool. These are cells that act like PacMen. Their job is actually to engulf the invaders and gobble them up, just like the little PacMen (or Ms. PacMen) in the old video game. Cells whose job description includes acting like PacMen are called *phagocytes*. Neutrophils (above) belong to this class, as do cells called *macrophages*. In talks I've given on nutritional immunity I show before and after pictures of macrophages, *before* they encounter an invader, and *afterward*. You can actually see the bloated macrophage after it gets hold of a pathogen and eats it up.

"WE ARE WHAT WE THINK ABOUT"

One of the most exciting new areas of research to emerge in the last few decades is the science of—get ready for a long word now—*psychoneuroimmunology*. Take it apart and it's not so daunting. *Psych* refers to psychology, what you and I might call the mind, with its entire constellation of thoughts and feelings. *Neuro* refers to what happens in the brain when you actually *think* those thoughts and feel those feelings—the release, for example, of neurotransmitters like serotonin and dopamine. And *immunology* is exactly what it sounds like—the study of the immune system.

Put them together and you get the fascinating study of the interaction between the brain and the immune system.

And what an interaction it is. As the great biologist and Stanford University researcher Robert Sapolsky, Ph.D., says, "The brain has a vast potential for sticking its nose into the immune system's business."

The real father of psychoneuroimmunology was the Buddha, who basically summed up the whole field of research even before it was invented with these words: "We are what we think about." You probably understand intuitively the connection between thoughts and physiology. Just think back to the last time you watched a horror movie or an exciting thriller. You sat in the theater (or in front of your wide-screen television), probably not moving very much, yet your heart was racing, your blood pressure was elevated, and if some mad scientist had hooked you up to a monitoring device to measure everything going on in your body, it would have shown that specific areas of the brain were lit up and that your body was pumping out increased levels of certain hormones (like cortisol and adrenaline) and certain neurotransmitters (like epinephrine).

The point is that what you *think about* and what you *feel* have far-ranging effects on your body.

As they do on your immune system.

USE LAUGHTER AS MEDICINE

Remember NK cells, one of the three types of lymphocytes and an important player in mounting an immune system attack on invading microbes? Those NK cells actually respond to your mood. You ready for how?

They increase when you're happy!

Yup, strange and counterintuitive as it may seem, when you're feeling good, optimistic, and happy, when you're pursuing your bliss, your NK cells multiply like rabbits. Why? Who knows? But they do. More than a few studies

ANTI-AGING ACTION PLAN:

Boost Your Immune System with these Techniques

Happiness and feeling good actually help multiply your NK cells, important players in mounting an immune system attack on invading microbes. Use these suggestions to help boost your immune system:

- → Be on the lookout for cynical thoughts.
- → Examine situations reasonably, from all angles.
- → Put yourself in other people's shoes.
- → Learn to laugh at yourself.

- → Learn to relax.
- → Practice trust.
- → Learn to listen.
- → Practice forgiveness.

have shown a relationship between, for example, optimism and immune system response—optimists have higher numbers of T-cells and a higher level of NK cell activity.[1]

Now I'm going to go out on a limb here and assume there are at least a few of you who might think: "But Dr. Jonny, I'm a confirmed pessimist. So what can I do about my immunity? How much of it is under my control?"

So glad you asked.

Japanese researchers recently designed an ingenious experiment that should be of interest to you. They made up what they called a "recreational music protocol" and tried it out in a corporate environment. Basically, they taught a group-drumming class. First, the researchers measured NK activity (as well as two important inflammatory markers, *interleukin-1* and *interleukin-10*) in two groups of Japanese executives. Then the execs got together and drummed for an hour, while a "control" group of execs spent the same amount of time reading leisurely. Afterward, the researchers measured NK activity again.

Act as if Life's a Stage and Boost Your Immune Responsiveness

A study done at the University of California, Los Angeles, showed that professional actors spending the day doing a depressing, negative scene had decreased immune responsiveness. However, actors who spent the day on an uplifting, euphoric scene had increased immune responsiveness. How does this apply to you: Fake it till you make it—if you don't feel happy, at least act like you do! Your body will respond accordingly.

The results? The drumming executives demonstrated enhanced mood, reduced levels of the inflammatory markers, and increased NK cell activity.[2] And lest you think that maybe the researchers just happened to accidentally pick happy guys for their drumming group who would have better immunity anyway, they came back six months later and reversed the groups. The previous drummers got to lay back and read for an hour while the previous readers got to drum. Same results—the drummers had improved immunity and lower inflammation.

So you may not be a natural optimist, but there are still plenty of things you can do to boost your immunity (and drumming is just one of them!).

Even the mere act of laughing can make a huge difference, something that was first discovered by a writer and editor named Norman Cousins.

If you don't know the story of Norman Cousins you're in for a treat, and I'm delighted to be the one to deliver it. Cousins was the editor of a once-legendary publication called *Saturday Evening Review*. In 1964, doctors discovered that he had *ankylosing spondylitis*, a condition that's as bad as it sounds—the connective tissue in the spine deteriorates. Doctors gave Cousins a one in five hundred chance of survival.

So here's what he did:

First he did his own research on all the drugs he was on and found that the drugs were totally depleting his body of vitamin C. Doctors agreed to take him off some of the drugs and inject him with massive doses of vitamin C, especially because Cousins believed this might be his last hope and the doctors didn't have much of anything else to offer.

The second thing he did—pay attention here, folks—was check himself out of the hospital. He reasoned that hospitals were probably the worst place to be for someone who was seriously ill, so he decided to check into a hotel.

The third thing he did was rent a bunch of Marx Brothers movies. (Okay, they didn't have rental back then, but Cousins was pretty famous and was able to get a supply from the distributors.) And then, he literally laughed his you-know-what off.

In a state of euphoria, Cousins basically laughed his way back to health. Within a month he was back to work at the *Saturday Evening Review,* and although he continued to have minor health problems, he lived another twenty years.

Cousins wrote about his experiences in *The Anatomy of an Illness,* considered one of the classic early works in psychoneuroimmunology.

Since then, there's been a ton of research on laughter and the immune system, notably by Lee Berk, Ph.D., and Stanley Tan, M.D., Ph.D., of the Center for Spiritual Life and Wholeness at Loma Linda University, California. Their studies have shown that laughter reduces blood pressure and stress hormones and increases immune function by raising both T-cell and B-cell numbers. They've also found that laughter triggers the release of endorphins, the body's natural painkillers, as well as the number and activity level of NK cells.[3]

NK cells are also protective against cancer. In one study of seventy-seven women with breast cancer, researchers took a sample of each woman's tumor at the time of diagnosis. They put these samples in test tubes, together with some NK cells taken from each of the women. Some women had NK cells that just kind of lay there and gave up, not doing much of anything. Other women had NK cells that were vital and alive and went on a cleanup mission, indicating a seriously active immune system. Then the researchers followed up with the women twelve years later. Almost half (47 percent) of the women whose NK cells were fairly inactive had died, but a whopping 95 percent of the women whose NK cells were tigers were still alive.[4]

Other studies have shown that the less active your NK cells are, the more rapid cancer progresses and the more it spreads throughout the body.[5] "Lively immune cells thus seem essential to countering the growth of tumors and the spread of metastases," writes David Servan-Schreiber, M.D., Ph.D. "Everything that strengthens our precious immune cells also impedes the growth of cancers."[6]

The moral of the story is that you may not be able to reprogram yourself to be a complete optimist at heart, but there are definitely things you can do—from making music to watching funny movies, from coloring in books to walking in the woods, from going to a comedy show to taking long, luxurious baths to spending time with friends—that can increase your sense of well-being.

Whatever increases your well-being also increases your immunity. And, incidentally, can extend your life!

THE STRESS CONNECTION

The connection between stress and immunity makes such intuitive sense that you'd think it wouldn't be necessary to demonstrate it scientifically. Nonetheless, a tremendous amount of research has been done and the results are pretty unequivocal.

"A period of stress will disrupt a wide variety of immune functions," says the internationally known biologist and stress physiologist Robert Sapolsky, Ph.D.. Among them: the formation of new lymphocytes, their release into the circulation, the amount of time preexisting lymphocytes stay in circulation, the manufacture of antibodies in response to an infectious agent, and even the way the lymphocytes communicate "trouble" to one another. These are just a few of the ways stress affects immunity, according to Sapolsky.

Take glucocorticoids. These are hormones produced in the adrenal gland that are chemically classed as steroids. The most important glucocorticoid is cortisol (aka "the stress hormone"), which goes around cleaning up a lot of the mess of inflammation. (This is why your physician may give you a shot of cortisone—the drug version of cortisol—for serious inflammation.) So the glucocorticoids (mainly cortisol) have important, even life-saving, functions in the body. However, they also produce a lot of collateral damage when they're in overdrive, which is what happens when you're in a state of chronic stress. Glucocorticoids can cause shrinking of the thymus gland, an important player in the immune system and the site of T-cell maturation.

"Before it was possible to measure directly the amount of glucocorticoids in the bloodstream, one indirect way of doing so was to see how much the thymus gland in an animal had shrunk," notes Sapolsky. Because the thymus gland is an important part of the immune system, this shrinkage has implications for immunity.

Glucocorticoids also stop the formation of new infection-fighting lymphocytes in the thymus. "They also make circulating lymphocytes less responsive to an infectious alarm," says Sapolsky, and cause lymphocytes to be yanked right out of circulation. "Most impressively, glucocorticoids actually kill lymphocytes," he says.

The interesting thing is that a little bit of stress actually gives a temporary boost to the immune system function. All stress isn't bad, and some small doses kind of "prime" the system, making it more rugged and able to take on bigger challenges. The problem arises with long-term, chronic stress. Remember from chapter 2, on inflammation, we talked about how adaptive it is to have a "turbo" pedal like stress hormones that help prepare the body for immediate action: fight or flight? Without the ability to turn those hormones on in response to an immediate stressor, you'd probably die. The problem is when the pedal is to the metal all the time.

Chronic, unrelenting stress ages us, exacerbates all the major diseases, lengthens the time we're sick when we're sick, and ultimately, left unchecked, can kill us altogether. Unfortunately, that's the kind of stress most of us live with, whether it be from traffic, commutes, family issues, job insecurity, unmet deadlines, lack of sleep, poor diet, environmental toxins or, more than likely, a combination of some or all of the above. The point here is simple and clear: Take stress seriously. And build some sort of steam escape valve into your daily life, whether it be in the form of deep breathing exercises, meditation, yoga, qi gong, tai chi, a warm bath, or a walk in the woods.

Those activities may seem like ones you "don't have time for," and if that's the case, let me describe an old *New Yorker* cartoon for you: A profoundly out-of-shape man is in the examination room with his doctor. The doctor gives him some simple advice about exercising a half hour a day. The man snaps that he hasn't got time in his busy schedule for something like that. At which point the doctor wryly replies: "Well then, can you find 24 hours a day in your busy schedule to be dead?"

Enough said. Find ten to thirty minutes a day to do something that lowers your stress and makes you feel good. That's it. Case closed. To quote the famous Nike slogan: "Just do it."

HOW SUPPLEMENTATION CAN HELP YOU

I'm about to make a completely unscientific statement that will get me banned from the society of smart academics who only believe double-blind studies. You ready? Here goes: *Many people who take vitamins on a regular basis don't get sick very often.* Whether that's because they're healthier to begin with or because the vitamins in some way support their immune system is an open question, but the fact is that there are probably many people reading this book who are nodding their heads in agreement. Vitamins aren't the only thing that can keep you healthy, but they may help. And I can tell you from personal experience that when I get sick—which is rarely—I have my "go-to" cocktail of immune-support nutrients that I find shorten the duration and intensity of anything I happen to come down with (I'll tell you about them in a minute).

Now for the science.

In a double-blind controlled trial, scientists studied a group of about a hundred people over sixty-five years of age in Newfoundland, Canada. Ranjit Chandra, M.D., of the Memorial University of Newfoundland and the World Health Organization Center for Nutritional Immunology, gave half the folks a basic multivitamin and mineral supplement and the other half a placebo. During the twelve months of the study, the supplemented group reported half as many sick days as the placebo group. And several of their biochemical measures of immune system function also improved.[7] Chandra has stated that his studies "indicate that a causal relationship does exist between under-nutrition and impaired immunity in many elderly individuals and that this is a correctable abnormality in the majority."[8]

A study of immune system functioning in elderly folks in New Jersey showed that taking a basic multivitamin for a year resulted in a stronger immune system. The researchers commented that the current recommendations for some nutrients may be too low to support optimal immune function in healthy older adults.[9]

Indeed. A survey of the dietary habits of more than 1,700 healthy adults over the age of forty showed that more than 60 percent had deficient dietary intakes of vitamin D, vitamin E, folic acid, and calcium. And their intakes were not just below recommended levels, they were below the average requirement. Plus only about *half* of them met the daily recommendation for eating fruits and vegetables.[10]

We can say a few things about nutritional deficiencies and the immune system that are incontrovertible facts:

1. Nutritional deficiencies make it easier for bacteria or a virus to invade the body.
2. Nutritional deficiencies have an effect on the bacteria or virus once it has established itself.
3. Nutritional deficiencies increase the susceptibility of secondary infection.
4. Nutritional deficiencies make convalescence longer.

According to no less a mainstream organization than the Cleveland Clinic, supplementing your diet with a balanced multivitamin is essential.[11] Read on for a list of the most important nutrients and herbs for immunity, any of which are worth taking on a regular basis.

GIVE YOUR IMMUNE SYSTEM A BOOST WITH ZINC

Zinc is present in every tissue, organ, fluid, and secretion of the body. In fact, it's present in every living cell. It plays a huge role in immunity (not to mention cell division, DNA synthesis, growth and development, and the activity of about a hundred different enzymes). And because the body has no specific storage sites for zinc, you need to consume it on a daily basis.

Many of us don't.

Sure, cereals and grains contain zinc, but that zinc is bound to phytates* which makes it unavailable for

---

* Phytates are a storage form of potassium found in plants; they bind to minerals and make them unavailable for digestion and assimilation. For this reason, they're sometimes described as "anti-nutrients."

Get Your Immune System In Sync with Zinc

Take a multivitamin with at least 15 milligrams of zinc every day. When you feel an illness coming on, boost your zinc intake to 50 milligrams daily.

Studies show that zinc supplementation helps fight illness. The body can't store zinc, so taking a daily supplement is important.

absorption by the body. Alcohol and other drugs may also reduce zinc absorption (or increase zinc excretion). And we really don't have consistently reliable measures of zinc deficiency, so we have to make guesstimates from our dietary intake. The average zinc intake of Americans from food is a measly 13 milligrams a day for men and 9 milligrams a day for women.[12] Yes, that just about meets the minimum daily requirement set by the Food and Nutrition Board at the Institute of Medicine, but barely. The symptoms of zinc deficiency include hair loss, delayed wound healing, apathy, and low energy.

And definitely depressed immune function.

Although the conservative *Physicians' Desk Reference for Nutritional Supplements* says "there is little evidence that zinc supplementation will enhance immune responses in those who are not zinc deficient," it also states clearly that "zinc deficiency has been shown to impair immunity in many ways." The question then becomes a philosophic one: What exactly is deficiency? Is it having less than the bare recommended daily allowance that will allow you to escape major disease? Or is it any amount that's less than optimal?

I'm going with the latter.

The body requires zinc to develop and activate T-cells. Low zinc levels are associated with increased susceptibility to pneumonia and other infections in the elderly. And even mild to moderate degrees of zinc deficiency can impair macrophage functions (the PacMen of the immune system), as well as NK cell activity.[13]

In one study on patients with HIV, zinc supplementation produced higher lymphocyte cell counts and reduced the incidence of bacterial infections. In another double-blind study, volunteers with colds were separated into two groups. One took zinc lozenges every two hours while awake while the other did not. The group taking zinc lozenges recovered from their cold symptoms in 4.4 days compared to 7.6 days for the group not taking the supplements. Another study, involving 273 participants with experimentally induced colds, found that zinc gluconate lozenges (providing 13.3 milligrams of zinc) significantly reduced the duration of illness compared with a placebo.[14]

The best food source of zinc is oysters. Six medium oysters give you 76.7 milligrams. Beef is another excellent

GREEN TEA AND GREEN TEA EXTRACT

Much research has pointed to the protective effects of green tea on the human body, including the ability of compounds in green tea (called catechins) to inhibit the growth of tumors. In fact, the evidence that green tea has a protective effect against cancer is so compelling that the chemoprevention branch of the National Cancer Institute has initiated a plan to develop tea compounds as cancer-chemopreventive agents in human trials. It's now fairly well established that green tea may help prevent a number of different cancers in humans, including bladder, colon, esophagus, pancreas, rectum, and stomach cancer. One Chinese study suggested that the mechanism for this anticancer activity included cellular immune function, and noted that animals treated with green tea extract had significantly greater NK cell activity.[15]

If "all" it did was help prevent cancer, green tea would be assured a place on the table of every meal designed to promote longevity. But its resume is hardly limited to fighting cancer (as if that weren't enough!). In a 2004 article titled "Effects of Green Tea Intake on the Development of Coronary Artery Disease," researchers writing in the Japanese medical publication *Circulation Journal* concluded that "the more green tea patients consume, the less likely they are to have coronary artery disease."[16]

Other research has shown that green tea helps fight oxidation and glycation, two of the Four Horsemen of Aging. It appears to help with stress as well. Green tea contains a substance called *theanine*, which is helpful in improving mood and increasing a sense of relaxation. Green tea also lowers a nasty compound in the blood called *fibrinogen*, which can contribute to clots and strokes. Finally, in several animal studies, green tea has

source; 3 ounces of cooked beef shanks gives you 8.9 milligrams, a distant second to oysters but still far ahead of everything else. Red meat and poultry provide the majority of zinc in the American diet, and with many people becoming vegetarians, there's reason to be concerned that we're consuming less than the optimal amount of this important immunity nutrient.

It's worth pointing out that high levels of zinc can inhibit copper absorption, sometimes producing copper deficiency. For this reason, dietary supplement formulations containing high levels of zinc sometimes include copper just for balance.

demonstrated the ability to lower blood sugar, and regular consumption of green tea can be a great help in the quest to maintain a healthy weight.

OLIVE LEAF EXTRACT: A BOUNTY OF GOODNESS

Open any basic nutrition textbook and you're sure to find a paean to the healthy Mediterranean diet, which features a generous amount of olive oil. But according to Nutrition *Research Reviews* in 2005,[17] the Mediterranean diet's healthy effects can be attributed not only to the high relationship between unsaturated and saturated fatty acids in olive oil but also to the antioxidant property of abundant plant chemicals in the olive called phenolic compounds.

The use of olive leaf for medicinal purposes goes all the way back to the ancient Egyptians. They believed that the olive leaf was a symbol of heavenly power, and they used the extracted oils from the leaf in the mummification rituals of their kings.

Olive leaf extract is a rich source of some of the most important phenolic compounds on earth, such as *oleuropein, hydroxytyrosol, tyrosol, rutin, luteolin, catechin,* and *apigenin,* which are believed to be responsible for most of the leaf's pharmacological effects. Olive leaf extract also contains various trace elements vital to good health, such as selenium, chromium, iron, zinc, vitamin C, beta-carotene, and a wide range of amino acids.

Olive phenolics have a powerful ability to eat up free radicals and are a tremendous weapon in the fight against oxidative damage. They also show a strong synergistic behavior when combined, as occurs naturally in the olive leaf, and concentrated, as in olive leaf extract. The most active flavonoids, rutin, catechin, and luteolin, exert antioxidant effects almost two and a half times greater than those of vitamin C and E and are comparable to those of lycopene, according to in vitro tests. The powerful antioxidant effect produced by high-quality olive leaf extract may also be due to the synergy of flavonoids, phenols, and a high oleuropein content.

Olive leaf extract can be a powerful weapon in the battle between your immune system and invading microbes. Compounds in the olive leaf have long been used to help fight illnesses brought on by microbes. The first formal mention of olive leaf, an account describing its ability to cure severe cases of fever and malaria, occurred in 1854, when the *Pharmaceutical*

"Boil a handful of (olive) leaves in a quart of water down to half its original volume. Then administer the liquid in the amount of a wineglass every three or four hours until the fever is cured."

— *Pharmaceutical Journal*, 1854

Extend the Olive Branch to Your Immune Cells

Take one to two capfuls of a high-quality olive leaf extract daily (such as Barlean's Olive Leaf Complex, available on my website, www.jonnybowden.com).

Olive leaf complex can help prevent the spread of viruses and may stimulate immune cells. It also eats up free radicals and fights oxidative damage.

Journal carried a report by one Daniel Hanbury, according to James R. Privitera, M.D.. The report contained the following simple healing recipe:

This method became popular in England for treating sick Englishmen returning from the tropical colonies, according to Hanbury. He believed that a bitter substance in the leaves was the healing ingredient. That substance in olive leaf extract, since identified as oleuropein, has been found to be particularly helpful in resisting bacterial damage. In fact, early research by the drug company Upjohn found olive leaf extract to be effective in treating infection by a large number of viruses, as well as bacteria and parasitic protozoans.

One of the active ingredients in oleuropein is a substance called *elenolic acid*. Research shows that Elenolic acid has an uncanny ability to inhibit the growth of viruses. And one form of elenolic acid, *calcium elenolate*, fights not only viruses but bacteria and parasitic agents as well, studies show.

According to Privitera, olive leaf extract directly penetrates infected cells and stops viral replication. And Privitera is not the only health expert who has taken note of the amazing antimicrobial properties of olive leaf extract.

Noted naturopath Jack Ritchason, N.D., in his excellent book on olive leaf extract, writes that compounds of olive leaf extract can "directly penetrate infected cells and inhibit further microbial reproduction." Ritchason also points out that olive leaf extract may also directly stimulate the formation of immune system cells that combat various types of microbes.

PROBIOTICS: GOOD FOR THE GUT

If you've never heard of probiotics or you're not entirely sure what they are, let me introduce you, as they play an important role in immunity.

Your gastrointestinal tract (i.e., your gut) basically functions as a barrier against stuff that doesn't belong, stuff (like microbes) that comes from microorganisms and food. In this sense, it's like a "second skin," only an internal one. The gut functions by providing a colony of live bacteria that have many functions, such as helping you digest and absorb important nutrients, helping alleviate intestinal inflammation, and helping maintain a balance between inflammatory and anti-inflammatory chemicals in the body (cytokines).[18]

The gut is like a garden, and like any garden it has both weeds and flowers. The weeds are the bad bacteria, such as *Candida albicans*, or yeast, which, when they overgrow, can create all kinds of problems in the body. The flowers are the good guys—healthy bacteria that protect your gut, help you digest food, and improve immunity. Those "good guy" bacteria we call probiotics.

"Probiotics are involved in controlling the inflammation of the intestinal system by promoting defense mechanisms and preventing bad microbes from growing there," says Allison Tannis, M.Sc., R.H.N., author of *Probiotic Rescue.*

One of the most famous probiotics is *Lactobacillus acidophilus,* a strain often found in yogurt with live cultures (the probiotics are the live cultures referred to on the label). But there are many other strains of probiotics as well. The point is that those healthy bacteria are a powerful weapon in the fight to improve immunity, resist infection and disease, and extend life.

In one study, New Zealand researchers wanted to see whether probiotic supplements could enhance mmunity in people aged sixty-three to eighty-four years old. Over nine weeks, the researchers looked at the activity of key immune system factors in samples of the patients' blood. They found that the bug-eating activity of phagocytes and the tumor-killing ability of NK cells improved, showing that probiotics do indeed support and improve immunity.[19]

In addition to helping you digest and assimilate nutrients needed for a long and healthy life, probiotics also make a serious dent in the ability of one of the four horsemen to age your body—inflammation. "A lack of probiotics in the intestinal tract allows bad microbes to grow and release toxins that cause intestinal inflammation," explains Tannis. "Probiotics may also help the immune system become strong enough to fight off viral infections."

MIXED ANTIOXIDANTS

No matter how well you design your diet, you can still augment it with supplemental antioxidants, according to the Cleveland Clinic website.[20]

Vitamin C, for example, though it may not necessarily prevent colds, definitely shortens their duration. It also increases antibodies, *phagocytosis* (the ability of the PacMen to eat up the bad guys), and *chemotaxis* (the speed with which white blood cells get to the infection or injury site). "The concentration of vitamin C in immune cells is twenty to a hundred times higher than in the rest of the blood," says Robert Rountree, M.D. "People who take vitamin C supplements see a measurable increase in NK activity within twenty-four hours."[21]

Selenium, one of the most important microminerals on the planet, is associated with higher rates of survival in AIDS patients and lower rates of cancer in general. According to Bert Berkson, M.D., Ph.D., selenium acts like "birth control" for the hepatitis C virus. It's important stuff!

ANTI–AGING ACTION PLAN:
Take an Immunity Cocktail

Sprinkle a spoonful of powdered probiotics on yogurt or fruit and consume every day. The powder has virtually no taste, and blends quite well into yogurt dishes. In my house, we put some Greek yogurt (higher in protein but lower in probiotics) on top of fruit (blueberries and cherries are my favorite), sprinkle with powdered probiotics (I use Designs for Health Probiotic Synergy Powder), and then top with some flaked coconut and slivered almonds. Mix it up and enjoy!

Alternately, take probiotic capsules (such as Vital Nutrients Acidophilus/ Bifidobacter/FOS) or the new, very effective Probiotic Pearls (which don't require refrigeration) with at least two meals per day. (All three products are available on my website, www.jonnybowden.com, under "P" in the shopping/ supplements section.)

On **beta-carotene,** the Cleveland Clinic has this to say: "You should add beta-carotene in a dose of 25,000 international units (IU) twice per day. Beta-carotene is one of the most potent nutrients and can protect the body from oxidative stress. Populations that have diets high in beta-carotene have a lower incidence of certain forms of cancer."[22] (Most experts now recommend "mixed carotenoids" (clearly visible on the label) rather than beta-carotene exclusively.

Vitamin E is one of the most important antioxidants on the planet, and it's especially critical for older people experiencing the typical slowdown in immune function, according to Rountree. In a study at the U.S. Department of Agriculture's Human Nutrition Center at Tufts University, eighty-eight people aged sixty-five and older were given either a placebo or vitamin E supplement daily for four months.[23] At the end of the four-month period, researchers reported an increase in both T-cell and B-cell activity among the vitamin E takers. The people taking vitamin E also had a more vigorous immune system response totetanus and hepatitis B vaccines, meaning their ability to produce antibodies had improved. "If you supplement the elderly with vitamin E, you can enhance their immune response," said lead researcher Simin Meydani, D.V.M., Ph.D.[24]

The general antioxidant protection formula I like best comes from my good friend Robert Rountree, M.D., whose excellent book, *Immunotics*, provides an in-depth exploration of many of the issues discussed in this chapter. "[Antioxidants are] a building block of a healthy immune system," he writes. "Everyone should take a daily antioxidant supplement, but it is especially important for people over fifty and endurance athletes."

Just as health experts now recommend mixed *carotenoids*, as opposed to just beta-carotene, we now strongly recommend that your vitamin E be from mixed *tocopherols*. Vitamin E actually has eight different components, and most early studies (and many health food stores) only sell vitamin E as "alpha-tocopherol" (one of the eight fractions). Emerging research is clear that *alpha*-tocopherol is not a particularly effective form of vitamin E and pales in comparison to *gamma*-tocopherol, which seems to do all the heavy lifting. Get a high-gamma formula or at least one where the vitamin E comes from "mixed tocopherols." Don't buy vitamin E supplements that are exclusively alpha-tocopherol. (I have high-gamma vitamin E available on my website, www.jonnybowden.com. Several reputable companies, such as Designs for Health and Crayhon Research, make this type of vitamin E, and it's worth getting.)

While the recommended nutrients (see page 199) constitute a "greatest hits" of the best supplements for immunity, it's very far from a complete list of immune-supportive compounds. You should also consider:

Quercetin is a member of the flavonoid family and found in apples and onions. It's known for it's powerful anti-inflammatory effect and also for its ability to block the action of many known cancer-producing substances. "Quercetin has strong antiviral activity, particularly against herpes, so I recommend it to people with serious viral infections," says Rountree.

Mushrooms have been used medicinally for centuries and are terrific immune boosters. Each of the "big three" has a special purpose, though they may overlap. According to Rountree, shiitake works for people at high risk for colds and flus, while reishi can help the body cope with physical or emotional stress. Maitake is the most potent, but also the most expensive. "Maitake is my choice for cancer prevention and chronic hepatitis," he says.

IMMUNITY AND AGING

So here's the bad news: All things being equal, as we age we have a reduced ability to fight off infection and other health challenges.[*]

In elderly people, the body's usual, innate response to infection, such as heating up with a fever, doesn't happen automatically. Twenty percent of adults over the age of sixty-five with serious bacterial infections don't have fevers at all, according to Edith Burns, M.D., associate professor of medicine at the Medical College of Wisconsin. "At this age [the body] probably still has the ability to generate fevers and other immunity weapons, but the central nervous system is simply less sensitive to immune signals and doesn't react as quickly or efficiently to infection," she writes.

Elderly adults are also less capable of producing lymphocytes. And the cells that they do produce are less vigorous and effective. The duration of antibody response is shorter in older adults, and fewer of them are made. In fact, warns Burns, elderly adults, particularly those older than seventy, are more likely to produce autoantibodies, which attack parts of the body itself rather than attacking infections. Autoantibodies are factors in causing rheumatoid arthritis as well as atherosclerosis.

Then there are the psychological components of immunity. "Older adults often experience loss and stress, and suppressed immunity has been associated with bereavement, depression, and poor social support," writes Burns.

Garlic is a wonderful immune system booster. It has antimicrobial properties and is able to kill or stop the growth of various types of bacteria. It also increases NK cell activity and stimulates T-cells. "For more than twenty years, garlic has been a mainstay of my medical practice," says Rountree.

---

[*] Of course, the key phrase here is "all things being equal," and the purpose of this book is to make sure all things are not equal; rather, that you've stacked the deck in your favor, increasing the odds that what usually happens in the course of aging will either not happen (loss of memory, for example) or happen significantly less or significantly later (if at all).

ANTI-AGING ACTION PLAN:
Take Antioxidant Supplements Daily for Immune System Support

Your daily supplements should include:

→ Vitamin E (from gamma-tocopherol or mixed tocopherols): 400 IU

→ Vitamin C: 1,000–2,000 mg

→ Zinc: 25–50 mg

→ Selenium: 100–200 mcg

→ Mixed carotenoids: 15,000–30,000 mg

Again, there's much you can do to increase the odds that your body will maintain healthy and robust immunity well into your ninth decade and beyond. Stress reduction and an active social life, the focus of the last section in this book, are certainly at the top of the list. Removing toxins, pesticides, and other physical stressors from your diet is another, as is eating a whole foods diet with plenty of protein and omega-3 fats. And exercising on a regular basis is another strong booster of immunity and general health. A recent study looked at all the available evidence on exercise and immunity and concluded that "aerobic exercise is a friend of the immune system," helping to balance diminished adaptive responses and reduce inflammation.[25]

And what does Burns, a mainstream doctor with academic ties who specializes in geriatrics, have to say about vitamins and supplements?

"In both healthy and nutritionally deficient older adults, vitamin and dietary supplements have been found to enhance the response of the immune system."[26]

That statement might not be any more scientific than the one I made earlier, but it's still the truth.

11

What You Should Know about Hormones

"It's my hormones!" says the woman suffering from a host of monthly related maladies sometimes known as PMS. "It's his hormones!" says the parent, describing the bafflingly stupid behavior of a teenage boy risking life and limb in the latest version of some extreme sport.

Are they right?

Hormones have been blamed for everything from groping backseat encounters in the teenage years to the purchase of a red Porsche at age fifty-five. But the idea that "it's all about hormones," like many clichés, has some grounding in fact. Hormones are absolutely essential messengers that tell cells, organs, tissues, muscles, and bones what to do. They are drivers of behavior and physiology. Many of them diminish with aging. And it's a reasonable question to ask how hormones change as we age, which ones change, how those changes affect our longevity, and what, if anything, we can or should do about it.

Let's start with one hormone over which we actually have some control. Compared to the sexy stuff (like testosterone and estrogen), it doesn't get a ton of attention from the media, but it's almost impossible to overstate its importance.

I'm talking about insulin.

INSULIN, LONGEVITY, AND HEALTH

In 1992, researchers collected data on people who were both mentally and physically fit and were at least one hundred years old.[1] They looked carefully at the factors these folks had in common to see whether they might turn out to be predictors for a long and healthy life.

They came up with three.

The first was low blood levels of triglycerides, a kind of fat found in the body and blood, high levels of which put you at risk for heart disease. The second was high blood levels of the so-called "good" cholesterol, HDL, the kind of cholesterol thought to be protective against heart disease. And the third was a low level of fasting insulin.

Let's take a look at this last factor.

Insulin: Sensitivity versus Resistance

Although there's not a whole lot you can do (short of recommended hormone replacement therapy) to change your levels of important hormones like testosterone, there's a *tremendous* amount you can do to modify your insulin levels. The cells' sensitivity to insulin—a property called (big surprise) *insulin sensitivity*—is turning out to be one of the most important predictors of overall health. "If there is a single marker for life span," says Ron Rosedale, M.D., author of *The Rosedale Diet*, "it's insulin sensitivity."

Insulin sensitivity? Aging?

Yup.

To understand this incredibly important phenomena and its effect on metabolism and longevity, let's start by looking at the metabolism of a five-year-old kid. Why? Because, theoretically at least, a five-year-old hasn't screwed up his metabolism yet. After all, if you want to know how something is supposed to work, it's good to look at how it performs before it gets screwed up. Hence, our mythical five-year-old.

So our five-year-old kid comes home from school and he eats an apple. The apple causes his blood sugar to rise just a bit, which is perfectly normal—when you eat food, especially carbohydrate and to a lesser extent protein, your blood sugar goes up. (It actually doesn't rise when you eat fat, but that's another discussion.) That slight rise in blood sugar is a good thing because our mythical five-year-old is now going to go outside and play. He's going to run, jump, slide, bike, and do all the things kids do—or at least what they did before the days when every playdate was micromanaged and video games replaced sandlot softball!

Now when blood sugar goes up, even a little, the pancreas jumps into action and releases a hormone that is the star of our discussion—insulin. Insulin has many jobs in the body, but first among them is to get that excess sugar out of the bloodstream and escort it into the muscle cells, where it can be used for energy. This is an important job, because excess sugar in the bloodstream is damaging to long-term health. And getting that sugar into the muscle cells not only removes it from the bloodstream, preventing damage and aging, but also delivers an important fuel to the muscle cells, which are going to need it if our kid's going to make it through his strenuous afternoon playtime.

So far, so good.

Insulin and its behavior are critically important for longevity. Although there's not a whole lot you can do (short of recommended hormone replacement therapy) to change your levels of important hormones like testosterone, there's a *tremendous* amount you can do to modify your insulin levels.

Eventually, insulin peacefully escorts that sugar into the muscles, and the muscles gratefully accept it and burn it, thus fueling our kid's activities. Gradually, his blood sugar returns to normal, even a little below (because he's been so active), which is a good thing because now it's dinnertime.

That's also pretty much the last time you'll see things work that well, at least in modern Western society.

Let's fast-forward thirty to forty years.

You wake up in the morning, probably tired and groggy from not having slept enough. Your stress hormones are immediately elevated as you ponder a ridiculously crowded day in which there's hardly enough time to do half the things you need to get done. You fly out of the house on the way to work, stop briefly at the local coffee emporium to grab a calorie-laden, sugar-loaded caffeinated beverage, perhaps accompanied by one of those 900-calorie healthy-looking "low-fat" muffins that also happen to be loaded with sugar and carbs. Now your blood sugar is through the roof. The pancreas jumps into action: "Oh my God, this dude just ate the equivalent of five Ding Dongs," it mumbles to itself while it starts pumping out insulin like crazy to deal with the enormous sugar load.

Insulin dutifully begins shoveling that excess sugar into the muscle cells, but this time the muscle cells are having none of it. "We don't *need* all that sugar," they say. "This guy is going to sit around at the computer all day and when he gets home, he's going to veg out on the couch. What do we need all that fuel for? Go take it somewhere else!" In technical terms, the cells become *resistant* to the actions of insulin—insulin resistance, get it?—and they lock their doors and essentially say, "We gave at the office."

What to do, what to do?

Well, insulin's got to take that sugar somewhere, so it starts knocking on the doors of the fat cells. "Hey, let us in! We've got all this sugar for you." And guess what? The fat cells are more than happy to open their doors (at least in the beginning. After a while, even they get resistant, leaving all that sugar to float around the bloodstream, causing all sorts of mischief). Eventually, insulin gets the sugar out of the bloodstream so effectively that your blood sugar plummets and you're starving. Now it's 11:00 in the morning and you'll kill someone if you don't get a candy bar.

Welcome to blood sugar hell.

Of course, that's just the beginning. Once on this terrible roller coaster you're caught in a cycle of low blood sugar, mood swings, cravings, carb overeating, and the resultant inevitable fat around your middle (or thighs, butt, or hips). I talk about this in detail in my book *Living Low Carb*, but the point here is that this phenomenon is about much more than unwanted weight gain. It's also about aging. And here's why.

Remember glycation? Let me refresh your memory: It's one of the Four Horsemen of Aging, and it happens when excess sugar gloms onto proteins in the blood, eventually causing them to become sticky and gooey and gum up circulation.

Excess sugar. Like the kind that's floating around in your bloodstream, all dressed up with nowhere to go. The kind that hooks a ride onto innocent proteins, like teenagers hopping on the outside of buses looking for a thrill ride.

From the point of view of aging, the results are disastrous.

Proteins that have become "glycated" (sticky with sugar) are too big and gummy to get through small blood vessels and capillaries, including the small vessels in the kidneys, eyes, and feet (which is why so many diabetics are at risk for kidney disease, vision problems, and amputations of toes and feet). The sugar-coated proteins become toxic, making cell machinery run less efficiently, damaging the body and exhausting the immune system. When cells become insulin resistant, the result is you now have way too much sugar in your bloodstream, which is a disaster just waiting to happen.

All this would be bad enough, but because of your elevated sugar you also have elevated levels of insulin, which is not a good thing from a longevity point of view. Insulin does many things besides acting as a sugar wrangler. For one thing, it sends a message to the kidneys to hold on to sodium, which drives your blood pressure up, increasing your risk for heart disease. For another, insulin turbo-charges the activity of a particular enzyme (with the unwieldy name of *HMG-coenzyme A reductase*, or *HMG-CoA reductase*) that runs the cholesterol-making machinery of the body. So high levels of insulin basically signal the liver to ramp up the production lines on cholesterol.

Meanwhile, high levels of sugar in the blood increase the production of triglycerides, another serious risk factor for heart disease. And elevated insulin makes losing weight fiendishly difficult—not for nothing is it nicknamed "the fat-storing hormone."

High-sugar diets are also a risk factor for cancer; cancer cells thrive on sugar, consuming far more of it than normal cells. Sugar is pure ecstasy for cancer cells, which chow down on it like hungry rabbits in a lettuce patch. Although the evidence is mixed, emerging research[2] suggests a link between high-sugar diets (technically known as *high-glycemic diets*) and different types of cancer—not exactly a great thing from the point of view of aging well!

Thoroughly depressed? Don't be. This one is easy to fix.

The absolute, number-one-with-a-bullet, easy-as-pie, quick fix for insulin resistance is—wait for it—a low-carb diet. In fact, a low-carb diet (and don't panic, I'll define what I mean by that in a minute) may be a fix for a number of issues that concern those of us who want to live long and well. With its reduced intake of processed carbs and sugar, a low-carb diet will drop your triglycerides like a rock, thereby reducing at least one major risk factor for heart disease. And there's no faster way to bring blood sugar down to normal levels, or keep insulin in its "happy" zone, where it can work for you instead of against you.

Now is it starting to make sense why the 1992 researchers found low fasting insulin to be one of the trademark blood measures of healthy centenarians? And why the famous Baltimore Longitudinal Study of Aging found the same thing?

The opposite of the dreaded insulin resistance is *insulin sensitivity*. Insulin sensitivity is *good*. You *want* your cells to be responsive to insulin. In fact, you want them super-responsive, you want them listening like crazy and opening

their doors when insulin comes knocking. This keeps glucose (sugar) metabolism working, keeps sugar from getting too high in the bloodstream, keeps the muscle cells fueled, and means that your pancreas doesn't have to work too hard overproducing insulin because a small amount gets the job done quite well. This is a perfect scenario for living longer!

And you can accomplish that with a few lifestyle modifications.

Number one with a bullet: exercise! Here's why.

Balance Your Diet with the Jonny Bowden Four Food Groups

Here are my four food groups: food you can hunt, fish, pluck, or gather. Make that the mainstay of your diet and you'll live a very long time. These foods are part of a low-carb, low-glycemic diet that won't raise your blood sugar, and thus keep you off the blood sugar roller coaster.

Every time you move around you create a demand for fuel. Your cells literally open up and say to insulin, "Come on in, the water's fine!" That allows insulin to remove excess sugar from the bloodstream and dump it into the receptive (sensitive) muscle cells, which are eager to have it.

Number two, and probably just as important: adjust your diet.

First, cut out the sugar. The more sugar you eat, the higher your blood sugar goes up, and the more insulin you secrete. For most people this is a disastrous scenario (I say

"most" to allow for the few, lucky individuals on the planet who can eat all the sugar they want and not have it hurt their health. And in any case, even if such people do exist, I guarantee you're not one of them. Neither am I!).

Second, reduce foods that the body treats as sugar. Unfortunately, it's not just plain ordinary white sugar that plays havoc with your metabolism and contributes to aging. It's anything the body *thinks* is sugar. The body treats most white foods—potatoes, breads, starches, rice, cakes, you name it—as nothing more than sugar, which is pretty much what they turn into once they leave your mouth and enter your stomach. One of the many reasons people who eat fewer carbs have such good results is that they eliminate many of the foods that put you on the hellish blood sugar roller coaster. (A great deal of research has shown that people on low-carb diets not only lose body fat and overall weight, but lower their triglycerides and often improve their cholesterol ratios as well.)

A low-carb diet does not have to mean the stringent first stage of the Atkins Diet (not that there's anything *wrong* with that). Remember, the average American consumes more than 300 grams of carbohydrate a day. You don't need anything like that amount. You can be a pretty active athlete on one-third of that amount, and many people flourish at even lower levels. And forget all the garbage you've heard about "needing carbs for energy." Most carbs that we eat will *sap* your energy, not add to it. The body's main source of fuel is fat, and we can get by quite nicely with fewer carbs—although how *much* less is an individual question and one best answered by another book (see my book *Living Low Carb*).

When I talk about this stuff in person at workshops, I usually put a PowerPoint slide up that has a person with a megaphone with the following talk balloon coming out of it so it comes across loud and clear: "He's not talking about fruits and vegetables!" So let me be clear: *I'm not talking about fruits and vegetables (especially vegetables!)*. When I talk about reducing carbs for longevity, I'm talking about *bar-code carbs*: processed cereals, pastas, breads, cakes, crackers, all that stuff. Eat all the vegetables you want, and add some healthy, low-sugar fruits, such as berries, apples, grapefruit, and the like. Send back the breadbasket at dinner (believe me, you don't need it) and get a second portion of salad or soup. There, wasn't that easy?

Insulin is one incredibly important hormone over which we have a lot of control. But what about the sexy stuff alluded to earlier, those other hormones that get the lion's share of attention in the media?

Let's take a look.

THE SEX HORMONES

With sex hormones (like testosterone and estrogen) and aging we're presented with something of a chicken-and-egg conundrum. Changes in hormone levels might well be the result of underlying changes that are associated with unhealthy aging rather than the cause. "Often, it is not possible to establish cause-effect relationships," write Jeffrey Bland, Ph.D., and David Jones, M.D., "but it is clear that changes in (hormones) throughout life are associated with significant changes in physiology and vitality."[3]

Then, for those of you who like to philosophically ponder these things, there's this: It's just possible that hormone levels at *one* stage of life are not necessarily the best levels to have at a *different* stage, at least from an evolutionary standpoint.

Take testosterone. Aggression is often associated with young males with raging levels of this much-maligned male hormone, levels that are typically way higher than

"Lower levels of testosterone are associated with greater risks for coronary heart disease and diabetes."

— David Leonardi, M.D.

those seen in older men. If you're a young caveman, a high level of testosterone (and even aggression) makes a lot of sense from an evolutionary perspective. It might give you an advantage in both reproduction and protecting your young or your village. But for older males, it's a whole different ballgame. For these guys, judgment, reason, and passion control are way more important for staying alive. After all, what eighty-year-old man is driven by "raging hormones"? Would he ever make it to ninety if he were?

But I digress. As a practical matter, we do not need to sit idly by and watch our passion hormones diminish

completely (okay, maybe just to the point where extreme skateboarding no longer seems like such a great idea). Testosterone replacement, for both men and women (yup, you read that right), is increasingly becoming part of an anti-aging strategy, for reasons that will become clear shortly. And other hormonal changes that take place over the years are modifiable by diet and lifestyle. Many of these can contribute to a much more youthful old age.

The Truth about Testosterone

Ah, testosterone. The much-maligned engine of male behavior, the one blamed for everything from grand theft auto to soccer riots. Never has one hormone gotten such a bad, and undeserved, rap. True, without it, we'd probably be spared the sight of football fans with painted faces waving big spongy fingers in the air, and the entire sport of NASCAR might not exist, but truth be told, testosterone has another, gentler side, and its decline has serious implications for aging well.

First, some definitions. Testosterone, the principle male sex hormone, is what's called a *steroid hormone*. It's primarily secreted in the testes of men and the ovaries of women. It's classed as an *androgen*, which means it controls the development and maintenance of masculine characteristics. It figures prominently in libido, energy, and well-being.

The bad news is it starts to decline around age thirty. So why should you care?

"Lower levels of testosterone are associated with greater risks for coronary heart disease and diabetes," says David Leonardi, M.D., medical director of the Leonardi Executive Health Institute in Denver, Colorado. "When you take a group of men of the same age and test them for cognitive function, mood, strength, speed, endurance, and markers

ANTI–AGING ACTION PLAN:

Boost Your Well Being and Get Your Testosterone Levels Checked

An estimated 13.9 million American men have low testosterone, yet only 9 percent of men are currently being treated with testosterone replacement therapy (according to a report at the 2009 annual meeting of the Endocrine Society). The condition takes a significant toll on men's lives. Among men polled, 97 percent said low testosterone had a somewhat or very negative impact on the sexual aspect of their lives, and 90 percent said it adversely affected their self-esteem.

"Low testosterone levels may have a marked impact on a man's sense of well-being," said Raymond Rosen, Ph.D., chief scientist of the New England Research Institutes in Watertown, Massachusetts. Among men polled, 61 percent said they were generally unsatisfied with their lives before being treated.

Low testosterone is associated with a broad range of physical, psychological, and sexual symptoms, including decreased energy and mood, fatigue, loss of muscle mass, depressed libido, and erectile dysfunction. In addition, low testosterone has been associated with other serious medical conditions, including diabetes, cardiovascular disease, and metabolic syndrome.

for disease risk, typically those with the lowest levels of testosterone also have lower markers for vitality, mental and physical vigor."

It's not an accident that there's a booming business these days in male hormone replacement therapy. Testosterone makes you feel good. It also makes it easier to gain muscle and lose body fat. People on testosterone replacement therapy commonly report feeling more youthful and more energized. And that's not all. "Testosterone replacement is strongly associated with improvement in mood," says Leonardi.

It also improves libido, for both men and women (which is why responsible, smart hormone-replacement docs who treat the "whole person" are now routinely including very small, physiologic amounts of testosterone in the hormone-replacement programs of their female clients).

Go on the Internet and look up "testosterone replacement" and you'll find hundreds, maybe thousands, of ads and claims for designer nutrient formulas and herbs (especially the herb *Tribulus terrestris*, which is frequently touted as "natural testosterone") that promise to raise testosterone levels naturally and provide the well-documented benefits of bringing testosterone back up to youthful levels. Don't believe them. In fact, read my lips: *None of them work*. Sorry.

"I have never seen one shred of valid data that any over-the-counter substance can raise testosterone," says Beth Traynor, M.D., an advocate of testosterone replacement and a physician at Cenegenics Medical Institute, a top anti-aging clinic in Henderson, Nevada.

You can only raise testosterone one way—with testosterone replacement therapy.

My personal opinion is that testosterone therapy is an effective anti-aging treatment that can significantly improve well-being, energy, and mood as well as body composition and libido.

It's also my strong opinion that if you're going to do this, you should consult with a highly knowledgeable doctor who knows what he or she is doing, knows what to measure, knows just how much to give you, and also monitors the levels of your hormones carefully.* (This goes for *all* hormone replacement programs, not just for testosterone replacement.)

Four examples of the doctors and clinics I'm talking about are listed in the resource section at the end of this book. If you don't happen to live in the cities in which they practice, it might be worth traveling to see them for an initial consultation. All of them have patients from around the country, and often all that's needed is an initial (or yearly) in-person visit. Lab tests can be done in your own town, and follow-ups are frequently done by phone.

The Estrogen Controversy

Years ago I attended a daylong seminar by the famous nutrition educator (and biochemist) Jeffrey Bland, Ph.D., who has taught health practitioners about nutrition for twenty-five years. The title of the event was "Female Endocrinology," and we were there to learn about the subject of women's hormones.

Bland started the day with the following statement: "Well, we're here to talk about female hormones, and we only have eight hours, so it's important that we get started because there's an awful lot to cover." Pause for effect. Then, deadpan, "If we were going to be talking about male hormones, we'd be out of here in forty-five minutes."

Female hormones are, to put it mildly, a complicated subject. But, like all hormones, they play a major part in the aging process and can dramatically affect a number of parameters (from the bones to the heart to the brain).

Take menopause, for example. Menopause is the permanent cessation of the female reproductive cycle. Technically, menopause is the date, fixed retrospectively, from which twelve months have passed when a woman experiences no menstrual periods, but in common usage

---

* Most doctors who specialize in this kind of work are members of the American Academy of Anti-Aging Medicine (www.worldhealth.net, 888.997.0112).

menopause is used to refer to the whole of the transition period (which can take a few years) from regular monthly cycles to the complete cessation of monthly periods. (When I was growing up, it used to be quaintly called "the change of life.")

A full discussion of menopause, with all its psychological, physical, and social ramifications, is several light years beyond the scope of this book, and it has been written about extensively (and sometimes brilliantly) from a number of different points of view. What I want to concentrate on here is the hormonal component and its implications for aging well.

"Up until 2002, it was absolutely routine that hormone replacement was *the* answer to menopause," said Traynor. "Every woman who became menopausal was put on HRT (*hormone replacement therapy*). Doctors believed it protected bone density, protected the heart, even protected against Alzheimer's."

So what happened in 2002?

Well, to answer that question you have to go back to the fall of 1997, when a landmark study called the Women's Health Initiative began. That study, known as the WHI, looked at more than 16,000 healthy, postmenopausal American women between the ages of fifty and seventy-nine. The purpose of the study was to evaluate the use of HRT by healthy women for the prevention of disease—to study the effect of HRT on all those things doctors believed it was good for, including the bones, heart, and brain. The study was scheduled to be completed eight years later in 2005.

It was stopped in 2002.

Yes, researchers stopped the study because apparently the hormone replacement therapy under investigation increased a woman's risk of breast cancer as well as heart disease, blood clots, and strokes. The media had a feeding frenzy, reduced a complicated issue to a few dramatic (and frightening) sound bites about hormones causing cancer, and thousands of women immediately ceased their use of hormone replacement therapy.

Okay, now listen up. The truth of what researchers found in that study, and who specifically those results apply to, is far more complicated.

As time went on and the data was picked apart, it became apparent that the effects of these replacement hormones differed greatly depending on whether you were an older woman who was long done with menopause or a younger woman just beginning menopause. To this day, opinion remains divided over how to balance the benefits of a few years of hormone replacement with the possible risks, though it seems to be accepted that the risks vary depending on the age of the woman, her health history, other lifestyle issues, and countless other variables.

If I tried to summarize all the data on hormone replacement, brain health, well-being, depression, heart health, and bone health, we'd be here all day, probably all month. (If you're interested, *The Hormone Decision* by Tara Parker-Pope is a great place to start.) But I do want to make two important points about female hormones and aging. The first has to do with the issue of "bioidenticals" and the second has to do with the method of delivery.

Let me explain.

Chemical versus Natural Estrogen

There has been much debate over "natural" or *bioidentical* hormones. The Women's Health Initiative, along with all the other major studies on hormone replacement, used pharmaceutical drugs that conventional doctors believe act the same as the hormones the body makes. (These drugs were also taken orally, an important point about which more later on.) The most common of these drugs are Premarin and Provera, both of which are made by Wyeth, which funded the WHI in the first place. (The actual drug used in the WHI was Prempro by Wyeth, a combo drug that consists of both Premarin and Provera in one capsule.)

"Premarin contains hormones that belong in a horse," scoffs Traynor. "It's not natural in the human body." Proponents of bioidentical hormones argue that it's highly unlikely that they would produce the increased risks to women seen with Premarin and Provera (Prempro). Of course, we don't know this for a fact, but it sure does pass the smell test. Virtually every doctor I talked with who deals responsibly with hormone replacement therapy and aging uses only bioidentical hormones and wouldn't be caught dead writing Premarin on their prescription pad.

The debate over whether bioidenticals are safer or different than the pharmaceutical drugs derived from the urine of horses will continue, but it may turn out that those on both sides of the debate are neglecting one important point. In fact, this point is so important that I continue to

be amazed that it has not taken center stage in the debate. What is this critical point?

Simple. The method of delivery.

When your conventional doctor gives you a prescription for hormone replacement drugs like Prempro, Premarin, or Provera, these drugs come in the form of pills that, of course, you swallow. When your integrative, anti-aging doc gives you a prescription for a bioidentical hormone made by a compounding pharmacy, it comes in the form of a cream or a patch that you put on your skin. This method of delivery (called *transdermal*, meaning "through the skin") may make all the difference in the world.

When you swallow an estrogen pill, the entire dose hits the liver. "Everything from the intestines goes from the portal vein to the liver before it goes anywhere else," explains Leonardi. "It's been shown that when you flood the liver with estrogen, you increase the production of clotting protein." Indeed, five of the six problems that occurred in the WHI—heart attack, stroke, blood clots in legs, blood clots in lungs, and dementia—are directly or indirectly related to blood clots.

To make matters worse, oral estrogens may interfere with thyroid function by increasing chemicals (thyroid-binding globulin) that make thyroid hormone less available. "And oral estrogens are pro-inflammatory," says Traynor.

So even if you were to grant the questionable argument that synthetic hormones are the same as bioidentical ones, you can't disregard the fact that oral hormones have a different effect than transdermal hormones do. "When you take estrogen through the skin, it's disseminated equally over the body, just as if the body made it. The liver doesn't get an 'extra' share," says Leonardi.

Adds Traynor, "Transdermal forms of hormones bypass many of the issues we're worried about with hormone replacement."

The "method of delivery" issue hasn't escaped the attention of researchers. In 2007, an important study from France, where transdermal estrogen is far more common than in the United States, compared patients on oral estrogen with patients on transdermal estrogen. The study found that oral estrogen therapy was associated with a fourfold increase in the risk of conditions associated with clotting (including pulmonary embolism) while transdermal estrogen presented no increased risks. The study also found that the type of progesterone used by women taking combination estrogen-progestin hormone therapy made a significant difference as well. [4]

In my view, if you're a candidate for hormone replacement therapy, transdermal hormones are the way to go, be they bioidentical or synthetic. (Even Premarin, the most common synthetic hormone drug for women, is now available in a transdermal form.) "It's conceivable that synthetic hormones applied through the skin might avoid some of the problems with synthetics that have been seen in the studies," admitted Leonardi. But that being said, the question remains whether taking hormones at all is necessary for successful, optimal, youthful aging.

On that all-important question, there continues to be passionate debate. "Women in my practice constantly tell me that they just feel better on hormones," Leonardi told me, a comment echoed by virtually all of the hormone docs I interviewed (see resources). "It's a quality of life issue." But others are more cautious. "When you look at centenarians in the so-called 'blue zones' you see that their longevity is all about the food they eat, the nontoxic environment they live in, their daily activities like gardening, their daily time in the sun, and their relationships with others," points out my friend Susanne Bennett, D.C., president of Wellness for Life in Santa Monica, California. Bennett advocates nutritional supplements and dietary changes rather than hormones of any kind.[*]

"We know that hormones are not a fountain of youth, nor are they as risky as they have been portrayed," writes Parker-Pope in *The Hormone Decision*. "Hormones are not good for all women, nor are they bad for all women. The question is whether they are right or wrong for *you*."

In fact, according to Parker-Pope, analysis of data from both the Nurses Health Study and the WHI found that the right lifestyle choices could have such a profound effect on health and aging that they dwarfed any protective (anti-aging) effects of hormone replacement. "The benefits of a healthy lifestyle were so powerful that they literally erased any impact of menopausal hormones," she writes. "This means that the health gains of exercise and healthful eating far exceed any potential benefit or any potential risk of hormone use."

As of this writing, we are far from knowing all the answers to balancing the risks and benefits of hormone replacement therapy for women. The best we can say for now is that the benefits and risks of estrogen (or combo estrogen/progesterone) therapy probably depend on the age of the patient, the route of administration, and individual factors best evaluated with your health professional.

It's worth pointing out, as Bennett did, that some of the longest-lived and healthiest societies in the world have

[*] Bennett will occasionally use DHEA in certain cases; see page 222.

never even heard of hormone replacement, and wouldn't even know how to pronounce Premarin, let alone what to do with it. That does not mean that hormone replacement can't improve mood and well-being and help you feel better, especially if used for a few years early in menopause. But it does mean that HRT isn't the end-all and be-all of an anti-aging strategy. At this point, the best advice seems to be to be a variation on the tired old mandate to "talk to your doctor," though I'd add that you'll want to do some due diligence in finding a specialist who's really familiar with all the issues.[*]

THE PROS AND CONS OF USING HUMAN GROWTH HORMONE

HGH, or *human growth hormone,* is (pardon the pun) a growth industry.

Although growth hormone was around for a long time as a treatment for kids whose growth was abnormally stunted, it achieved quite a bit of media attention after *The New England Journal of Medicine* published a study in 1990 that attracted mainstream media attention.

The study looked at healthy men, aged sixty-one to eighty-one, who had IGF-1 levels below those found in normal young men. (*IGF-1* is a hormone that is stimulated by growth hormone and believed to be responsible for much of growth hormone's effects. It's much easier to measure IGF-1 in the bloodstream than it is to measure growth hormone itself, so docs use IGF-1 measurements as a surrogate marker for actual growth hormone levels.) The men received growth hormone injections three times a week for six months and were compared with a group of men who received no treatment.

The treatment resulted in a decrease in fat and an increase in lean body (muscle) mass and bone density.

This study eventually gave birth to the industry that is now growth hormone replacement and ranges from highly respected anti-aging doctors doing responsible hormone testing/replacement to every scam artist on the Internet selling pills and potions that promise to "raise growth hormone naturally at a fraction of the cost!" (*Note:* As of this writing, none of them work.)

The whole growth hormone thing is somewhat (okay, a lot) controversial. Proponents swear by it. "Patients tell me they get a substantial boost in energy that's very noticeable," says Leonardi.

But it's expensive, and it requires that you inject yourself several times a week. Most important, the elephant in the growth-hormone room is the fact that anything that makes *good* stuff grow (like muscles) or makes things reproduce (like cells) might also make *bad* stuff do the same thing (like cancer). I don't think for a minute that growth hormone causes cancer, but I *do* think there's a disturbing possibility that if you *already have* a slow-growing cancer it might speed things along. We just don't know.

You can raise growth hormone levels (IGF-1 levels) on your own (although not nearly as much as by using the real thing). It's released during deep sleep, so anything that helps you sleep more deeply and restfully may have an effect (see melatonin, below). And very strenuous exercise will also raise it.

Although my anti-aging doctor friends will disagree with me on this, my personal opinion on growth hormone replacement is that it's a fairly minor weapon in the anti-aging strategy. However, if you're interested, all of the docs

---

[*] I've listed some of the best in the resource section, but you can also check the "Find a FM Practitioner" tab on the website for the Institute for Functional Medicine (www.functionalmedicine.org).

and clinics listed on page 272 provide growth hormone therapy. Just don't waste your money on any of the "natural" replacements.

IT COULD BE YOUR THYROID

Probably no one did more to bring the issue of thyroid problems to the attention of the American public than Oprah Winfrey.

In October 2007, the wildly popular talk show host discussed her bout of exhaustion and weight gain that was ultimately diagnosed as a thyroid condition. She followed up with an article in her magazine, and before you could say "Dr. Phil," thyroid problems went from relative obscurity to the top of the pile on Google searches.

Hypothyroidism, a condition in which your body does not make enough thyroid hormone, is one of the most underdiagnosed diseases of the aging population. Why? One reason is that the symptoms are a bit ambiguous— weight gain, depression, fatigue. Another reason is that the symptoms are frequently written off as simply stress, overeating, menopausal, or a part of "normal" aging. Thyroid disorders are much more common in women (let's not even talk about the number of women who've been told by their doctors that the symptoms are "all in their head"). And finally, for reasons we'll talk about in a minute, the tests that many docs use are not necessarily the best ones; the results can be vague and misleading, especially for a doc who doesn't specialize in this kind of thing.

The third U.S. National Health and Nutrition Examination Survey (NHANES III) of people aged twelve and older reports that nearly 6 percent of the U.S. population has thyroid disease. As the population ages, the proportion of people with thyroid conditions increases.

Vladimir Korenchevsky was one of the first scientists to document similarities between hypothyroidism and aging.[5] His list of similarities shared between aging and low thyroid included:

- Low metabolism
- Low body temperature, (i.e., chilliness, such as cold hands and feet)
- Obesity
- Elevated cholesterol
- Poor skin elasticity with increased wrinkling
- Dry skin
- Constipation
- Brittle nails
- Poor muscle tone
- Arthritis
- Easy fatigability (physical and mental)
- Depression

Korenchevsky died in 1959, but many of his observations were prescient. The thoroughly modern *Textbook for Functional Medicine* lists as typical symptoms of low thyroid function the following: low energy, cold hands and feet, fatigue, elevated cholesterol, muscle pain, depression, and cognitive defects.

You get the idea.

Although Korenchevsky stated that thyroid hormone replacement was no "cure" for aging, he found it highly effective in reversing many of the above-listed aging and thyroid-related signs and symptoms. "Maintaining thyroid hormone function throughout the aging process may be an important hallmark of healthy aging," write Bland and Jones.[6]

ANTI-AGING ACTION PLAN:

Feel Better and Get Your Thyroid Checked!

At the very least, have your doc order a *TSH (thyroid-stimulating hormone)* test. In 2002, the American Association of Clinical Endocrinologists (AACE) changed the recommended values of TSH to 0.3 to 3.0, but many labs (and docs) continue to use the old reference levels of 0.5 to 5.0, meaning thousands of people are walking around with undiagnosed sub-par thyroid function. Most knowledgeable experts now consider a TSH of 1.0 to 2.0 to be optimal. And many knowledgeable docs will not stop with a TSH test, but will also look at total T4, free T3, and total T3.

"Estrogen will make thyroid hormone tests even more unreliable than they are," writes thyroid expert Richard Shames, M.D., which might explain why so many women have thyroid issues. According to a 2001 report in *The Journal of Epidemiology*, as many as 26 percent of menopausal women were hypothyroid, making their menopause years worse.

CROSS YOUR T'S WHEN IT COMES TO THYROID MEDICATION

The normal thyroid secretes way more T4 than T3. But the T4 hormone doesn't do all that much. The T3 is where the action is—it's about four times stronger than T4. This is important.

The popular thyroid medicines (Synthroid, Levothryoxin, Levothroid, Levoxyl) are all pure T4. It used to be thought that simply giving people T4 would correct any thyroid problem because the body converts T4 into the active form T3. But in a substantial number of people, that conversion doesn't take place very well. And, here's something your doc may not know: Converting T4 into T3 depends on the presence of a mineral called *selenium*. If you're not getting enough selenium in your diet (through food or supplements) your body is going to have an even harder time converting that T4 into T3 and you're not going to feel great, even with the standard thyroid meds.

An important study in the *Journal of Clinical Investigation* showed that merely replacing thyroid hormone with the inactive T4 hormone did not ensure normal thyroid activity in all tissues.[7] That was followed by a landmark study in the *New England Journal of Medicine*[8] showing that the vast majority of people felt considerably better, especially in terms of mental functioning, when they were given a combination of T4 and T3 (T3 is commonly known as *Cytomel*). *Armour Thyroid*, which is a more natural thyroid med that contains both T4 and T3, is often used by holistic doctors.

THE IODINE CONNECTION

Thyroid cells are the only cells in the body that can absorb iodine. Thyroid cells combine iodine with an amino acid called tyrosine to make the two major thyroid hormones—T3 and T4. So iodine is critical for thyroid health, but that doesn't necessarily mean you should take iodine supplements. You do absolutely need iodine, of that there is no doubt, but you don't need too much of it.

About 10 percent of men and 20 percent of women are iodine deficient, according to thyroid experts Richard Shames, M.D., and Karilee Shames, Ph.D., R.N., authors of *Thyroid Power*.

"If you are a person who never consumes fast food, avoids salt like the plague, doesn't eat much seafood, and feels that sea vegetables are for fish, and especially if you live more than 100 miles from any coast, then you might well consider supplementation with iodine, the key mineral in thyroid hormone production," say the Shames. "If you are not in this category, you would probably do well to not take extra iodine, as you're likely to be getting more than enough from other sources, such as iodized salt and the natural sources of fish and sea vegetables."[9]

Although I'm a huge fan of the Shames, it's worth noting that there are dissenting views.

One who says "not so fast" is David Brownstein, M.D., author of *Iodine: Why You Need It, Why You Can't Live Without It* and *Overcoming Thyroid Disorders*. In Brownstein's view, iodine levels in American soil have fallen 50 percent over the past fifty years. Iodine deficiency is the most common preventable cause of mental disability in the world, resulting in a huge movement to consume iodized salt.

But with all the public health warnings to reduce salt, it's just possible we may be throwing out the baby with the bathwater, and may be consuming a lot less of one of our most important sources of iodine. (If you eat a ton of seaweed, this doesn't apply to you, but not many people I know do that.)

And there's another potential fly in the ointment. Iodized salt (and even most iodine supplements) contain iodine in the form of *iodide* (I can see your eyes glazing over, but stay with me for a moment). Brownstein hasn't had a lot of success treating patients with iodide alone. Rather, he uses an easily available over-the-counter (or over-the-Internet)

supplement called Iodoral that contains both the iodine and the iodide forms of iodine—he believes the body needs both.

If you want to try iodine supplements, a mixed form like this is probably a good way to go. Another easily available supplement that combines the two forms is Iosol Iodine by TPCS. For those interested in learning more about Brownstein's views on the importance of iodine for a variety of health conditions, his excellent short videos are available on the Vitamin C Foundation's website (www.vitamincfoundation .org/videos).

GET YOUR THYROID LEVELS TESTED

The role of thyroid in aging has not gone unnoticed or unresearched. In 1992, Italian researchers performed a series of studies examining the importance of the thyroid during aging. They looked at thyroid function in thirty-four healthy centenarians, the youngest of whom was one hundred and the oldest of whom was—wait for it—108! They compared the results to tests for thyroid functions in a bunch of "youngsters" aged seventy to eighty-five.

One of the measures the researchers looked at was the presence of thyroid antibodies. See, in some people, the immune system is overly vigilant and will mistake our own tissues for foreign invaders, mounting an attack. (This is usually what happens in autoimmune diseases.) When the body creates antibodies that attack our thyroid, it's a condition known as *Hashimoto's Thyroiditis*—the body actually creates thyroid antibodies (also known as *anti-thyroid antibodies*). It was these antibodies, which ultimately wind up seriously compromising thyroid function, that the researchers tested for.

They found a significantly lower level of thyroid antibodies running around the bodies of the healthy centenarians. In fact, these one-hundred-plus-year-old folks had much lower levels of thyroid antibodies (and presumably a much better performing thyroid) than any of the seventy to eighty-five-year-olds who had varying levels of chronic diseases.[10]

Now granted, not everyone with low thyroid has Hashimoto's. But it's way more common than you might think, and its diagnosis tells us a lot about the misdiagnosis of thyroid problems in general.

Most conventional docs do not test for thyroid antibodies. Instead, they simply use the TSH (*thyroid stimulating hormone*) test, which, while a useful piece of data, does not tell the whole picture on how the thyroid is performing. Indeed, for a period of time, your TSH test may be "normal" while your thyroid is under attack and well on the way to failing.

"If you've tested positive for antibodies, and have a TSH in the 'normal range' but still don't feel well, you may wish to consult with a practitioner who believes that the presence of thyroid antibodies alone is enough to warrant treatment with small amounts of thyroid hormone," advises About.com's highly regarded thyroid expert Mary Shomon, author of *Living Well with Hypothyroidism: What Your Doctor Doesn't Tell You . . . That You Need to Know.*

Elizabeth Vliet, M.D., author of *Screaming to Be Heard: Hormonal Connections Women Suspect . . . and Doctors Still Ignore,* is a doctor who believes exactly that. Here's what she says:

"The problem I have found is that too often women are told their thyroid is normal without having the complete thyroid tests done. Of course, what most people, and many physicians, don't realize is that . . . a 'normal range' on a laboratory report is just that: a range. A given person may require higher or lower levels to feel well and to function optimally. I think we must look at the lab results along with the clinical picture described by the patient . . . I have a series of more than a hundred patients, all but two are women, who had a normal TSH and turned out to have significantly elevated thyroid antibodies that meant they needed thyroid medication in order to feel normal. This type of oversight is particularly common with a type of thyroid disease called thyroiditis, which is about 25 times more common in females than males . . . a woman may experience the symptoms of disease months to years before TSH goes up . . ."[11]

Low thyroid is one of those conditions in which how you actually feel may be as important as the lab test results. (Having all the symptoms of a low thyroid without confirmation from a lab test is often referred to as *subclinical thyroid dysfunction*.) More and more integrative medicine practitioners or holistic health care providers now treat the classic symptoms of low thyroid with thyroid meds regardless of whether the tests come back "normal."

But here's what's even more important: Low thyroid function, even in the absence of an abnormal standard test result, may be a sign that the complicated signaling processes and feedback loops in the endocrine (hormonal) systems are not working properly. In fact, it might even be the first sign you notice. (You will never "notice" high blood pressure, but it's hard to ignore feeling fatigued, cold, constipated, or depressed.) And these imbalances or dysfunctions in the hormone signaling systems in your body just might put you at risk for the conditions of aging.

THE DARK SIDE OF SOY

So why does there seem to be such an epidemic of low thyroid levels these days?

The environment we all live in clearly contributes to aging in a lot of insidious ways, some of which are obvious (stress, pollutants, toxins) and some of which aren't. One of the less obvious ways is in connection to thyroid function.

Exposure to toxic levels of heavy metals can interfere with thyroid function.[12] "Lead and mercury invade the thyroid gland and disrupt the production of thyroid hormones," write Laura Pizzorno, M.A., and William Ferril, M.D., in the *Textbook of Functional Medicine*.[13] Pesticides can interfere with thyroid function, as can weed killers, artificial fertilizers, and who knows what other chemicals we're exposed to on a daily basis.

"Hormone and antibiotic residues in meat and dairy products, foodborne bacteria, chemicals in cleaning products, food additives, cosmetics, and the metabolic byproducts of unfriendly gut bacteria can [interfere with] thyroid hormones," the authors point out. These things can also wreak havoc with liver function, potentially decreasing the conversion of the inactive T4 thyroid hormone into the active T3 hormone, another elegant demonstration of how "everything is related to everything" and how detoxification and a "clean" diet can have multiple beneficial effects on aging.

Another possible reason for thyroid malfunction is the fact that up until recently, practically every woman who became menopausal was put on standard hormone replacement therapy, consisting of synthetic estrogen and progesterone (Premarin and Provera). Why would this matter? "Oral estrogens like Premarin induce thyroid-binding globulin," explains endocrinologist Traynor.

Thyroid-binding globulin grabs up circulating thyroid hormones, making them unavailable for use by the tissues. Wouldn't it be ironic if the very type of hormone replacement therapy that was widely thought to be so protective for women wound up being a cause of thyroid issues for so many women?

Even foods can have a negative effect, including some that you would never suspect. The much ballyhooed health benefits of soy, for example, have come under attack by a vocal minority of holistic health practitioners who point out that soybeans contain *goitrogens*, which suppress thyroid function by interfering with iodine uptake.

"More than seventy years of studies link soy to thyroid disorders," says Kaayla Daniel, Ph.D., C.C.N., author of the book *The Whole Soy Story: The Dark Side of America's Favorite Health Food*. "The myth that soy is a healthy food has had tragic consequences, especially for women in the throes of menopause," Daniel told me, adding that *phytoestrogens* (plant chemicals that have weak estrogenic activity) found in soy products inhibit enzymes needed to produce essential thyroid hormones.

Daniel is one of a growing number of leading scientists, physicians, and toxicologists who have raised alarms about consumption of soy products high in phytoestrogens causing significant endocrine disruption and thyroid damage. "Women in midlife are already at risk for developing thyroid problems," she says. "To make matters worse, the soy industry heavily markets soymilk and other soy products to women who are menopausal as an effective and safe method of hormone replacement therapy. The truth is that it is neither effective nor safe."

Although this view remains controversial, there's pretty universal agreement, even among the "soy-hating" set, that authentic *fermented* soy products are not the problem. Tempeh, miso, and real fermented soy sauce are quite different than the hundreds of soy-based products flooding the marketplace. Fermented soy products are the kind of soy that Asians eat, and they're also the kind of soy foods eaten by some of the long-lived societies studied throughout the world. What those folks don't stock up on is soy chips, soy ice cream, soy milk, soybean oil, and other pretenders that line the shelves of the typical Western supermarket.

The United Kingdom's Committee on Toxicity of Chemicals in Food, Consumer Products and the Environment has identified several populations at special risk for soy-induced thyroid disease: infants on soy formula, vegans who use soy as their principle meat and dairy replacement, and men and women who use isoflavone supplements to prevent or protect against cancer. And even if a certain minimum amount of soy in the diet weren't the worst thing in the world, even the "pro-soy" set no longer recommends supplementation with concentrated soy isoflavones, though these supplements remain popular and are sold everywhere. Don't take them.

Goitrogens are even found in the royalty of the vegetable kingdom— the brassica family (cabbage, broccoli, brussels sprouts). "However, few adults and even fewer children eat these foods in excess," points out Daniel. Light cooking will neutralize most of the goitrogens in these valuable vegetables. Boiling cruciferous vegetables also reduces the goitrogens, but you'll lose a ton of important nutrients. "Patients for whom goitrogens may be problematic can be advised to briefly steam these vegetables and consume them in modest amounts," advise Pizzorno and Ferril.

Don't let the fact that cruciferous vegetables contain goitrogens stop you from eating them. Cruciferous

BRODA BARNES'S BASAL TEMPERATURE TEST FOR THYROID

Broda Barnes was an American doctor who spent his life researching endocrine disorders and specialized in the thyroid. He is widely credited with exposing the inadequacy of most thyroid tests and discovering that undiagnosed hypothyroidism may affect as much as 50 percent of the American population. He also linked hypothyroidism to other diseases of aging, including heart disease, hypertension, and depression.

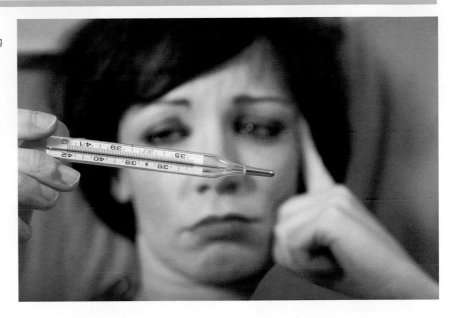

Barnes developed a simple, at-home, low-tech test for thyroid function that many holistic practitioners still use.[14] The test measures basal body temperature, which the thyroid controls, and is an excellent way of assessing how much T3 (the active thyroid hormone) is actually working inside cells. Here's how to do it:

1. Shake down a thermometer to below 95°F (35°C) and place it by the bed before going to sleep.

2. Upon waking, place the thermometer under your armpit for a full ten minutes. Remain as still as possible, resting with your eyes closed.

3. Record the temperature for at least three consecutive mornings, preferably at the same time of day. (It's important that you write it down because many people don't think clearly upon waking and may well forget the reading.)

If you're menstruating, check your temperature on the second, third, and fourth day of menstruation. Men and postmenopausal women can check on any three consecutive days.

The average of the three days is what's known as your early morning basal body temperature, and it should be between 97.8°F and 98.2°F (36.55°C and 36.77°C). If it's lower, there's more than a good chance that you're hypothyroid.

The details of this test were published in the *Journal of the American Medical Association* as well as the prestigious journal *Lancet*.

Although the traditional medical establishment has not widely adopted it, the method continues to have enthusiastic support among many holistic practitioners. Some of the doctors I most respect, including Alan Gaby, M.D., Jonathan Wright, M.D., and Erika Schwartz, M.D., are big supporters. Although Barnes never claimed the test was 100 percent accurate, it is a wonderful, noninvasive, and painless way to get a valuable piece of data.

vegetables also contain powerful plant chemicals that have a positive effect on estrogen metabolism. These plant chemicals, called *indoles*, are considered to be cancer-protective. Just be aware that if you have a thyroid problem, you might want to make sure that you steam them lightly before eating them, thus reducing the amount of thyroid disrupters while preserving the enormous nutritional benefits.

EAT YOUR WAY TO A HEALTHY THYROID

Thyroid is one of the hormones that you can definitely support with the proper diet and supplements. You may not be able to make more testosterone just by eating certain foods, but you will surely not make enough thyroid hormones if you're not providing the nutrients needed for its manufacture. Those nutrients and their best sources include:

- Iodine: Sea vegetables such as nori, arame, wakame, kombu, and kelp; sardines; eggs; haddock; shrimp; clams; oysters; and sardines
- Zinc: Fresh oysters, Brazil nuts, lamb chops, pecans, split peas, almonds, walnuts, and sardines

- Vitamin E: Mainly found in wheat germ oil (or supplements)
- Vitamin A: Liver, red chili peppers, collard greens, turnips, kale, Swiss chard, beet greens, apricots, winter squash, cantaloupe, papaya, and nectarines. The precursors to vitamin A, the things your body makes vitamin A from, are found in yellow and orange/green vegetables as well as some green ones.
- Vitamin B2 (riboflavin): Almonds, wheat germ, wild rice, mushrooms, and egg yolks
- Vitamin B3 (niacin): Bran, peanuts (with skin), and the light meat of turkey and chicken
- Vitamin B6: Sunflower seeds, tuna, liver, walnuts, salmon, trout, lentils, lima beans, navy beans, garbanzo beans, pinto beans, brown rice, and bananas

In addition, the Shames recommend vitamin D (necessary for thyroid hormone production) and essential fatty acids (needed to have your thyroid hormones get to where they need to go), which I've covered extensively in this book.

DHEA: THE MOTHER HORMONE

Throughout this book I've emphasized the interaction between the inner environment (hormones, neurotransmitters, immunity) and the external environment. As I've said before, "Genetics loads the gun, but environment pulls the trigger." Nowhere is this more evident than in the case of stress hormones.

Long-term, unremitting stress results in a loss of the ability of the adrenal glands to put out important stress hormones, a phenomenon that's becoming increasingly well known and is popularly characterized as "adrenal burnout."

The adrenal glands, two little walnut-shaped glands that sit on top of the kidneys, are responsible for secreting the stress hormones cortisol and adrenaline. But that's not all they do. They also produce an important hormone called *DHEA* (*dehydroepiandrosterone*) as well as a related compound called DHEA-S. And DHEA is a hormone that may have important implications for aging.

DHEA is the most prevalent hormone in the human body. And many researchers consider it a "mother hormone" because of the important role it plays in producing other hormones. The body can convert DHEA into testosterone, estrogen, progesterone, and a whole bunch of other hormones collectively called "steroid" hormones (the kind your body makes, not the kind baseball players shoot up with). Although it is considered a "minor" hormone in the scheme of things, low levels of it can result in mood changes, fatigue, and weight gain.

In normal folks, DHEA concentrations are highest around age thirty, after which they gradually decrease. By age seventy or eighty, the values are about 20 percent of peak values in men and 30 percent of peak values in women.[15]

But folks with a condition known as *adrenal insufficiency* don't produce enough of the important adrenal hormones. Studies of people with this condition provide some of the strongest evidence for a beneficial effect of DHEA replacement.

The most well known of the adrenal insufficiency conditions is Addison's disease, from which President John F. Kennedy famously suffered. When women with adrenal insufficiency received 50 milligrams of DHEA daily, they experienced improved overall well-being, mood, and sexual activity.[16] In another study of fifteen women and twenty-four men with Addison's disease, three months of 50 milligrams a day of DHEA corrected the hormonal deficiency and improved self-esteem, while it also tended to enhance overall well-being, mood, and energy.[17]

So now of course the question is: Will it benefit people without adrenal insufficiency? Although there isn't a definitive answer yet, emerging evidence suggests that it might.

Epidemiological studies suggest an association between decreasing levels of DHEA (and DHEA-S) and the adverse effects of aging. One large observational study

DHEA is the most prevalent hormone in the human body. And many researchers consider it a "mother hormone" because of the important role it plays in producing other hormones.

Adrenal Gland

Cortex

Medulla

Renal Artery

Renal Vein

Ureter

Kidney

showed a small but meaningful relationship between low DHEA levels and the risk of cardiovascular mortality in men.[18] Another study of more than two thousand people (men and women) younger than sixty-five found that both "all-cause" and cardiovascular mortality were highest in men with the lowest levels of DHEA (though there was no significant relationship for women).[19] Other studies have associated low DHEA levels with depressed mood and bone loss in women.[20]

So is low DHEA simply a biomarker of aging, or is it causally related to mortality in the elderly? Hard to say. One research study investigated the effect of giving 50 milligrams of DHEA a day to men and women forty to seventy years old and found that they improved in

measures of both physical and psychological well-being.[21] Another study used 100 milligrams daily (a very large dose) for men and women fifty to sixty-five years of age and found that the men had decreased fat mass and enhanced muscle strength.[22] And in a study of 280 men and women sixty to seventy-nine years old, 50 milligrams of DHEA a day increased the women's libido and sexual function (as well as slightly increased their bone mineral density).[23]

As mentioned above, the adrenals produce both cortisol and DHEA, but here's the thing: The relationship is like that of sharks and dolphins. Where you see a lot of sharks in the water, you won't see Flipper and his crew, and when you see a lot of dolphins, Jaws is nowhere to be found. Cortisol and DHEA have a kind of seesaw relationship; when one is up, the other tends to be down. Unfortunately, in modern life, it's cortisol that's usually elevated and DHEA that's down. An increased cortisol/DHEA ratio seems to be a contributing factor to an aging immune system, according to the *Physician's Desk Reference for Nutritional Supplements*. In general terms, cortisol tends to suppress immunity while DHEA enhances it. DHEA is a powerful immune-system stimulant that can improve your metabolism, energy levels, mood, memory, and sexual function, according to Linda Ojeda, Ph.D., of the Institute for Functional Medicine. Studies show that seniors who maintain a higher level of DHEA do, in fact, experience a longer and healthier life.

DHEA is available over-the-counter and I almost wish it weren't. When all is said, it's still a hormone, and though replacement of some hormones can be a powerful anti-aging strategy, it should still be done under the supervision of health practitioners who know what they are doing. You wouldn't fill up the gas tank in your car with a set amount of gas; you'd let the amount you put in be determined by how full (or empty) the tank was in the first place. So why would you replace hormones in your body without measuring them first, so you can know how much you need?

"It's very important to precede the administration of DHEA with salivary or serum tests for DHEA and DHEA-S, as well as testosterone and estradiol," write Bland and Jones. "A baseline hormone analysis is critical to establish the overall influence of DHEA on [hormone] balance." Most anti-aging docs use DHEA regularly as part of an overall anti-aging strategy that involves monitoring various hormones and replacing as needed to levels that make sense. Anything else is throwing darts at a dartboard blindfolded.

Because DHEA is a slight mood elevator, it could potentially—I repeat, potentially—clash with antidepressants, according to Michael Lam, M.D., M.P.H. Theoretically, the dose of antidepressants might be lowered if you took DHEA, but check with your health care practitioner.

Worth noting: In a laboratory, test-tube situation, DHEA can be synthesized from substances in wild yams, which has led to a persistent myth that if you buy an over-the-counter product made from wild yams, the body will naturally convert this into DHEA. Most health food store clerks will tell you that. This is precisely why you should not get your nutrition information from health food store clerks. Your body can't synthesize DHEA from natural wild yams. Save your money, and if you decide DHEA is worth a try, go to an anti-aging doc and get the real thing. Getting a hormone panel done by a doctor versed in anti-aging medicine (see page 272) makes a lot of sense, and it's likely that DHEA will be on the list of hormones the doc recommends. The evidence is pretty strong that DHEA can help, and it appears to elicit few short-term side effects when used in the recommended doses.

MELATONIN: BUSTING THE AGE-ROBBERS

A few years ago I wrote about the many benefits of melatonin in my book, *The Most Effective Natural Cures on Earth*. But I also wrote the following sentence: "Though claims have been made for melatonin as an anti-aging supplement, those claims are bogus."

Okay, maybe that's technically true. It's not a magic bullet, but the real role of melatonin and longevity may be a bit more nuanced than I implied.

Melatonin is a potent antioxidant and may therefore help protect the brain against one of the Four Horsemen of Aging: oxidative damage. It protects cell membranes even more than vitamin E does, and is more effective than glutathione (an important antioxidant in the body) at neutralizing a deadly free radical that causes oxidative damage, *hydroxyl radicals.* Melatonin also supports immune function in a number of ways, and may even play a role in protecting against cancer. (One reason scientists believe that blind women have significantly less breast cancer risk is because blind women, with their reduced exposure to light, presumably make a greater amount of melatonin.) So although melatonin is not by itself a miracle anti-aging supplement, it helps protect against a number of age-robbers.

Take sleep, for example. During sleep, a great deal of cellular damage that occurs during the day is repaired, and that repair process is initiated by secretions of melatonin.[24] And because disturbed sleep so often accompanies aging, anything that can help us sleep better (with ancillary benefits to boot and no side effects) might be something to take note of. Melatonin definitely fits the bill.

Poor sleep quality reduces the growth hormone, an important (though minor) hormone that helps us keep muscle and lose fat. It may also raise levels of stress hormones such as cortisol. "This may argue strongly for sleep therapy and/or melatonin being of primary importance in the management of some symptoms associated with . . . aging," write Bland and Jones.

And because melatonin plays an important role in setting our "biological clock," it influences metabolism. Just as this was being written, researchers at the University of California, Irvine discovered that proteins involved with circadian rhythms and metabolism are in fact intrinsically linked with and dependent upon each other.[25] "Our circadian rhythms and metabolism are closely partnered to ensure that cells function properly and remain healthy," said researcher Paolo Sassone-Corsi, distinguished professor and chair of pharmacology.[26]

Circadian rhythms are twenty-four-hour cycles that govern fundamental processes in the body. They operate like an inner clock, respond to light and darkness, and anticipate environmental changes. When these rhythms are disturbed, serious health consequences can result. In fact, disruption of these internal rhythms has been linked to diabetes, depression, heart disease, and cancer.

According to Sassone-Corsi, when the balance between circadian rhythms and metabolism is upset it can ultimately lead to illness and disease. Lack of rest or disruption of normal sleep patterns can increase hunger, leading to obesity-related illnesses and accelerated aging. Because melatonin is so helpful in getting a good night's sleep, the use of melatonin as a supplement may have far-reaching consequences for many of the conditions that interfere with healthy aging.

And if all of this weren't enough, melatonin may also be good for the heart. Researchers tested melatonin supplements on women aged forty-seven to sixty-three and found that supplementation improved the "day-night" rhythm of blood pressure, significantly decreasing nighttime blood pressure.[27] "Melatonin, in addition to being an incredibly powerful antioxidant, may well turn out to be cardio-protective," says Traynor.

Melatonin is available over-the-counter. You might think after all I said that I wouldn't be hugely happy about its over-the-counter status.

Actually, I think it's fine and here's why: Melatonin is a hugely important hormone with many overlapping benefits. Virtually everyone over the age of forty doesn't make enough, and taking extra doesn't seem to have any negative side effects. So I'm comfortable with people trying it on their own.

Melatonin has been used successfully as a supplement for sleep in doses from as low as 0.1 milligram to as much as 10 milligrams (which, if you're curious, is what I take nightly).

The Secrets of Emotional Intelligence:
Underrated and Ignored—Until Now

· ·

I want to start by telling a little story about fish.* Two young fish are swimming along and they happen upon an older fish swimming the other way. The older fish nods hello and says, "Morning boys, how's the water?" The two young fish keep swimming on for a bit, and eventually one of them turns to the other and says, "What the hell is water?"

To some extent, every one of us is like those young fish, swimming in a milieu, inside a perspective that we take so for granted we can't actually reflect upon it. In popular parlance, it's where we're coming from. It's our way of being, and it's so much a part of us that we don't even notice it. Our "water" is our personal perspective—it's the self-evident fact that we see everything through the view of "me."

* This story comes from the writer David Foster Wallace's 2005 commencement address at Kenyon College in Ohio. If you haven't read this legendary gem, I highly recommend it; simply Google "David Foster Wallace commencement speech." *The Wall Street Journal* published an excellent adaptation on September 19, 2008, which you can find online as well.

nd when you think about it, how could we not? Every single thing that happens to you is experienced through the filter of your own brain, eyes, experience, and history. From the news you watch on television to the color of a flower you notice in a garden to the relationships that form the fabric of your life, all are filtered through your eyes and your experience of them. When we begin to look beyond that view, then we begin to see (and hopefully appreciate) how others view things. And that ability is a cornerstone of anti-aging.

If you have kids, you have a living, breathing laboratory to observe how this works. One of the stages of infant development is when babies begin to realize that there's another person in the room. Slowly, over time, they begin to anticipate another person's perspective. When that perspective expands, you can actually see how others might see something, what it's like to live in their shoes, what it's like to see things from their perspective. We call that being well adjusted. You've adjusted your natural, personal "me" perspective to one that incorporates other people and other things.

The fish story is a good starting point for what I want to talk about in this section of the book, and the term I've chosen to use for what I'm going to talk about is *emotional intelligence*. Emotional intelligence is what happens when you adjust and expand that "me" perspective—when you're able to take on another person's perspective and, ultimately, the community's perspective. With that achievement comes empathy, sympathy, altruism, the reduction of stress, and a kind of wisdom that in many ways is far more important than IQ. That "adjustment and expansion," or emotional intelligence, is the key (perhaps the most important key) to aging well and living long.

Now that might seem like a radical concept. But consider this: The longest-lived societies in the world (and we're going to talk about a few of those) don't take supplements. They don't have "designer genes." They're not the beneficiaries of stem cell treatments. They don't have *nanobots* (microscopic electronic devices envisioned by the pioneers of anti-aging medicine) circulating in their bloodstream. They don't go to the gym. Yet in many of these societies it's not uncommon to see ninety-four-year-olds out tilling the fields, or shepherds in their late eighties climbing mountains with their sheep, or people in their late nineties milking cows before dawn.

How do they do it?

ANOTHER KIND OF STRENGTH

One thing every one of them has is this ambiguous, hard-to-define, amorphous set of qualities that, for want of a better term, I call emotional intelligence. For the purpose of this book, I'm defining emotional intelligence as everything

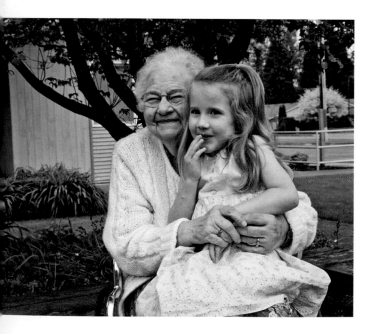

that comes under the heading of relationships, community, and contribution. That includes relationships with self (being at peace, contented, and satisfied) and relationships with others. In fact, a fast definition of emotional intelligence is the ability to deal with people effectively from a place of integrity and self-awareness.

We can trace the most distant roots of the whole concept of emotional intelligence to Darwin, who discovered that there was an evolutionary purpose in having a developed emotional intelligence, even though he didn't call it that. Why? Because you needed to be able to read cues from other people to survive. You needed to know right away: Is this guy friendly? Is he dangerous? Is this wildebeest staring me down on the African Serengeti wanting to be petted, or is he about to make me lunch? Life-and-death decisions hinged on the ability to read others' signals. Am I food for this creature, or is he food for me? Is this tribesman friend or foe? This kind of intelligence is not the sort that lets you win a chess game or perform brain surgery, but it's an intelligence that's necessary for survival, and as we'll see, it's vital for living well and living long.

Around the 1920s, a psychologist named E. L. Thorndike started to use the term *social intelligence* to describe the skill of understanding and managing other people. Decades later, in 1983, a psychologist named Howard Gardner put forth a theory of multiple intelligences. He defined interpersonal intelligence as the capacity to understand the intentions and motivations of other people, whereas intrapersonal intelligence was the capacity to understand ourselves; it was the ability to look inward and appreciate our own feelings, fears, and motivations.

In 1990, psychologists Peter Salovey and John Mayer published their landmark article "Emotional Intelligence" in the journal *Imagination, Cognition and Personality*. They basically defined the term as a part of social intelligence that involves "the ability to monitor one's own and others' feelings and emotions," and to discriminate among them and use this information as a guide to our own feelings and actions. Emotional intelligence involves the perception of emotion, the ability to reason using emotions, the ability to understand emotion, and the ability to manage emotion, according to Salovey and Mayer. (The term *emotional intelligence* burst through into the popular consciousness with the 1995 release of psychologist and *New York Times* science writer Daniel Goleman's seminal book, *Emotional Intelligence: Why It Matters More Than IQ*, which currently has more than five million copies in print worldwide in thirty languages!)

What's important to remember is that despite differences in approach, all of the writers on emotional intelligence talk about the same thing: how you relate; how you adapt; how you handle your own feelings; and how you manage your relationships with others, the wider community, and in fact, the whole planet.

THE FABRIC OF LIFE

Remember those long-lived societies? These are the healthy civilizations that we keep going back to in order to get the secrets of a long and healthy life. These folks have never heard of this peculiarly academic and Western concept of emotional intelligence. If we went and asked them about this they'd look at us like we were crazy. Emotional intelligence is just something that they live with.

They don't have a word for it, or books about it, or even a definition of it. It's part of their lives—like exercise, healthy food, and sleep—there for us to observe (and hopefully emulate, or at least adapt to our own circumstances).

If you asked them about emotional intelligence, they'd respond just like those two young fish: "What the heck is emotional intelligence?" It's so much a fabric of their lives that to question or label it would be like asking a fish about water or a person about air.

So if you look at every one of the longest-lived and healthiest people on the planet, what would you see? What patterns would emerge from their daily activities? What could you say about their relationships to themselves, each other, and their community?

As it turns out, quite a lot.

First and foremost, every one of them has firm family and community connections. Every single study of healthy centenarians shows that the number one thing about them is that they're connected. There is no such thing as a healthy one-hundred-year-old who is isolated. Scientists would be happy to study any such person or people, but the problem is they just don't exist. There are people who defy every other "rule" of long living; those who, for whatever strange reason, are able to smoke, not exercise, take lousy care of their bodies, and somehow, by some miracle of the genetic lottery, live long and seem to be healthy.

But there's not a single person on the planet who has been able to do that in isolation, sans connections to family, community, social group, religious institution, or some other entity that gives their life meaning and purpose.

Not one.

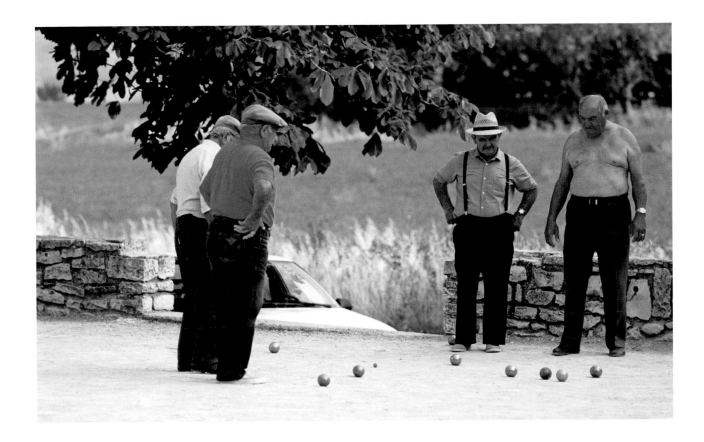

THE ROSETO EFFECT

To give you an idea of the true power of community and connectedness, you need to look no further than Roseto, a close-knit little town of Italian immigrants in Pennsylvania.

The study of the Roseto Effect began quite by accident in the 1960s. A local doctor was having a couple of beers with the head of medicine at the University of Oklahoma and casually mentioned something he'd noticed: that heart disease in Roseto seemed to be far less prevalent than in the adjoining towns. Word of this spread among the doctor rumor mill and eventually captured the attention of some scientists, who began to seriously study cardiac mortality in Roseto. And what they found was astonishing.

It's well known that the frequency of death from heart disease rises with age, but in Roseto, the rate of death from heart disease was near zero for men aged fifty-five to sixty-four. And for men over sixty-five, the rate of death from heart disease was about half of the national average.[1] Scientists quickly began poking around, extensively interviewing the Rosetans, but this simply deepened the mystery. All the data ruled out any genetic or physical cause of the apparent resistance to heart disease among the people of Roseto.

To make matters worse, or shall we say, more maddening to the conventional medical thinkers, these people had the worst lifestyle imaginable. They smoked like chimneys. They drank. They spent their days in what has been described as "backbreaking, hazardous labor," working underground in the slate mines. Their traditional Italian food was modified and Americanized in a way that would drive a dietitian nuts. Not able to afford the traditional olive oil, for example, they simply fried everything in lard.

So why weren't they dropping like flies from heart disease?

Subsequent research uncovered some very interesting facts. Number one, nearly all the houses in Roseto contained three—count 'em, three—generations of the family. Rosetans didn't put their elderly out to pasture; they incorporated them into community life, treating them as the wise village elders. Those enormous lard-ridden dinner tables offered nourishment and nurturing for the human spirit. The villagers took evening strolls, belonged to numerous social clubs, and participated in church festivals in which the whole community was engaged. And, by the way, both the crime rate in Roseto and the applications for public assistance were zero.

The Roseto Effect seemed to be caused by something that escaped traditional investigations.

In their book, *The Power of Clan*, Stewart Wolf, M.D., and sociologist John Bruhn speak about the phenomena seen in Roseto (and elsewhere). They talk of the mutual respect and cooperation that contribute to the health and welfare of a community and also note that lack of concern for others and self-indulgence in general seem to exert the exact opposite influence.

"People are nourished by other people," says Wolf, adding that the characteristics of tight-knit communities predict heart health better than cholesterol or even tobacco use. According to Wolf, an isolated and unconnected person is far more likely to be overwhelmed by the problems of everyday life than someone who is connected in the way the Rosetans are connected. Being overwhelmed then turns into stress, which, as we've seen in this book, is arguably the most destructive of the Four Horsemen of Aging.

"We looked at the social structure of healthy communities," Wolf said, "and found that they are characterized by stability and predictability. In those communities, each person has a clearly defined role in the social scheme."[2]

Now there are things about life in Roseto in the 1960s that most people reading this book might find suffocating. It was a town based on predictability and conformity (characteristics it seemed to share with many of the modern long-lived societies like those in Okinawa, Sardinia, and Loma Linda, California). Display of wealth was taboo. People knew from early on what they would be doing. If you were a boy and your father worked in the mine, so would you, and if you were a girl and your mother worked in one of the small blouse factories found in the village, that was likely to be where you'd wind up as well.

Even meals were somewhat ritualized. "Monday," recalled sixty-six-year-old Angie Martocci, "almost everyone in town ate *spezzati* (a spinach and egg soup). Tuesdays, it was spaghetti and gravy (tomato sauce). Wednesday was roast chicken and potatoes. Thursday, spaghetti again. Fish on Fridays, of course. Veal and peppers on Saturday; and antipasto, meatballs, and spaghetti on Sunday."

And always, there was the work ethic. Virtually everyone worked, and they worked toward the shared communal goal of creating a better life for their children. This work ethic and shared goal was part of the fabric of Roseto life, virtually from the town's beginnings. The very first priest in Roseto, Father Pasquale de Nisco, who arrived in 1896, took up a pick and shovel and started breaking ground next to the church to build a graveyard.

TOO MUCH TO CHOOSE FROM

The absence of choice and the emphasis on conformity and the social order is anathema to today's generation, where choices are limitless (and overwhelming) and attention is limited. (It's interesting that until recently, such emphasis on conformity and community was deeply embedded in Japanese life, where people smoke like chimneys and live longer than we do!) But that enormous buffet of choices that we enjoy, in everything from jeans to colleges to mates, comes with a price.

There's a great deal of stress involved in choosing among hundreds of options, a phenomena that has been noted time and again, notably in Barry Schwartz's brilliant book, *The Paradox of Choice: Why More Is Less.*[*] And although none of us would probably be willing to go back to a time when everything was static and predictable, it's worth considering some of the positive aspects of communities where regularity and predictability are the norm, and seeing whether we can adapt some of those good things to a more modern life. Especially because whatever those folks are doing seems to be life-extending.

First let me give you the executive summary on the above-mentioned good things (and then we'll get into the details). Every long-lived society on earth has several things in common: sleep, friends, community, exercise, and a diet absent of processed foods.

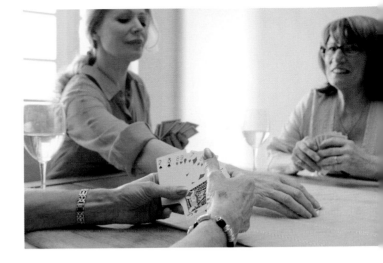

Sure, their career and lifestyle choices might be limited. They might not be able to access the Internet, or buy any of the two hundred styles of jeans available in any mall. They might not have Facebook and MySpace, or endless channels of digital cable. In fact, life in these places might even seem downright boring compared to what we're used to in modern Western societies. But let's face it—we're not doing so great when it comes to living long and well, and they are. Maybe we can dig a little deeper to find out exactly what works so well for these people and then find a way to graft some of our modern amenities onto those basics that seem to produce such robust health for people in several hidden corners of the globe. Maybe there's a way to have our organic whole grain cake—and eat it, too. (Hopefully, you'll agree after finishing this book.)

GREEK PARADISE

One of those places where people live longer, healthier lives is the Greek island of Ikaria. Ikaria is the ultimate

---

[*] You can watch the twenty-minute video of Schwartz's entertaining presentation on choice all over the Internet, notably on the www.TED.com site or on YouTube. Or you can Google "Schwartz video paradox of choice." Highly recommended!

Mediterranean paradise. It's ninety-nine square miles of mountainous terrain, filled with gorgeous green valleys and eye-popping beaches. (The more I read about Ikaria while researching this book, the harder it was to resist booking a vacation there immediately!) The people of Ikaria routinely live into their nineties and beyond. In fact, they reach the age of ninety at four times the rate that we do in the United States! More important, they have far fewer years of disease and poor health (remember "rectangularizing the curve"?). As Anderson Cooper put it on his CNN special on Ikaria, "I'm guessing [that] living on a Greek island doesn't exactly lead to depression, but for those of us who can't pack up and move to a Mediterranean paradise, we can reap the benefits of Ikarian culture at home."

My sentiments exactly.

One person who knows firsthand what it looks like to "transport" the best of Ikarian culture to America is chef and author Diane Kochilas. Kochilas's Ikarian mom (and aunt on her dad's side) lived to age ninety-five, and her husband's paternal Ikarian grandmother lived to age ninety-eight! Diane herself grew up in an Ikarian home in Queens, New York. Here's how she describes growing up:

"We always had a stream of guests dropping in and our kitchen table was always ready to accommodate them. The foods were usually simple: a salad, boiled greens (picked in the New York of the 1960s during countless Sunday outings to Long Island), some cheese, bread, olives, some bean dish or other that was my father's specialty. Maybe a savory pie filled with more greens, usually spinach. Olive oil was part of every dish, even many of the sweets we ate, even then, before the Mediterranean Diet was discovered. But most of all, it was the conviviality of it all I remember, the open hospitality, the de rigueur offering of food and wine to anyone who came through our door."

We've covered foods for longevity elsewhere in this book, so let's concentrate on those other aspects of how Ikarians live. As we'll see, the lifestyle of the Ikarians has a lot in common with the lifestyle of the other longest-lived peoples in the world. And that isn't an accident.

Take, for example, Okinawa.

This little Pacific archipelago is about a thousand miles from Tokyo and has been described by explorer and researcher Dan Buettner as a "Japanese Hawaii" with a "warm, temperate climate, palm trees, and sugar-sand beaches hemming a turquoise sea."[4] Okinawans have one of the highest life expectancies on the planet and one of highest centenarian rates (about 5 per 10,000 people). Compared to the United States, they have one-fifth the rate of cardiovascular disease, one-fourth the rate of breast and prostate cancer, and one-third of the rate of dementia.

One Okinawa senior, Fumiyasu Yamakawa, cycles to the beach every morning at 4:30, swims for a half hour, runs for a half hour, does yoga, and then meets with a group of other seniors. They stand in a circle and laugh.

"Why is that?" asked Buettner.

"It's vitamin S," replied Yamakawa. "You smile in the morning and it fortifies you all day."

No kidding.

There's something in Okinawan life called a *moai*, which, according to Buettner, means "meeting for a common purpose." It could be a group of lifelong friends or it could be a social support network. Doesn't matter. It's the fabric of social connection that's important here, and it appears to be central to Okinawan longevity. It might not be the single cause of long life—after all, Okinawans also

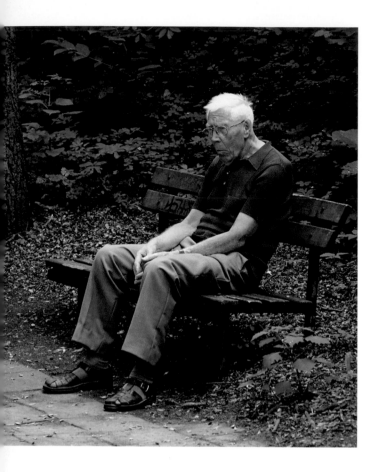

the fourth of Buettner's "Blue Zones," where people live the longest and maintain their health into their ninth and tenth decades, the oldest people live with their families, not by themselves or in assisted living homes. Their children and grandchildren provide support and a sense of belonging and purpose. Their neighbors visit frequently. They find joy in the physical chores of everyday life. "They know how to listen, laugh, and appreciate what they have," says Buettner.

What all these folks have in common is emotional intelligence. It's their "water." It's their way of being. It's what keeps them "young" even when, as so many of them have, they reach the age of one hundred.

If there's any one take-away message that stands out in the studies of all these robust and healthy older people it's this—social connections matter. Social connections are life extending and health promoting. This has been demonstrated in virtually every study of centenarians or of long-lived societies like the ones in Okinawa and Ikaria.

YOU'VE GOT TO HAVE FRIENDS

Closer to home, one of the most famous studies of successful aging is the MacArthur Foundation Study, which is widely believed to be the most comprehensive and extensive study on aging in America. Many of the healthy, long-lived people in the MacArthur Foundation Study report that they thrive because of social bonds with family and friends. Many credit friendship with being the single most important factor in keeping their lives active and emotionally stable.

Geriatrician John Rowe, M.D., of Mount Sinai Medical Center, is the chair of the MacArthur Foundation Research Network on Successful Aging. Here's what he had to say about social connections:

eat in a healthy way and exercise regularly—but it sure is a big part of the secret of living longer and better.

And it's not just the Okinawans. In every area of the globe where people live long, robust lives, social connections are essential. In Sardinia, for example, Buettner tells us that men gather in the street each afternoon to laugh with and at each other. (There aren't too many better ways to reduce stress than that.) The Adventists in Loma Linda, California, are encouraged to volunteer through their church and consistently told Buettner that they found a sense of purpose doing just that, often staving off depression by focusing on helping other people. And in the Nicoya Peninsula off Costa Rica,

THE RIGHT OF KIND OF EMOTIONAL SUPPORT

Nearly all the research on robust aging has found an interesting distinction between emotional support and direct assistance. And the best way to illustrate that distinction is to remind you of when you learned to ride a bike.

Most of us can remember the exact moment when we were able to remove those training wheels and feel the exhilaration of being able to balance on the two-wheeler. I know I do. It was a Sunday night in front of our apartment in Jackson Heights, Queens, New York. I was about eight years old and my father took off the training wheels and began to run alongside the bike, helping to balance it from behind as I pedaled with some uncertainty and wobbliness, slowly picking up speed, until he was finally able to let go as I shrieked, "I can do it!"

That moment of autonomy, which most of us have experienced, at least those of us who learned to ride a two-wheeler, is significant. And it has a lot to teach us about aging well. My father provided emotional support, but he also knew when to let go and let me do it myself. In research on aging, it's been shown time and again that emotional support fosters autonomy and well-being, but the kind of direct assistance (helping someone with a task or doing it for him) is associated with the exact opposite.

"Even if that assistance were given with the best intentions, providing *more assistance than people really need* can reduce their belief in themselves, as well as their ability to function," says geriatrician John Rowe, M.D.. "Giving direct assistance in excess of what people need or perhaps want is a frequent, well-meant, but mistaken form of support" (italics mine).

"The current slogan of 'use it or lose it' applies not only to exercise and athletic ability, but to basic physical and cognitive function as well," says Rowe. Or as Tennyson put it in his classic poem *Ulysses*, "Shine in use!"

People feel best when they're self-sufficient and making a contribution to others, when they're participating in life, and we don't really need a scientific study to prove that (although we have plenty of them). Nothing extends life and well-being like the feeling of competence, and nothing destroys it like a lack of autonomy. Support is one thing; dependence is another.

"We know four important things about the connection between social relations and health, and all apply to older people. First, isolation, a lack of social ties however measured, is a powerful risk factor for poor health. Second, social support in its many forms—emotional, actual physical assistance, and so on—has direct positive effects on health. Equally important, but less widely known, social support can buffer or reduce some of the health-related effects of aging. Finally, and perhaps most important, no single type of support is uniformly effective for all people and all situations."[5]

As the song famously says, "You've got to have friends."

"Human beings are not meant to live solitary lives," adds Rowe. "Talking, touch, and relating to others are essential to our well-being."

Caring for others extends to the nonhuman universe as well. In a classic experiment in 1977, researchers gave each resident of a nursing home a plant. Half the residents were told the plant would be cared for by the staff while the other half were told that the plant was their responsibility. The people who took care of their plant had better medical outcomes, better blood tests, fewer visits to the doctor, and higher scores on virtually every measure of well-being that the researchers could come up with. Just caring for a plant improved their health measurably and significantly! And that's a plant![6]

One of the participants in the MacArthur Foundation Study was eighty-two-year-old Stanley, who told the researchers that, besides his many human connections, his nonhuman social bonds were also vitally important in keeping him healthy and happy. Gardening, for example. "If you're involved in the garden, you're involved in living things that depend on you, and you're in a sense in a spiritual relationship with them—you do for them and

they do for you," he told them. "I have a dog, too, and the same can be said for her, even more so. The joy is rather like friendship, and keeps you young, because you keep concerned and healthy."

Rowe sums it up perfectly: "Loneliness breeds both illness and early death," he says. "As a rule, people whose connections with others are relatively strong—through family (including marriage), friendships, and organizational memberships—live longer."[7]

In fact, for people who have few relationships, or whose relationships with others are weak, the risk of death is between two and four times greater than it is for those who have strong social bonds. This is regardless of age, race, socioeconomic status, physical health, smoking, alcohol use, physical activity, or even obesity. "The bottom line is we do not outgrow our need for others," Rowe says. "The life-giving effect of close social relationships holds throughout the life course."

Having friends, community, and social relationships even protects your brain and helps preserve your memory. Harvard researchers looked at data from 16,000 study participants from the Health and Retirement Study. The researchers checked for marital status, volunteer activity, and frequency of contact with children, neighbors, and parents. Based on this information they assigned each participant a "social integration" score. (Those with the most contact with others received the highest scores, and those with the least contact received the lowest.)

Then the researchers gave the participants a standard battery of memory tests. Those with the lowest "social integration" scores had much greater loss of memory than those with the highest scores. In fact, their memory declined at twice the rate as those who had the most social connections! "Our study provides evidence that social integration delays memory loss among elderly Americans," the researchers concluded.[8]

The protective effects of social relationships aren't just limited to the brain. In a classic 1979 study[9] of the residents of Alameda County, California, researchers found that people who lacked social and community ties were far more likely to die during a nine-year follow-up period than those who had more extensive and meaningful contact with others, regardless of any other health practices, including smoking.

David Snowdon, Ph.D., author of *Aging with Grace*, puts it quite well: "It has now been convincingly demonstrated," he writes, "that marriage, membership in churches, clubs or other social groups and regular contact with family and friends all reduce the risk of death from the major killers, coronary heart disease and stroke."[10]

John Rowe (of the MacArthur Foundation Study) agrees: "The more [that] older people participate in social relationships, the better their overall health," he says. Rowe points out that there are all kinds of venues for social contact and support that promote healthy and successful aging, such as phone conversations, visits from family, neighbors, and friends, participation in religious groups, and attendance at meetings of organizations. In fact, the two strongest predictors of well-being, according to Rowe's research, are frequency of visits with friends and frequency of attending meetings of organizations. "All these interactions [predict] robust aging," Rowe writes, "an index of overall well-being that includes involvement in productive activity, emotional and mental status and functional level."[11] "Interestingly," he adds, "the more meaningful the contribution in a given activity, the greater its impact on health."

So if there is something you care about passionately and that has deep personal meaning to you—volunteering at an animal shelter or participating in Habit for Humanity, for example—you get double the life-extending benefit!

The bottom line: Get involved. It's a good bet it will extend your life.

A WORD FROM THE WISE

At this point, we've come full circle. We've discussed the goal of longevity that is to "square the curve," making old age so healthy and robust that it no longer seems like anything we need to dread and doesn't even look like anything our parents would recognize as old age. Not only that, but the goal is to keep it that way right up to the very end. We've discussed the major systems of the body, how they (typically) break down, and how they can be protected, even enhanced! And finally, in this section, we've discussed the personal and social aspects of living well and long: emotional intelligence, social connectedness, and the inevitable wisdom and peace that come with both.

And here's a little secret: It's all pretty simple.

Dan Buettner interviewed many extraordinary people for his research on healthy aging, but one of the wonderful folks he spoke to stands out: Kamada.

Kamada is 102 years old, healthy, active, serene, and beautiful. Surely she knows something about living long and well. Not surprisingly, Buettner asked her what the secret was to living to 102. Here's what she said:

"Eat your vegetables, have a positive outlook, be kind to people, and smile."

As a simple prescription for a long life, and, as a bonus, for wisdom, it doesn't get much better than that.

The take-home message of this chapter is pretty simple: Live life well, reduce stress by simplifying your life, keep your friends and families close, and contribute to others.

It's hard to come up with a scientifically accurate prescription that dictates how you might accomplish all that, but I'm going to give you my own personal take on how to develop a program for emotional intelligence. Think of it as a personal training program for developing both inner peace and social connectedness. I can't claim that this list of suggestions is either perfect or complete, but it's what I would personally suggest if you were my client and I were your personal trainer in the field of longevity and robust living.

Developing EI: Your Personal Training Program for Extending Life

Shakespeare's famous words "know thyself" were never more appropriate, because emotional intelligence begins with self-awareness. (Self-awareness morphs easily into empathy, and from there into compassion, caring, and contribution.) By developing an inner sense of peace and contentment you will not only reduce stress and increase well-being, but you will also develop precisely the kinds of social connections that have been found to extend life in virtually every study of healthy robust aging that's ever been done.

This is my personal training program for developing both. My Emotional Intelligence Workbook on page 260 may help you get the ball rolling.

1. Acknowledge Someone

An acknowledgement is a simple statement of another's value. It's a small act that can contribute enormously to the well-being of another and will also make you feel good at the same time (trust me on this one). You can acknowledge the most significant person in your life, or you can acknowledge a stranger, or both. Just tell them what they mean to you.

How about thanking a waiter for excellent service and for making your dinner a pleasant experience? Or telling your partner how much his or her smile lights up the room? Approach the world with new eyes and look for an opportunity where you can express even a small amount of thanks to someone every single day. Look for opportunities where you can acknowledge somebody's worth, especially when there are no strings attached. Think about how you feel when somebody tells you what a great job you're doing or what a difference you make in that person's life. We don't get acknowledged enough, and more important, we don't give enough acknowledgments. Acknowledge somebody on a daily basis. It takes

virtually no time or effort and repays in dividends that would make Wall Street blush.

2. Practice Forgiveness

Full disclosure: I actually think that forgiveness (together with the next item I'm going to talk about, gratitude) is the key to happiness and longevity.

In my very, very first book, *Shape Up* (it's out of print, you'll never find it), I told the story of a young New York City cop named Terry McDonald. McDonald was on patrol in New York City during the early 1990s, when crime was at an all-time high in the city. He got shot in a gunfight during a robbery attempt and was paralyzed. The bullet went into his spine and he never was able to walk again.

I remember this story when it happened. I lived in New York at the time and it was headline news, particularly in the *New York Post* and the *New York Daily News* for several days. People were outraged and angry about the injustice of it all, and there was an outpouring of sympathy for McDonald and his family.

McDonald had every reason to be bitter and hateful. He was cut down in the prime of his life by a heartless young punk, confined to a wheelchair in his thirties, and unable to live a normal life with his wife and two kids (with a third on the way, thank you very much). Who would blame him for being bitter and angry? McDonald, however, didn't quite see it that way.

He decided to forgive.

It wasn't easy. But he did it. Somehow, over time, he decided to forgive the person who shot him and release the anger he felt. He decided to find the opportunity in his tragedy and he wound up taking his experience and turning it into a career about bringing people together. When last heard from, he was leading peace marches in Ireland between the two warring factions there—in his wheelchair.

Here's what forgiveness is not: It's not about making it be "okay" that someone did something really horrible and unforgivable. It is about releasing something that is poisoning you. If you think of anger as a little ball of fire that you're holding on to in your hand, consider who's getting burned. Who does anger and resentment ultimately hurt?

Exactly.

Anger takes up psychic space and it drives your stress hormones through the roof. Stress, as we've seen throughout this book, shortens your life. On a more metaphysical level, anger and resentment poison and pollute your soul. Who needs them? And one thing can be said clearly and unequivocally about the long-lived people mentioned throughout this book: They are not angry. Not even a little.

Forgiveness is an art, and like any art it needs practice. It's also a muscle, and like a muscle, it needs training. A good way to start is by making a list of everyone for whom you feel any anger or resentment.

Then forgive someone on the list.

As an exercise, put yourself in that person's place and try to see the world through his eyes. What would it have been like to be that person while he was doing whatever he was doing that made you feel angry? Maybe whatever he did to you was born of his own fear or frustration or ignorance. Whatever. Remember this is not about "excusing" him or making him "right"; it's about you letting go of the disappointment, rage, frustration, or anger that you're left with.

I don't recommend that you start practicing your forgiveness muscle by trying to forgive the worst offender on your list. (That would be like a beginning golfer taking on Tiger Woods!) So you may not be able to forgive the stepdad who abused you, but you may be able to forgive the person who cut in front of you in line at the cafeteria, or the waitress who brought the wrong dish, or the coworker who didn't thank you for the work you did that saved his butt. The important thing is to start practicing with something you can actually manage. Remember, it's a muscle. It needs practice. You don't start doing bicep curls with fifty-pound weights; you start with little hand weights. And it's the same with forgiveness.

Forgiveness is an amazing "muscle." If you develop it, it will extend your life and your well-being, and those of everybody around you as well.

(continued on page 224)

3. Volunteer

"Volunteering makes the heart grow stronger," says David Eisner, CEO of the Corporation for National and Community Service.

He's absolutely right. A boatload of research has found a significant connection between volunteering and good health. Volunteers have lower mortality rates, greater functional ability, and lower rates of depression later in life than those who do not volunteer, according to a comprehensive 2007 report.[12] Here are a few of the findings from the report, titled *Health Benefits of Volunteering: A Review of Recent Research*:

- Older volunteers are most likely to receive the most health benefits from volunteering. These benefits include improved physical and mental health.

- Volunteering leads to greater life satisfaction and lower rates of depression.

- Volunteering and physical well-being are part of a positive reinforcing cycle.

- Individuals who volunteer live longer.

It's more than a little interesting that the rate of volunteering in any given state in the United States is strongly correlated with the physical health of that state's population!

And no wonder. A study of longitudinal data from the Americans' Changing Lives survey[13] found that those who volunteered reported higher levels of happiness, life satisfaction, self-esteem, sense of control over life, and general physical health.

Not a bad group of benefits just for helping other people.

If you've spent any time at all around what is unfortunately called *the self-help movement* (what I would prefer to call the *personal growth movement*), you may have attended a weekend seminar by one of the great motivational leaders, such as my friends Mark Victor Hansen, Jack Canfield, or T. Harv Eker. At any one of these seminars, you can find dozens of volunteers who do all these amazing things for the participants. These guys arrive early and stay late, working insanely long hours for . . . let's see now . . . no pay. Zero. Nada. Zilch.

Why do they do it?

Well, it may have started back in the 1970s with the brilliant teacher and innovator Werner Erhard. (Sharp-eyed readers may have noted that Werner is thanked in every book that I've ever written, and will continue to be for as long as I'm writing.) When Werner had a weekend seminar called *EST training* (which later evolved into what is now *The Forum*) he began the concept of assisting at seminars, and he did it with a very simple rule. He told volunteers at his centers that the value they created for the organization by assisting had to be bettered by the value they created for themselves by doing it. He demanded that the situation be not only a win-win for the assistant volunteers, but also that the assistants win even more!

This philosophy has permeated every personal growth organization I've ever seen in action, and the energetic volunteers who "work the room" at all those weekend events will be the first to tell you what a gift and a privilege it is to do so.

Why?

Because contributing to the world feels good.

Remember those long-lived societies we keep coming back to? They don't have personal growth seminars, nor do they have formal organizations for volunteering, and many of them don't even know how to spell the word *charity*, let alone what it means.

But every one of them volunteers on a regular basis. They may not call it volunteering, preferring to consider it just the part of life when you help out where needed. But help out they do, whether through their church, community, *maoi*, or circle of friends, or just by bringing a dish to the village potluck dinner. "Volunteering" is simply a way of life for them; it's their "water."

Volunteering lets you focus on something other than yourself, at least for a while, providing a kind of therapeutic "time-out" from self-involvement. And that's something from which most of us who grew up as part of the "me" generation could well benefit.

It allows us to feel we're contributing and that we're productive, and that is one of the most life-extending, life-enhancing feelings on the planet. It produces feelings of accomplishment, it engages our compassion and empathy circuits, and—although this hasn't been tested—I'm absolutely sure it produces beneficial biochemical changes in our brain.

And of course, it reduces our stress hormones.

4. Make a Gratitude List

Gratitude is the other side of forgiveness, and together they are the cornerstones of any youthful, energetic, happy life.

Most of us don't spend nearly enough time actually focusing on what we have and what we're grateful for.

Years ago, Steven Sills recorded a song called "Love the One You're With" that spoke to a generation of baby boomers. Maybe it's time to recall the metaphysical sentiment of that song, which was that we would all be better off celebrating what we have instead of always questing after something that we don't have.

We live in a very acquisitive, materialistic society and it's easy to get caught up in aspiring to "something better." Although there's nothing wrong with wanting more out of life, what often happens is that we focus so intensely on what we want (and what, by definition, we don't have) that we forget what we do have.

Gratitude is the enemy of stress. It's hard to be angry, frustrated, or resentful—all emotions that produce bucketfuls of stress hormones—when you're taking a deep breath and thanking the universe for the gifts you've been given.

The thing of it is, when people begin the exercise of making a gratitude list, something profoundly changes for them. I've seen it countless times. You can even try it for yourself (and I hope you do). Simply make a list of any ten things you're grateful for. They can range from the seemingly insignificant (like your new wide-screen TV) to the profoundly important (your relationship with your son).

You can be grateful for the ability to see or hear, for the ability to smell a rose outside your dining room window, for your new computer, for the good health of your loyal ferret. Doesn't matter. Just focusing on gratitude and satisfaction will reduce your stress hormones, brighten your day, and increase your well-being.

Studies on gratitude suggest that subjects who were instructed to keep gratitude journals actually showed higher levels of positive emotions, more life satisfaction, more vitality, lower levels of depression, and lower levels of stress.[14] You get better quality sleep. You have less pain. You're more likely to exercise, and you're more likely to actually make progress toward important personal goals. That sure

sounds to me like the beginnings of a prescription for longevity.

I can't prove it, but my guess from reading interviews with dozens of folks in the long-lived "Blue Zones" of the planet is that gratitude is a deep and persistent part of their lives and that they feel it profoundly on a daily basis. Innkeeper Ishikichi Tanaka, for example, ninety-nine years young, summed it up wonderfully:

"I never pray for a long life, but I just express my gratitude for another day. It reminds me that every day is important."

Make that list, and then read it every single morning for thirty days.

Conclusion
A Plan for You: The 7 × 3 Matrix of Healthy Aging

Thank goodness for the vision of three young guys named Steve Chen, Chad Hurley, and Jawed Karim working out of a garage in Menlo Park, California, in 2005. Because without them, we wouldn't have YouTube and I wouldn't be able to start this chapter with the following request:

1. Go to your computer.
2. Go to either Google or YouTube and type in: "Never Underestimate an Old Gal."
3. Watch.
4. Return to this book.

Okay, on the off-chance that you might not have followed my directions to the T or would prefer to watch the video another time, let me give you the summary of what happens on that clip, which, as of this writing, is sweeping the Internet.

The video was made during the finals of a salsa dance test in a big auditorium somewhere in South America. A handsome, fit Latin man in a white suit enters from one side of the stage while his female partner, dressed in sequins, enters from the other. Over the course of the next 4 minutes and 45 seconds they put on a dazzling display of classic salsa. There's attitude, sexiness, athleticism, and dazzling technique, some of which includes leg extensions, lifts, spins, and dips that produce jaw-dropping amazement in the audience and result in a tumultuous standing ovation at the end of the routine. It is, to be blunt, awe-inspiring.

Oh, I forgot to mention: The female partner in this duo is eighty-seven years old.

Now let's be clear: Following every piece of advice in this book doesn't guarantee you'll be performing world-class salsa routines in your ninth decade. Or that you'll be conducting grueling workouts in Malibu like our friend Don Wildman. Or still teaching and training jujitsu like ninety-year old Helio Gracie, or choreographing until her death at age ninety-six like the great modern dancer Martha Graham, or painting "Young Bather with Sand Shovel" at the age of ninety like Pablo Picasso, or even shepherding flocks in the mountains like many of the ninety-plus-year-old citizens in Sardinia. Fact is, we don't completely understand why some people are vital and robust and still having fun forty years after some of their contemporaries can barely drag themselves off their recliners.

But we've got some ideas.

This concluding chapter is, in some ways, the most personal chapter in the book because the opinions expressed here are solely my own. These are the core strategies that seem to me, after reading as much research as I could get my hands on about living long and well, to be the most important things you can do to increase the odds of a long and healthy life.

Remember, we don't have any multi-decade studies that examine the precise effect of each one of these strategies, and we probably never will. (We also don't have any double-blind studies that "prove" water puts out fire, but the fire department of every major city acts on the assumption that it's true!) So here, for what it's worth, is my own "water puts out fire" theory, boiled down into a matrix I call the "7 x 3 Matrix of Healthy Aging." These are the strategies I try to follow, and although I can't prove it to the satisfaction of the most hard-nosed scientists in the world of academia, it's a good bet that these strategies will increase the odds that you'll be among those left standing, jogging, shepherding, painting, dancing the salsa, or just plain having fun long after many of your contemporaries have sadly departed this universe.

And one more thing, a footnote, if you will: If you happen to be reading this book and your age has any number less than four as the first digit, congratulations. Here's what I've discovered about anti-aging strategies and life: They parallel what happens with a car.

Let me explain.

I drive a really nifty little two-seater car that never breaks down. But it only has 30,000 miles on it. When a car has low mileage, you will not usually see the result of poor car maintenance. You can lease a car and totally neglect it for the first three years of its life (and the length of the typical lease) and nothing will happen. Ignore the oil changes, drive it into the ground, don't rotate the tires—it doesn't much matter because the car's youth will ensure that it can weather the damage (which is, after all, cumulative). By the time you trade in the car, it will still perform pretty much the way it was when you drove it off the lot. You won't notice a difference in performance at all.

But the next owner will.

Most damage, to cars and to the human body, is cumulative. So the person who takes up smoking a pack of cigarettes a day doesn't notice a change in his health for the first year, maybe even the first twenty, except perhaps an annoying hacking cough when he wakes up that usually goes away by midday. His first wakeup call is when he gets that X-ray with a suspicious spot on it, and that might well be twenty years down the road. The first "symptom" of heart disease is often death, and high blood pressure, which seriously increases the risk, usually has no symptoms at all. The same with diabetes.

But back to the car.

So my lovely little convertible performs great at 30,000 miles, and you would expect that it would no matter how it was taken care of. But the fact is I take great care of it. It never misses a service or an oil change. It's garaged. The tires are changed regularly and even rotated pretty much on schedule. So why do I do that?

Because when the car has 75,000 miles, or 175,000 miles, I expect it will still run great.

I have good reason to suspect that. Because my *other* car, a fifteen-year-old version of the new one, has nearly 180,000 miles and I've taken care of it in the same way as I take care of the newer car, and guess what—it never breaks down. It runs like a dream, and except for a little aging of the mechanical parts, it's almost as good as new. Sure, it creaks a bit here and there, but it's certainly as good as cars

half its age, and it still elicits smiles and waves when I drive it with the top down on the Pacific Coast Highway.

I was thinking about that this morning as I got off the tennis court. I feel the way I felt when I was in my thirties, maybe better. Of the major complaints that are a daily occurrence in people my age—constipation, low back pain, joint aches, inflexibility, low energy—I have none. (The sound you hear is me knocking wood—I never said I wasn't suspicious or grateful!)

When I fill out those medical questionnaires (e.g., "have you ever had …"), I draw a big circle around all the "no's" on the page. And I'm 100 percent convinced that the reason that is so is because I do most of what I've talked about in this book. I started at age thirty-eight, but I know people who've started a lot later than that. (Friends of mine, like the fit and muscular Jeff Life, M.D., the "poster boy" for the anti-aging clinic Cenegenics in Las Vegas, started at fifty-seven.) The point is, start now. Even if you don't notice the results while you're young, look around you in your decades that start with five, six, and seven and beyond, and wonder why everyone else looks and sounds and feels old and you don't.

And trust me with one more thing—it's worth it.

TWENTY-ONE STRATEGIES FOR AGING WELL

So here's the 7 x 3 Matrix of Healthy Aging. The "7 x 3" comes from the fact that there are three categories—food, supplements, and lifestyle—each of which contains seven simple strategies. It's the program I try to follow on a daily basis and I hope you will, too.

1. Food: Age Well with the Right Foods

Hippocrates, the father of modern medicine, said, "Let food be thy medicine and medicine be thy food." How right he was. Remember, heart disease isn't a Lipitor deficiency. If you give the body what it needs in the way of fuel, it will make everything it needs to keep you healthy, glowing, and robust for decades. And though there are probably hundreds of different diets (or eating styles), there are a few standout foods and beverages that seem to be found in the diets of the healthiest people on earth. These are the ones that form the core seven strategies below.

Green tea: Arguably the healthiest beverage in the world, or at least one of the top five, green tea contains compounds that have been found to reduce the risk of esophageal cancer,[1] breast cancer,[2] and heart disease.[3,4] Mayo Clinic scientists found that components in green tea kill human prostate cancer cells in test tubes.[5] Green tea may also help you lose weight. Emerging research suggests that the chemicals found in green tea may also protect the brain against Alzheimer's and Parkinson's diseases.[6] I recommend a minimum of two cups a day and think that if you can drink five you're golden!

Nuts: Some of the largest and most important long-term studies of diet and health have shown a consistent 30 to 50 percent lower risk of heart attacks or heart disease associated with eating nuts several times each week.[7] Nuts are a regular part of the daily menu in virtually every one of the Blue Zones. "We don't know if it's the omega-3s in the nuts or the fact that by eating nuts they're not eating salty chips, but we do know that people who eat a handful of nuts four times a week live on average two years longer than those who don't," *The Blue Zones* author Dan Buettner told Diane Sawyer on *Good Morning America.*

The magic number from the research seems to be one ounce four to five times a week. Enjoy! (And it doesn't much matter which kinds of nuts you choose.)

Beans: Beans are the cornerstone of every one of the diets in the Blue Zones. They reduce the risk of cancer, heart disease, and diabetes. One study found that women who eat the most beans had a 38 percent reduction in the risk for diabetes,[8] not surprising because beans are one of the greatest sources of fiber on the planet and fiber helps stabilize blood sugar. (A high-fiber intake is also associated with a lower risk of colon cancer.) When it comes to antioxidants, beans are among the richest sources, with red beans, red kidney beans, and pinto beans being particularly outstanding. And in one major research study,[9] four or more one-cup servings of cooked legumes per week was enough to decrease the risk of heart disease by 22 percent. I recommend four servings per week.

Grass-fed meat: As of this writing, the controversies and misunderstandings about meat and health continue to rage. (We won't resolve the debate here.) It's worth noting, however, that even in the Blue Zones, people eat meat. They just don't eat it that often and they don't eat the processed, factory-farmed junk that we routinely consume in Western societies. Grass-fed meat is absent of steroids, antibiotics, and growth hormones, and the fat is rich in omega-3 properties and cancer-fighting conjugated linolenic acid (CLA). And meat remains one of the best sources of protein and vitamin B_{12}. My recommendation: Eat grass-fed red meat once a week.

Fish: Fish is a major component in the diet of virtually every long-lived society. Fish is the ultimate anti-aging food. High in protein, low in calories, it's a nutritional bonanza. Cold-water fatty fish like (wild) salmon, sardines, mackerel, and herring contain omega-3 fats that protect the brain and the heart, improve mood, and lower blood pressure and triglycerides. I recommend a minimum of two servings per week, but there's no problem with eating it more often than that!

Berries (and other fruits): I can't say enough good things about berries, but I'll mention just a few, starting with my favorite, blueberries. In a series of remarkable experiments, James Joseph, Ph.D., of the U.S. Department of Agriculture Human Nutrition Center on Aging at Tufts University found that when you feed animals blueberries, they behave like young stud muffins. Motor function, memory, and performance on assorted tests for muscle coordination and strength all improve. Cranberries are high in *phenolic acids*, plant chemicals known to protect against a wide range of health conditions. Raspberries are loaded with fiber, calcium, magnesium, phosphorus, potassium, vitamin C … should I go on? And they're also one of the best sources in the world of a plant chemical known as *ellagic acid* (also found in strawberries), which has been shown to inhibit the growth of tumors. I recommend a cup of berries every day, or at least five days a week. But don't neglect other great anti-aging fruits like apples, grapefruit, and cherries. A twenty-six-year prospective study of men in Sweden provided evidence that fruit intake in general is associated with greater longevity.[10]

Vegetables: You can't find a Blue Zone where vegetables aren't a big part of every meal. The vegetable kingdom is rich in antioxidants and anti-inflammatories, not to mention cancer-fighting plant compounds like indoles (found in the cabbage family), carotenoids, fiber, vitamins, minerals, and phytochemicals, all of which have substantial health benefits and can reasonably be assumed to keep you alive and disease-free for a long time. Data from two of the longest running studies of diet and health ever done—the Nurses Health Study and the Health Professionals Follow-Up Study—showed that men and women who ate the most vegetables (nine or ten servings a day) had a 20 percent lower risk of coronary artery disease compared to those who ate the least (only two or three servings a day).[11] Other studies have shown an even greater reduction in risk of heart attacks (38 percent),[12] and still others have shown decreased risk for stroke, diabetes, and a variety of cancers.

You don't have to be vegetarian to get the benefits of a high-vegetable intake—just eat them at every single meal. There's no maximum recommendation, but at minimum try for seven servings a day (nine is even better). It's not as much as you might think considering that one serving is only a half a cup.

So there you have it, and it winds up being pretty simple: green tea, nuts, beans, grass-fed meat, fish, berries and fruits, and vegetables. A glass of wine here and there wouldn't hurt either, nor would a square or two of dark chocolate. With minor variations, those foods seem to be part of the diet of just about every place on earth where folks live a long time in good health.

2. Get Nutritional Insurance with the Right Supplements

Okay, I can easily imagine the obvious question—if most of the people who live long and healthy lives don't even know what a supplement is, why would nutritional supplements be on the short list of strategies for a life-extension program? Can't you manage perfectly well without them?

Well, yes, you can. Especially if you live in the lush paradise of a Greek Isle and walk ten miles a day and eat only organic, locally grown food, breathe clean air, and enjoy low levels of stress.

Unfortunately, most of us don't.

I look at supplements as a high-tech delivery system for the nutrients that, in the best of all possible worlds, we would get from food. But most of us don't get anything like the optimal doses of certain nutrients from our food, even when we're eating really, really well.

There are two major reasons for this—besides the fact that most of us don't eat all that terrifically in the first place. One, nutrient levels in food have fallen over the years, due in large part to the way food is grown, processed, and prepared.[13] Important nutrients have declined between 5 and 40 percent, according to comprehensive research by professor Donald Davis, Ph.D..[14] Other researchers have shown even greater losses. David Thomas, D.C., analyzed and compared government tables for food composition in 1940 and 2002 and found losses of 55 to 60 percent in iron and 60 percent in copper just in meat alone, largely due to intensive farming methods.[15]

Two, optimal doses are far from adequate doses. It's hard to get 400 IUs of vitamin E from food, for example, and next to impossible to get any meaningful dose of such important nutrients as alpha-lipoic acid or coenzyme Q10. But it's easy to get them through supplements.

So even if you followed the above dietary recommendations to the letter, you might still benefit from additional quantities of certain nutrients. In previous chapters we've discussed how certain supplements can provide added protection for specific organs or systems in the body (the brain, heart, and bones), and you can certainly expand the following list of supplements with any of the ones mentioned in those chapters. But here, for what it's worth, is my list of seven supplements that seem to have demonstrated the most bang for the buck when it comes to protecting your body, brain, and heart, and which have the strongest likelihood of ensuring a longer life.*

Omega-3 fatty acids (fish oil): Throughout this book you've heard references to omega-3s, those fatty acids found in fish and flax. They protect the heart and brain and improve mood.[16, 17, 18, 19, 20] They keep you young. They are arguably the most important supplement you should take for a long and healthy life.

The ratio of omega-6s (vegetable oils) to omega-3s (fish oil, flax) is thought by most people who know what they're talking about to have a tremendous influence on human health. The ideal ratio is about 1:1; we typically consume about 16:1 or more in favor of the pro-inflammatory omega-6s. Omega-3s lower inflammation, blood pressure, and triglycerides.

Omega-3s are the one supplement I wouldn't be without no matter what. I recommend at least 1 gram a day of DHA and EPA, the two important fatty acids found in fish oil. (I personally take 2 grams a day.) If for some reason you can't or won't take fish oil or fish oil capsules, you can take flax oil instead but you'll need to take substantially more to get enough EPA and DHA in your system—at least 2 to 4 tablespoons a day. Only a relatively small portion of the omega-3 fatty acid in flaxseed converts in the body to the two omega-3 fatty acids, EPA and DHA, which are most important for human health.

Selenium: Selenium might just be the most important mineral you've never heard of. It's absolutely essential for your immune system,[21] and without a healthy immune system you are at a big disadvantage when it comes to healthy aging. When animals are deficient in selenium and exposed to a flu virus, the virus mutates into a much worse (and more life-threatening) form,

---

* Especially if taken as part of an overall plan like the one described in this chapter.

which is then passed on to other animals, research has found. A decline in selenium levels is a hallmark of AIDS progression,[22] but studies have found that selenium supplementation can suppress HIV-1.[23]

But bolstering your immune system is hardly the only thing selenium does (although if it was, it would be reason enough to take it!). Mortality rates are significantly higher in individuals with low selenium levels.[24] And, according to a study in the journal *Epidemiology*,[25] selenium may help slow cognitive decline. "Selenium status decreases with age and may contribute to declines in neuropsychologic[al] functions among aging people," concluded the researchers.

Finally, selenium has a clear anticancer effect. In one classic study published in the *Journal of the American Medical Association*, 1,312 patients with a history of skin cancer were treated for an average of four and a half years with either 200 micrograms of selenium or a placebo. The total cancer incidence was reduced by 37 percent in the selenium group, which also had 63 percent less prostate cancer, 58 percent less colorectal cancer, and 46 percent less lung cancer.[26]

There's a lot of hoopla about selenium toxicity, but most of it is nonsense. The "toxic symptoms" (garlic breath, brittle fingernails) occur at huge doses. Studies in China have found that nail and hair problems occur at the level of 4,990 micrograms a day (about twenty-four to forty-eight selenium capsules daily). I recommend 200 to 400 micrograms of selenium every day.

Worth noting: There's currently a phase 3 study of 32,500 men, funded by the National Cancer Institute, testing the benefits of selenium and vitamin E on preventing prostate cancer. The results will be released after the 2013 completion date of the study, but don't expect much. In fact, I suspect the antisupplement forces will use the outcome of this study to promote their "vitamins are worthless" agenda. Why? Because the U.S. Food and Drug Administration chose a ridiculously low dose of selenium, 55 micrograms per day, to test in the study. It's next to impossible that 55 micrograms of selenium a day will do very much to prevent cancer, so expect the media to report that this study "proves" selenium is worthless. Don't believe it for a second. Take my advice and take 200 to 400 micrograms a day as part of your supplement strategy program for a long and healthy life.

Vitamin D: If you had to pick one vitamin that achieved superstar status in the decade from 2000 to 2010, it would have to be vitamin D. The resume of health and potentially life-extending (and quality-of-life-improving) benefits of this long underappreciated vitamin is simply stunning. The conservative *Physicians' Desk Reference for Nutritional Supplements* summed it up best: "Over the past several years, studies have indicated that vitamin D may play beneficial roles in a wide range of disease and disorders, including osteoporosis, cancer, multiple sclerosis, heart disease, psoriasis, and Alzheimer's disease."[27]

A 2008 study showed that people with low levels of vitamin D are significantly more likely to die for *any* reason than are people with higher levels.[28] A diet lacking in adequate vitamin D may increase the risk for cancer.[29] And the definition of "adequate" intake is rapidly changing, especially because clinical experience shows that far more people than you might imagine have much lower than optimal levels of this vitamin.

"We found a marked increase in vitamin D deficiency over the past two decades," said vitamin D researcher Adit Ginde, M.D., assistant professor of surgery at the University of Colorado Denver School of Medicine.

"Over three out of four Americans now have vitamin D levels below what we believe is necessary for optimal health. African-Americans and Hispanics are at particularly high risk—nearly all have suboptimal levels."

Indeed. Vitamin D may help prevent diabetes[30] and heart attacks,[31] and people with higher levels of vitamin D have a significantly lower risk of cognitive impairment when they get older.[32] Vitamin D also improves physical performance in older adults.[33] It's also absolutely essential for strong bones, an important concern as we get older. For goodness sake, it may even help prevent colds.[34]

There are few food sources of vitamin D, which is one reason I strongly recommend this vitamin in your 7 x 3 strategy for robust aging. In 2008, several health organizations, including the American Pediatrics Association, recommended doubling the recommended daily allowance for vitamin D, but they're being conservative. I recommend 2,000 IUs of vitamin D on a daily basis. If you're in the sun, a source of vitamin D, for hours on end, you could reduce that to 1,000 IUs, but you're probably not in the sun for that long anyway.

Don't worry about toxicity. Your body makes many times that amount when you're in the sun all day, and studies have shown that up to 2,000 IUs a day is perfectly safe. Noted researcher Michael F. Holick, M.D., director of the Vitamin D Laboratory at Boston University, says, "We are in desperate need to have a marked increase in the adequate intake recommendation, and hopefully that will be 1,000 to 2,000 IUs per day—and raise the safe upper limit to at least 10,000 IUs a day."[35]

Folic acid: Here's a prediction: Folic acid is poised to become the "next" vitamin D, in the sense that researchers are still discovering the huge benefits of this nutrient and that we have woefully underestimated the optimal daily intake of this member of the B vitamin family.

We don't get enough folic acid in our diet, or at least not nearly the optimal amount. To make matters worse, the body doesn't absorb folate, the form of folic acid found in food, all that well. Folic acid, the form used in supplements, is actually much better absorbed. But none of this would make much difference if it weren't for what's been learned about low folate (folic acid) status and its impact on human health and longevity.

Low concentrations of folate in the blood have been associated with poor cognitive function, dementia, and Alzheimer's disease,[36] not to mention a higher risk for colorectal, lung, esophageal, brain, cervical, and breast cancers.[37] The *Encyclopedia of Dietary Supplements*, which was written by a blue-ribbon panel of scientists from the National Institutes of Health, says, "Observational studies continue to indicate an inverse relationship between folate (folic acid) intake . . . and the risk of developing certain common cancers."[38] Low intake has also been associated with depression and other psychiatric symptoms.[39] And let's not forget about homocysteine (see page 104), a risk factor for both heart disease and stroke. Folic acid is a key player in lowering this toxic compound in the blood.

But the main thing that convinced me to put folic acid on the short list of essential supplements for a long and healthy life was the Nun Study.

The Nun Study is a longitudinal study of aging and Alzheimer's disease funded by the National Institute on Aging. The participants are members of the School Sisters of Notre Dame and are between 75 and 106(!) years old. The idea was to look at this homogenous population of women, all of whom pretty much lead the same lifestyle, eat the same food, and have similar patterns of alcohol and cigarette use (which would be zero), and to determine which factors might account for the fact that some of them develop Alzheimer's and some don't. Good idea, right?

Here's what David Snowdon, Ph.D., the lead researcher in the Nun Study, had to say: "Nine years into the Nun Study, we finally found a nutrient that appeared to stave off the brain-damaging effects of Alzheimer's disease in the sisters."[40]

That nutrient? Folic acid.

I recommend taking 1,000 to 5,000 micrograms (1 to 5 grams) of folic acid daily.

Worth knowing: The current recommended dietary intake is 400 micrograms (about ½ gram), which is very low. The National Academy of Sciences' Food and Nutrition Board recommends 1,000 micrograms as a safe upper limit, but what's important to know is that number is not related to any possible toxicity of folic acid. Folic acid is not toxic or dangerous; doses of up to 15,000 micrograms (15 grams) in healthy adults have not produced any reported serious adverse effects.[41]

In my opinion, the only reason the recommendations for folic acid haven't been higher is that the people who make these recommendations are concerned about the fact that folic acid can mask vitamin B_{12} deficiency, which is something you definitely *don't* want. My solution to that is simple: Just make sure you get adequate levels of B_{12} (which you will get from grass-fed meat and many kinds of fish). Taking a multiple vitamin or a B complex should clear up any concerns about getting enough B_{12}.

Probiotics: When you think about it, all the food and supplement recommendations we've made so far are only beneficial to you if you are able to digest and absorb them. Probiotics, the "good" bacteria that live in your gut, help make digestion and absorption possible.

Your gut is teeming with bacteria, some of it good (probiotics), some of it not so good (*Candida albicans*, or "yeast"). There's a constant turf battle going on, and you want the good guys to win. Not only does a good balance of "good" to "bad" bacteria in the gut help with digestion and absorption, but growing evidence suggests that it may support the immune system as well. And emerging research is showing that probiotic benefits, including lowering inflammation, may extend to the whole body.

"If I could only get people to take one supplement a day, it would be a probiotic," says my friend and nutritionist Allison Tannis, M.Sc., R.H.N., author of *Probiotic Rescue: How You Can Use Probiotics to Fight Cholesterol, Cancer, Superbugs, Digestive Complaints, and More.* "The benefits of probiotics are so far-reaching it's mind-boggling."

Many people in countries where fermented food is routinely consumed get plenty of probiotics in their diet. Traditionally fermented sauerkraut, for example, or olives, or the Korean dish kimchi are all wonderful sources of these beneficial bacteria. But unless you're eating fermented food or a ton of yogurt that contains active cultures, you probably could use some extra help. Many health professionals are beginning to put probiotics on their short list of the most important supplements for general health. I agree.

Get a good brand that mixes various "families" of probiotics (like *lactobaccillus* and *bifidobacteria*) and take it daily, with food or just after a meal. (Note: The dose per enteric-coated capsule is given in billions of organisms— remember, these bacteria are really, really tiny!) You can also get probiotics in a powder, which is both convenient and effective. Sprinkle it on yogurt, fruit, or any cold dish. And unless the package says it's "shelf stable," remember to refrigerate it; the bacteria are alive and you want to keep them that way for as long as possible—until they hit your gut, where they can do some good!

Resveratrol: The fact that red wine is good for you is hardly news. For years we've heard about wine, which contains hundreds of chemical compounds that fall into the family of polyphenols. And the polyphenol that's gotten the lion's share of attention, at least when it comes to wine and grapes, is resveratrol.

Resveratrol is found in the skin of dark grapes. In every species studied, from yeast cells to fruit flies to mice, resveratrol seems to extend life. Research by Harvard Medical School professor of pathology David Sinclair, M.D., has shown that resveratrol extends the life span of mice by up to 24 percent and the life span of other animals by as much as 59 percent.

It's believed that resveratrol exerts its magic by turning on the SIRT genes, which are involved in longevity. (Some SIRT genes are turned on by caloric restriction, another well-known age-extending strategy, albeit a difficult one to follow.) Scientists are hard at work to develop a drug that turns on the SIRT genes, which, if successful, may be the pharmaceutical equivalent of the Fountain of Youth.

And many are counting on resveratrol to be the main ingredient. (You can be sure that just as soon as the pharmaceutical companies come up with a way to work it into a patented medicine, they'll not only do so, but they'll also make a killing.)

Resveratrol is also a powerful antioxidant. And it's been found to inhibit the growth of several cancer cell lines and tumors, "suggesting," according to the *Physicians' Desk Reference for Nutritional Supplements,* "that it has an inhibitory effect on cancer promotion [and] progression."[42]

You'd have to drink an enormous amount of wine to get the amount of resveratrol available in a single supplement pill. I recommend you take at least 250 milligrams a day, although many of the experts I spoke to take a lot more.

Worth noting: The only form of resveratrol shown to be effective so far is the *trans*-resveratrol form. The label on the bottle will tell you exactly how much trans-resveratrol you're getting. If, for example, you have a 500 milligram capsule of resveratrol "standardized for 20 percent trans-resveratrol," that means it contains 100 milligrams of tran-resveratrol (20 percent of 500 milligrams). Calculate your dose based on the trans-resveratrol each pill provides, not on the total amount of resveratrol per pill.

Coenzyme Q10: A healthy heart is a great thing to have if you want to live long and well, and coenzyme Q10 is one of the greatest nutrients for the heart on the planet.

Coenzyme Q10, or CoQ10 for short, is a vitally important nutrient for energy. It literally recharges the energy production furnaces in the cells (called the *mitochondria*). The heart cells produce more energy than any other organ, so CoQ10 and the heart are a natural fit. Indeed, CoQ10 is given as a prescription drug for congestive heart failure in Japan—it's that effective at helping the heart produce energy.

Our bodies make CoQ10, but as we age we produce substantially less. And don't think you're going to make up the difference with food—CoQ10 is found mainly in organ meats (heart, liver, and kidney). Other foods that have it, like sardines and beef, contain paltry amounts, and you'd need a ton of them to get even 30 milligrams a day, the absolute minimum dose for healthy folks looking for general protection.

Emerging evidence suggests that CoQ10 may be helpful in preventing certain neurodegenerative diseases.[43] It also helps prevent migraines[44] and lowers blood pressure.[45] And if that weren't enough, it's also a powerful antioxidant. I recommend at least 60 to 100 milligrams of CoQ10 daily for anyone over forty.

3. Adopt the Age-Management Lifestyle

The best foods in the world and the most potent supplements will not make you happy. They will give your body everything it needs in the way of fuel, but that's not enough. You could put the highest quality gas in a Ferrari, but to get the fun from a Ferrari you still have to take it out of the garage and drive it! (Well, I assume you do. I personally never have, but you get the point.)

The following strategies are drawn from themes I've discussed in these pages. They're the same themes that come up in every single piece of research I've seen on successful aging, whether it's the MacArthur Foundation Study, the Nun Study, the Baltimore Longitudinal Study of Aging, the Adventist Study, or in Dan Buettner's book, *The Blue Zones*. I've taken what I think to be the most important common denominators and put them together in seven basic strategies. Obviously, you can argue that not every healthy centenarian does every one of these things. But if I were a betting man, I'd bet the family farm that the following strategies represent an effective program for aging well that is bound to keep you active and happy for a long time.

Walk thirty minutes every day. I'm not saying you'll lose a ton of weight with this strategy, but that's not why it's on the list. Walking at a moderate clip has been shown to grow new brain cells in both animals[46] and humans.[47] It's the perfect natural antidepressant and mood elevator. Duke University researchers found that over sixteen weeks, walking (or jogging) for thirty minutes (plus warming up and cooling down) worked as well as antidepressant medications in improving mood.[48] And the American

Cancer Society's cancer prevention guidelines state that at least thirty minutes a day of dedicated exercise (like brisk walking) is needed to reduce cancer risk. Walking is good for the heart, the lungs, the brain, and, especially if you do it outside amid greenery and beauty, the soul.

Weight train twice a week. Walking is great, but you also need muscular strength if you're going to navigate through life effortlessly. I'm not necessarily talking about bench-pressing four hundred pounds here; I'm talking about keeping your muscles strong and useful so that you can do the daily tasks of life without any great problem. And muscles are the truest example of the old adage "use it or lose it." You lose about half a pound of muscle a year if you don't do anything to stop the loss. And it's not just muscle you lose. Because calories are burned primarily in the muscle cells, losing muscle means you lose calorie-burning ability and gain fat much more easily.

Weight training can significantly slow that loss of muscle to a negligible amount. You may not win the Mr. Universe contest at eighty, but you'll be strong as an ox and look pretty darn good to boot. And don't believe for a second that you're too old to start. Noted strength researcher Wayne Wescott, Ph.D., has done a number of studies on weight training with elderly people, some of whom were in wheelchairs, and nearly all of them improved in strength and autonomy. Ronald Reagan started using weights when he was eighty-two and even he gained some muscle!

The good news is that you don't have to train all that hard or all that frequently. Twice a week for a half hour or so is all you need to make sure those muscles don't atrophy.

Breathe—deeply! You can substitute mediation for this if you like, or stick with the basics of deep breathing (see below). Breathing deeply gets oxygen to the brain, calms the mind and the soul, lowers stress hormones, and is incompatible with anger and other destructive emotions. In case you don't want to look it up, here's how to do it in the simplest possible way:

1. Sit comfortably with your eyes closed.
2. Pay attention to your breathing and repeat a word, phrase, or prayer silently to yourself as you exhale.
3. Slowly fill your lungs up deeply and exhale fully.
4. When you notice your mind wandering, which it most definitely will, passively bring your attention back to your breathing.
5. Practice for approximately twenty minutes every day (or at least three or four times a week).

Although sitting quietly and meditating (or breathing deeply) is one way to reduce stress and calm the brain, don't rule out a more structured approach like gentle yoga, tai chi, or qi gong. All accomplish the same thing. It's probably no accident that most of the healthy people you see in parks doing tai chi are over seventy!

Get out in the sun for at least ten minutes a day. Not only does it give you some vitamin D the natural way, but sunshine is also a great mood enhancer. It's no accident that seasonal affective disorder (SAD) hits people most in winter or in the darker, colder months. It's also no accident that the tropics are frequently called paradises; you don't see too many people enjoying carefree vacations in Antarctica.

Remember that deeply etched into our DNA is a whole cascade of hormonal and biochemical responses that are regulated by light and dark. We ignore these at our peril. The sun is our original source of light, and it's no accident that so many of the longest-lived people in the world spend a lot of time outdoors and are probably much more in tune with the natural rhythms of light and dark produced by the cycle of night and day.

The importance of these rhythms was underscored recently in a surprising study of suicide in Greenland. Greenland has one of the highest suicide rates in the world, and researchers have found that suicides are far more pronounced during the periods in which the sun never sets—the months known as "constant day." In the north of the country, 82 percent of the suicides occurred during these months, and these suicides were almost exclusively violent. The researchers speculate that light-generated imbalances in the brain chemical serotonin may be responsible.[49]

The point is that light and darkness form an exquisite balance that has profound effects on our well-being. To paraphrase Goldilocks, when it comes to sun we need "not too much, not too little, but just enough." Don't be sun phobic. The sun is your friend, but so (as we'll see below) is darkness. Embrace both.

Sleep well! Prior to the invention of electricity, our sleep patterns were pretty stable. After all, we had no options to override the natural rhythm of light and dark. We went to bed in darkness when the sun set and woke up with the light, when the sun rose. There's a deep and abiding wisdom in this, one we would do well to copy in our modern life, especially if we want to live long and feel good!

How well you sleep has an enormous and sometimes underappreciated relationship to how good you feel. Undersleeping elevates stress hormones, increasing blood pressure, inflammation, irritability, and weight gain and decreasing energy. (Point of interest: People who sleep fewer than seven or eight hours a night are more likely to be overweight or obese, possibly because undersleeping disrupts hormones like leptin and ghrelin, which have a significant effect on appetite.)

Recent research has linked sleep and longevity. In 2007, researchers from the University College London Medical School studied 10,308 British civil servants to try to find out whether there was any link between the number of hours slept per night and what is technically called "all-cause mortality"—the likelihood of dying for any reason. They looked at the civil servants at two points in their lives: 1985 to 1988, and those still alive in 1992 and 1993. The researchers statistically adjusted for all the important factors, such as age, sex, smoking, alcohol use, weight, and physical illness, and were then able to isolate the effect that changes in sleep patterns over five years had on mortality rates eleven to seventeen years later.

The results were eye-opening. Those who had cut their sleeping from seven hours to five hours or fewer had a 1.7-fold increase in the risk of dying from any cause, and twice the likelihood of dying from a cardiovascular problem.[50]

"In terms of prevention, our findings indicate that consistently sleeping around seven hours per night is optimal for health and a sustained reduction may predispose to ill health," said the researchers.

During sleep, important biochemicals are replaced, hormones are released, and the body is rejuvenated and refreshed. Sleeping well and soundly makes you feel energized, increases well-being, and helps you maintain your weight at a healthy level. It also bolsters your memory.

Make getting a good night's sleep—every night of the year—a priority. It's one of the cornerstones of living well and living long. Although there are definitely individual variations, all indications point to seven hours a night as being the magic number needed for optimal health. (Full disclosure: I sleep six hours a night, but I'd worry if it were consistently less than that.)

Practice *hara hatchi bu*. With all the hundreds of books' worth of information on what to eat, what tends to get lost is this simple truth: Eating less extends life.

Clearly what you eat matters greatly—I wouldn't have written several books on the subject if I didn't think it was important. But what's also important is how you eat (relaxed, without stress, and mindfully) and how much you eat.

In every species studied so far, calorie restriction extends life. Seriously. But don't let the term *restriction* scare you. You don't have to join one of those calorie-restriction societies and count every single calorie every day of your life. Just eat about one-third to one-fourth less than you normally would. The benefits are enormous. (Though no authoritative figures are available, most estimates put the "average" daily caloric intake of Americans in the 3,600 range, with many people eating far more than that.)

The long-lived folks on Okinawa eat up to 40 percent fewer calories than Americans do[51] and 17 percent less than the Japanese average.[52] Seems to be working. Not only do they have one of the highest life spans of any group ever studied, but, compared to Americans, Okinawa elders are 75 percent more likely to retain their cognitive ability, develop 80 percent fewer breast and prostate cancers, have 50 percent fewer ovarian and colon cancers, experience 50 percent fewer hip fractures, and suffer 80 percent fewer heart attacks.[53]

The Confucian saying *"Hara hatchi bu"* sums it up best—"Eat until you are 80 percent full." The folks in the Okinawa peninsula live by this mantra.

You and I should do the same.

Connect. I've saved the best and most important part for last. Connect—that simple word sums up the most important message in this entire book. More than food, more than supplements, more than exercise, more than virtually any other strategy I can think of to extend both the length and the quality of life, connecting with others is the most important thing you can possibly do if you want to live long and well.

I've said it before, but it bears repeating. People have lived a very long time with some very unhealthy habits. I don't think it makes a lot of sense to risk the odds on this, but still, it's worth noting that every family has an Uncle Jack who smoked two packs a day and drank a fifth of Jack Daniels and lived to a hundred.

But no family has an Uncle Jack who lived to a hundred in isolation.

Whether it's friends, family, or extended family, whether it's church, temple, mosque, or charity, connection to something or someone outside of you is a prerequisite for living well and seems to be a prerequisite for living long.

Every society studied has intricate social networks where people offer help, assistance, companionship, friendship, and outreach. As we've seen in this book, even taking care of a houseplant improves medical outcomes substantially. If taking care of a plant, and paying attention to something outside yourself, improves medical outcomes that much, imagine what taking care of—or contributing to   people, animals, and causes can do. People who volunteer live longer and healthier lives. People who are connected to others thrive; people who don't, wither away.

IKAGI

On a personal note: I've spent most of my life studying human beings, and the more I learn the more I profoundly understand how little I know. I've changed what I believe about food and exercise (or at least modified it) many times over the two decades I've been in the health and wellness field. But one belief I've never changed is this: People want to contribute. Many people on this planet want nothing more than to contribute, be heard, make a difference, and have a meaningful life. No matter whether we are conscious of it or not, and regardless of whether we express it or not, the desire to contribute and make a difference is at the core of what every human being truly wants. It is what makes us human. It is what makes life both beautiful and fulfilling.

I hope the suggestions offered in this book help you live the longest and most productive life possible. I hope they make it possible for you to live a life you love, with purpose and meaning, and to fulfill your every dream— and even dreams you didn't know you had.

I started this book by saying that if you didn't have a purpose, all the anti-aging strategies in the world wouldn't mean much. So if I had but one "anti-aging" strategy to leave you with it would be this: Find your purpose.

And then live in accordance with it. Every single day.

With a purpose, an *"ikagi,"* as the Okinawans say, you have a reason for staying alive.

I hope this book has given you the tools to do exactly that.

Enjoy the journey.

My Emotional Intelligence Workbook

. . . .

Emotional intelligence is the ability to be both personal and interpersonal, to have relationships, community, and contribution, and deal with people from a place of integrity and self-awareness.

Working through the steps in this workbook will increase your awareness of yourself and your relationship to others. Copy these questions onto another piece of paper or other journal format of your choice.

Emotional intelligence encompasses most areas of our connection to other people (and our ability to be at peace with ourselves). Remember that one of the defining characteristics of the longest-lived and healthiest people on the planet—a characteristic that consistently shows up in every study of people around the globe who live extremely long and healthy lives—is connection to others. This includes friendships, marriages, relatives, community, and church or spiritual groups.

In this workbook, I've broken down the components of emotional intelligence into specific categories that allow you to focus on the little steps you could take to increase the enormous sense of well-being that comes with reaching out to other people and taking attention off yourself. Use this as a way to take inventory of where you are in your relationships, and where you would like to go. Consider it a working, breathing document, always subject to revision, and notice the effect taking these (sometimes small) actions have on your overall well-being, vitality, and longevity!

ACKNOWLEDGMENT (STATEMENT OF ANOTHER'S VALUE)

You can acknowledge the most significant person in your life or share with an acquaintance. You can even make a difference to a stranger. How about thanking a waiter for excellent service and for making your dinner a pleasant experience? Approach the world and look at where you can thank someone, where can you acknowledge somebody's worth. Bonus points if you acknowledge someone and expect nothing in return.

Who did I acknowledge?
How did that make me feel?
Who could I acknowledge?
Who will I acknowledge?

PRACTICE FORGIVENESS

Forgiveness is an emotional muscle. It needs practice. You may not be able to forgive the stepdad who abused you. You want to start with the person who cut you off on the highway. Start with something small that you can manage. Practice this idea of letting go of anger and forgiving.

Who did I forgive?
Who *could* I forgive?
Who *will* I forgive? (And by when?)

VOLUNTEERING YOUR SERVICES

Helping other people *actually* makes you healthier and happier. You will get more satisfaction out of life and experience better health and less depression. Volunteering is an enormous thing that you can do, not only for the world, but also for yourself, and there are many ways to do it.

Where did I volunteer?
How did it make *me* feel?
Where could I volunteer?
Where *will* I volunteer? (And by when?)

MAKE A GRATITUDE LIST

Make a list of some of the things you're grateful for in life. It can be your relationship, it can be the dogs that you're lucky enough to share space with, it can your home, or the vegetables you grow in your garden. It can be *anything*.

What am I grateful for?
Expand your list … What else am I grateful for?

Read this list *and the expanded list* every day for thirty days. This keeps your mental focus on things that are actually peaceful and happy. You will focus on things that you care about and things that you're grateful for rather than on things you don't have. It's a powerful healing technique.

PERFORM A RANDOM ACT OF KINDNESS

Perform a random act of kindness. *Bonus points if the act of kindness is completely anonymous.* Put a quarter in somebody's meter. Go on the Internet and make a donation to something. Giving back is rewarding to the person doing the giving, as well as the person receiving it.

Where did I perform a random act of kindness?
How did that make *me* feel?
How could I perform a random act of kindness? *Get creative!*
How *will* I manifest a random act of kindness?

PRACTICE MINDFULNESS

Mindfulness is the key to everything from relationships to safety. Practice *noticing*. Practice being mindful. Be present for your life and present in the moment.

In what areas of my life did I stay present and mindful?
What did I notice that was different about this experience?
In what areas of my life could I stay present and mindful?
In what areas of my life will I stay present and mindful?

STAY CONNECTED

Stay connected. *Face-to-face connection.* Nurture your social ties. These can be religious or spiritual affiliations, social groups, family, friends, and animals. It's all about connections.

Who did I connect with?
Who *could* I connect with?
Who *will* I connect with? (And by when?)

Remember to use this workbook as a living, breathing document. It's a work in progress, just like our lives! Use it to monitor what you're doing for yourself (and others) and notice how these steps, taken or intended, can benefit your well-being, energy, vitality, and longevity!

My Longevity Journal

Use these prompts to keep track of the changes you're making in your life in your journal.

Sometimes we're actually taking steps to being healthier without giving ourselves full credit for it. Writing down each thing you're doing helps make it more concrete and real for you. Acknowledge how far you've come—and use this journal as a springboard to go even further, one step at a time.

You can also use this journal to plan future steps you might take in each of the seven key areas of longevity. You may find that small actions might occur to you that would be worth jotting down as goals, such as a one-day fast. Even if you haven't done it yet, put it down in the *future goals* section, and make a game of moving items from the "to-do in the future" list to the "actions accomplished" list!

FIRST PILLAR OF LONGEVITY: FOOD

What things have I done today (or this week) to improve my diet and increase my longevity? These items could be foods that you've added to your diet, changes you've made to your protein intake or calorie consumption, foods that you've eliminated, or any other dietary improvements.

What things might I do in the *near future* that would make a difference in my diet and would increase my energy, vitality, and longevity? (This could be foods you're planning to eat more of, fast food meals you're planning to eliminate, or any other dietary strategy that would represent a step forward.)

SECOND PILLAR OF LONGEVITY: SUPPLEMENTS

What supplements am I taking now on a regular basis? Include everything, even if you're only taking a simple one-a-day formula.

What supplements might I add in the *near future* that would make a difference in my health and overall longevity on a long-term basis? Consider the basic ones discussed in this book, especially in section II, and others that seem like they make sense. Think about any supplements you may have taken in the past and whether they made you feel better. If so, in what way? Include those as well.

THIRD PILLAR OF LONGEVITY: DETOXIFICATION

What things have I done today (or this week) to reduce my exposure to toxins? This could include switching to a "green" laundry detergent or organic strawberries, for example. Think about the various toxins you are exposed to on a daily basis—food, water, air, even relationships!—and see what steps you've already taken to reduce their effects.

What things might I do in the *near future* that would further reduce my exposure to toxins, or that would support detoxification pathways in my own body? This could include things like dry skin brushing, an infrared sauna, or going on a one-week detox diet. It could also include taking liver support supplements such as milk thistle or alpha-lipoic acid. What might I do that could increase my energy, vitality, and longevity?

FOURTH PILLAR OF LONGEVITY: EXERCISE

What things have I done today (or this week) for exercise? You can include any activity at all; remember, it all starts with small steps. If you walked from the bus stop, put it in. If you gardened today, put it in. Or, if you're already a "gym rat," put down what you've done. Be specific. How many minutes did you walk/jog? Did you lift weights? What exercises? How many reps? Did you play tennis? You may find that you actually spend more time away from your desk than you thought. Use this part of the journal to acknowledge that.

What things might I do in the *near future* that would make a difference in my exercise or activity level and would increase my energy, vitality, and longevity? This could be anything from "park farther from the office and walk across the parking lot" to "run a marathon." It could be an extra ten pounds on your bench press or an extra fifteen minutes of gardening. Anything that adds to the total load of activity could be used in this section as a future goal. Have fun!

FIFTH PILLAR OF LONGEVITY: SLEEP

What things have I done today (or this week) to improve the quality of my sleep? This can include going to bed an hour earlier, banning the computer from the bedroom, or any other strategy to increase the quality (and quantity) of your sleep.

What things might I do in the *near future* that would improve my sleep? This could include anything from buying a new mattress to banning the television from the bedroom, or any other strategy to increase the quantity and quality of your sleep and increase your energy, vitality, and longevity.

SIXTH PILLAR OF LONGEVITY: STRESS REDUCTION

What things have I done today (or this week) to reduce my stress? This can include anything from organizing your inbox to taking a five-minute deep breathing break. It can also include bigger things such as removing a toxic relationship from your life or setting boundaries on one that's causing you stress.

What things might I do in the *near future* that would reduce my stress and increase my energy, vitality, and longevity?

SEVENTH PILLAR OF LONGEVITY: EMOTIONAL INTELLIGENCE

What things have I done today (or this week) that have the potential to improve the quality of my relationships—with people, my community, and the world around me—and ultimately improve my well-being?

What things might I do in the *near future* that would improve my relationships with others, myself, my community, and the world around me? This could include anything from donating time (or money) to volunteering. It can also include any increased efforts to reach out to other people in your life—be they family, friends, strangers, or animals!

Remember to use this workbook as a living, breathing document. It's a work in progress, just like our lives! Use it to monitor what you're doing for yourself or, in some cases, others, and notice how these steps, taken or intended, can benefit your well-being, energy, vitality, and longevity!

Resources

· ·

BRAIN

Amen, Daniel. *Change Your Brain, Change Your Life*. New York: Three Rivers Press, 1999.

Amen, Daniel. *Magnificent Mind at Any Age*. New York: Harmony, 2008.

Khalsa, M.D., Dharma Singh and Cameron Stauth. *Brain Longevity*. New York: Grand Central Publishing, 1999.

McCleary, Larry. *The Brain Trust Program*. New York: Perigee Trade, 2007.

Perlmutter, David, and Carol Colman. *The Better Brain Book*. New York: Riverhead, 2005.

EMOTIONAL INTELLIGENCE

Buettner, Dan. *The Blue Zones*. National Geographic, 2009. www.bluezone.com

HEART

Houston, M.D., Mark with Barry Fox, Ph.D. and Nadine Taylor, M.S., R.D. *What Your Doctor May Not Tell You About Hypertension*. Warner Books, 2003.

Sinatra, M.D., Stephen and James Roberts M.D. *Reverse Heart Disease Now*. Hoboken, NJ: Wiley and Sons, 2007.

Stoll, M.D., Andrew L. *The Omega-3 Connection*. New York: Fireside, 2001.

Oz, M.D., Mehmet C. and Dean Ornish. *Healing from the Heart*. New York: Plume, 1999.

HORMONES

Bowden, Jonny. *Living Low Carb*. New York: Sterling, 2010.

Brownstein, David. *Overcoming Thyroid Disorders*. West Bloomfield, MI: Medical Alternatives Press, 2002.

Daniel, Kaayla T. *The Whole Soy Story*. Winona Lake, IN: New Trends, 2005.

Gittleman, Ann Louise. *Before the Change*. Harper Collins, 1998

Northrup, Christiane. *The Wisdom of Menopause*. New York: Bantam, 2001.

Parker-Pope, Tara. *The Hormone Decision*. Emmaus, PA: Rodale, 2007.

Reiss, Uzzi. *Natural Hormone Balance for Women*. New York: Atria, 2002.

Sarrel, Philip. "Women's Health Initiative Study on HRT Stopped: What the News Means to You." He@lthLINK, Yale-New Haven Hospital.

Schwartz, Erika. *The 30-Day Natural Hormone Plan*. New York: Grand Central Publishing, 2005.

Schwartz, Erika. *The Hormone Solution*. New York: Grand Central Publishing, 2002.

Shames, Richard, and Karilee H. Shames. *Thyroid Power*. New York: Collins Living, 2002.

Sholomon, Mary. *Living Well with Hypothyroidism*. New York: HarperCollins, 2000.

INFLAMATION

Cannon, Christopher P. and Elizabeth Vierck. *The Complete Idiot's Guide to the Anti-Inflammation Diet*. Alpha, 2006.

Sears, Barry. *The Anti-Inflammation Zone*. Harper Paperbacks, 2005.

THE MEDITERRANEAN DIET

Acquista, Angelo. *The Mediterranean Prescription*. New York: Ballantine, 2006.

Schulman, Martha Rose. *Mediterranean Light*. New York: William Morrow, 2000.

Simopoulos, Artemis P. and Jo Robinson. *The Omega Diet*. New York: Collins Living, 1999.

MUSCLES, BONES, AND JOINTS

Knopf, Karl. *Stretching for 50+*. Berkeley, CA: Ulysses Press, 2005.

Knopf, Karl. *Weights for 50+*. Berkeley, CA: Ulysses Press, 2005.

Lanou, Ph.D., Amy and Michael Castleman. *Building Bone Vitality*. McGraw-Hill, 2009.

McCormick, R. Keith. *The Whole-Body Approach to Osteoporosis*. Oakland, CA: New Harbinger, 2009.

Nelson, Miriam. *Strong Women, Strong Bones*, updated edition. New York: Perigee, 2006.

Neporent, Liz, Suzanne Schlosberg, and Shirley Archer. *Weight Training for Dummies*. Indianapolis, IN: Wiley, 2006.

Sanson, Gillian. *The Myth of Osteoporosis*. Ann Arbor, MI: MCD Century Publications, 2003.

Schlosberg, Suzanne and Liz Neporent. *Fitness for Dummies*. Hoboken, NJ: Wiley, 2005.

Weatherby, Craig, and Leonid Gordin. *The Arthritis Bible*. Rochester, VT: Healing Arts Press, 1999.

Westcott, Wayne, and Thomas R. Baechle. *Strength Training Past 50*. Champaign, IL: Human Kinetics, 1997.

Doctors and Clinics Specializing in Hormone Replacement and Anti-Aging

Ann Louise Gittleman, Ph.D., C.N.S
UniKey Health Systems, Inc.
181 West Commerce Drive
Hayden, ID 83835
800-888-4353, www.unikeyhealth.com

David Leonardi, M.D.
Leonardi Executive Health Institute
8400 E. Prentice Avenue, Suite 700
Greenwood Village, CO 80111
303-462-5344, www.go2lehi.com

Prudence Hall, M.D.
The Hall Center
1148 4th Street
Santa Monica, CA 90403
866-933-HALL, www.thehallcenter.com

Preventative Medical Center of Marin
Elson M. Haas, M.D.
25 Mitchell Blvd., Suite 8
San Rafael, CA 94903
415-472-2343, www.pmcmarin.com, www.elsonhaas.com
(This is an Integrated Medicine Clinic that accepts insurance.)

Erika Schwartz, M.D.
10 West 74th Street
New York City, NY 10023
866-373-7452, www.drerika.com

Beth Traynor, M.D.
Cenegenics Medical Institute
851 South Rampart Boulevard, Suite 100
Las Vegas, NV 89145
866-694-1080
www.cenegenics.com

For more recommendations, go to the Institute for
    Functional Medicine (ww.ifm.org) and click "find
    a practitioner."

Endnotes

· ·

Section I: Rein in the Four Horsemen of Aging

1. U.S. Centers for Disease Control and Prevention, *National Vital Statistics Reports* 54, no. 13 (April 19, 2006).

2. Yusuf, S., S. Hawken, S. Ounpuu, et al. on behalf of the INTERHEART Study Investigators. Effect of potentially modifiable risk factors associated with myocardial infarction in 52 countries (the INTERHEART study): case-control study. *Lancet* 364 (2004): 937–952.

3. Doll, R. and R. Peto. The causes of cancer: Quantitative estimates of avoidable risks of cancer in the United States today. *J Natl Cancer Inst* 66, no. 6 (1981): 1191–1308.

4. "Cancer Prevention Tied to Diet and Way of Life," *New York Times,* Nov. 20, 1996.

5. "Diet and Cancer Research," The Cancer Project, www.cancerproject.org/diet_cancer/facts/major_killers.php.

6. "Heart Disease and Stroke," Canadian Diabetes Association, www.diabetes.ca/about-diabetes/living/complications/heart-disease-stroke.

7. Stampfer, M., F. Hu, J. E. Manson, E. B. Rimm, and W. C. Willett. Primary prevention of coronary heart disease in women through diet and lifestyle. *N Eng J Med* 343, no. 1 (July 6, 2000): 16–22.

8. Institute for Functional Medicine. *Textbook of Functional Medicine,* 2005.

9. Vita, A. J., R. B. Terry, H. B. Hubert, and J. F. Fries. Aging, health risks, and cumulative disability. *N Eng J Med* 338, no. 15 (1998): 1035–41.

10. Campion, E.W. Aging better. *N Eng J Med* 338, no. 15 (1998): 1064–66.

Chapter 1: Fight the First Horseman of Aging—Free Radicals

1. McCall, M. R., and B. Frei. Can antioxidant vitamins materially reduce oxidative damage in humans? *Free Radic Biol Med* 26 no. 7-8 (1999): 1034–53.

2. Halliwell, B. Oxygen and nitrogen are pro-carcinogens. Damage to DNA by reactive oxygen, chlorine and nitrogen species: measurement, mechanism and effects of nutrition. *Mutat Res* 443 (1999): 37–52.

3. Valkon M., M. Izakovic, M. Mazur, C. J. Rhodes, and J. Telser. Role of oxygen radicals in DNA damage and cancer incidence. *Mol Cell Biochem* 266 (2004): 37–56.

4. Aslan, M., and T. Ozben. Reactive oxygen and nitrogen species in Alzheimer's disease. *Curr Alzheimer Res.* 1 (2004): 111–119.

5. Ryan-Harshman, M., and W. Aldoori. The relevance of selenium to immunity, cancer, and infectious/inflammatory diseases. *Can J Diet Prac Res* 66 (2005): 98–102.

6. Harman, D. Nutritional implications of the free-radical theory of aging. *J Am Coll Nutr* 1 (1982): 27–34.

7. Pesticide Data Program, Annual Summary: Calendar Year 2005, United States Department of Agriculture, 2006.

8. Blatt, Harvey. *America's Food: What You Don't Know About What You Eat.* MIT Press, 2008.

9. "National Report on Human Exposure to Environmental Chemicals," Centers for Disease Control and Prevention, http://www.cdc.gov/exposurereport.

10. "Pesticides in Produce," Environmental Working Group, 2006, foodnews.org/walletguide.php.

11. Knight, J. A. The biochemistry of aging. *Adv Clin Chem* 35 (2000): 1–62.

12. Polidori, M. C., E. Mariani, G. Baggio, et al. Different antioxidant profiles in Italian centenarians: the Sardinian peculiarity. *Eur J Clin Nutr* 61, no. 7 (Jul 2007): 922–4.

13. Mecocci, P., M. C. Polidori, L. Troiano, et al. Plasma antioxidants and longevity: A study on healthy centenarians. *Free Radic Biol Med* 29, no. 5 (Sep 1, 2000): 486.

14. McBride, Judy. "High-ORAC Foods May Slow Aging," USDA Agriculture Research Service.

15. Pelligrini, N., M. Seafini, B. Colombi, et al. Antioxidant capacity of plant foods, beverages and oils consumed in Italy assessed by three different assays. *J Nutr* 133 (September 2003): 2812–2819.

16. Prior, R.L., L. Gu, et al. Plasma antioxidant capacity changes following a meal as a measure of the ability to alter in vivo antioxidant status. *J Am Coll Nutr* 26 (2): 170–181.

Chapter 2: Put out the Fire of the Second Horseman of Aging—Inflammation

1. Mora, S., and P. M. Ridker. Justification for the use of statins in primary prevention. *Am J Cardiol* 97, no. 2A (2006): 33A–41A.

2. Simopoulos, A. P. Evolutionary aspects of diet, the omega-6/omega-3 ratio and genetic variation: Nutritional implications for chronic diseases. *Biomed Pharmacother* 60, no. 9 (November 2006): 502–07.

3. Knight, J. A. The biochemistry of aging. *Adv Clin Chem* 35 (2000): 1–62.

4. Brod, S. A. Unregulated inflammation shortens human functional longevity. *Inflamm Res* 49, no. 11 (November 2000): 561–70. Review.

5. Stanner, Sara, Keith N. Frayn, and British Nutrition Foundation. *Cardiovascular Disease: Diet Nutrition and Emerging Risk Factors: The Report of A British Nutrition Foundation Task Force,* Blackwell, 2005.

6. Ibid.

7. "Inflammation, Heart Disease and Stroke: The Role of C-Reactive Protein," American Heart Association.

Chapter 3: Avoid the Damage of the Third Horseman of Aging—Glycation

1. Vlassara, H., W. Cai, J. Crandall, et al. Inflammatory mediators are induced by dietary glycotoxins, a major risk factor for diabetic angiopathy. *Proc Natl Acad Sci USA* 99, no. 24 (Nov. 26, 2002): 15596–601.

2. "Why Antioxidants Aren't Enough," *Life Extension Magazine*, January 2002.

3. "Carnosine: Nature's pluripotent life extension agent," *Life Extension Magazine*, January 2001.

Chapter 5: How Much Influence Do Genes Have on the Four Horsemen of Aging?

1. Zhang, J., J. Asin-Cayuela, J. Fish, et al. Strikingly higher frequency in centenarians and twins of mtDNA mutation causing remodeling of replication origin in leukocytes. *Proc Natl Acad Sci USA* 100, no. 3 (Feb 4, 2003): 1116–1121.

2. Yu, B. P., E. J. Masoro, I. Murata, et al. Life span study of SPF Fischer 344 male rats fed ad libitum or restricted diets: Longevity, growth, lean body mass and disease. *J Gerontol* 37, no. 2 (March 1982): 130–41.

3. Hursting, S. D., J. A. Lavigne, D. Berrigan, et al. Calorie restriction, aging, and cancer prevention: Mechanisms of action and applicability to humans. *Annu Rev Med* 54 (2003): 131–152.

Section II: How to Keep the Key Players in Your Body Fit

1. Carey, Benedict. "At the Bridge Table, Clues to a Lucid Old Age," *New York Times*, May 22, 2009.

Chapter 6: Start with the Seven Pillars of Longevity

1. Dauchet, L., P. Amouyel, S. Hercberg, and J. Dallongeville. Fruit and vegetable consumption and risk of coronary heart disease: A meta-analysis of cohort studies. *J Nutr* 136 (October 2006): 2588–2593.

2. *The World Health Report 2002: Reducing Risks, Promoting Health.* Geneva: World Health Organization, 2002.

3. "Diet, Nutrition and the Prevention of Chronic Diseases." Report of a Joint FAO/WHO Expert Consultation. Geneva World Health Organization, 2003 (WHO Technical Report Series No. 916).

4. Jiamton, S., J. Pepin, R. Suttent, et al. A randomized trial of the impact of multiple micronutrient supplementation on mortality among HIV-infected individuals living in Bangkok. *AIDS* 17, no. 17 (2003): 2461–9.

5. Watkins, M. L., J. D. Erickson, M. J. Thun, et al. Multivitamin use and mortality in a large prospective study. *Am J Epidemiol* 152, no. 2 (Jul. 15, 2000): 149–162.

6. Dickerson, Annette. "Benefits of Nutritional Supplements," Council for Responsible Nutrition, 2002, www.crnusa.org/benefits.html.

7. Fletcher, R. H. and K. M. Fairfield. Vitamins for chronic disease prevention in adults: Clinical applications. *JAMA* 287 (2002): 3127–3129.

8. Shankle, W. R. and D. G. Amen. *Preventing Alzheimer's: Ways to Help Prevent, Delay, Detect, and Even Halt Alzheimer's Disease and Other Forms of Memory Loss.* New York: G. P. Putnam's Sons, 2004.

9. Bartholomew, J. B., D. Morrison, and J. T. Ciccolo. Effects of acute exercise on mood and well-being in patients with major depressive disorder. *Med Sci Sports Exer* 37, no. 12 (December 2005): 2032–7.

10. Pereira, A. C., D. E. Huddleston, A. M. Brickman, et al. An in vivo correlate of exercise-induced neurogenesis in the adult dentate gyrus. *Proc Natl Acad Sci USA* 104, no. 13 (March 27, 2007): 5638–5643.

11. Erickson, K. I., R. S. Prakash, M. W. Voss, et al. Aerobic fitness is associated with hippocampal volume in elderly humans. *Hippocampus*, Jan 2, 2009.

12. Demet, W. C. and C. C. Vaughan. *The Promise of Sleep.* New York: Delacorte Press, 1999: 274.

13. Spiegel, K., R. Leproult, and E. Van Cauter. Impact of sleep debt on metabolic and endocrine function. *Lancet.* 354, no. 9188 (1999): 1425–9.

14. Taheri, S., L. Lin, D. Austin, et al. Short sleep duration is associated with reduced leptin, elevated ghrelin, and increased body mass index. *PLoS Med* 1, no. 3 (December 2004): e62.

15. Spiegel, K., J. F. Sheridan, and E. Van Cauter. Effect of sleep deprivation on response to immunization. *JAMA* 288 (2002): 1471–2.

Chapter 7: Keep Your Heart in Shape

1. "Top 10 Causes of Death," WHO (World Health Organization), 2005.

2. "Leading Causes of Death," Centers for Disease Control and Prevention, 2005.

3. Kris-Etherton, P., R. Eckel, B. Howard, et al. Lyon Diet Heart Study. *Circulation* 103 (2001): 1823.

4. Panagiotakos, D., C. Pitsavos, and C. Stefanadis. Inclusion of dietary evaluation in cardiovascular disease risk prediction models increases accuracy and reduces bias of the estimations. *Risk Analysis* 29, no. 2 (2009).

5. Hu, Willet. Optimal diets for prevention of coronary heart disease. *JAMA* 288 (2002): 2569–2578.

6. "Stick To Wild Salmon Unless Heart Disease Is A Risk Factor, Risk-Benefit Analysis Of Farmed And Wild Fish Shows," Science Daily, www.sciencedaily.com/releases/2005/12/051226100222.htm.

7. "Results from Tests of Store-bought Farmed Salmon Show Seven of 10 Fish were so Contaminated with PCBs that they Raise Cancer Risk," Environmental Working Group, http://www.ewg.org/reports/farmedpcbs.

8. "Stick To Wild Salmon Unless Heart Disease Is A Risk Factor, Risk-Benefit Analysis Of Farmed And Wild Fish Shows," Science Daily, www.sciencedaily.com/releases/2005/12/051226100222.htm.

9. "Omega 3 in Fish: How Eating Fish Helps Your Heart," Mayo Clinic website, www.mayoclinic.com/health/omega-3/HB00087

10. Xue, M., Q. Qian, A. Adaikalakoteswari, et al. Activation of NF-E2-related factor-2 reverses biochemical dysfunction of endothelial cells induced by hyperglycemia linked to vascular disease. *Diabetes* 57, no. 10 (2008): 2809-17.

11. Menotti, A., D. Kromhout, H. Blackburn, et al. Food intake patterns and 25-year mortality from coronary heart disease: Cross-cultural correlations in the seven countries study. The Seven Countries Study Research Group. *European Journal of Epidemiology* 15, no. 6 (July 1999): 507–15.

12. Bazzano, L. A., J. He, L. G. Ogden, et al. Dietary fiber intake and reduced risk of coronary heart disease in U.S. men and women: the National Health and Nutrition Examination Survey I Epidemiologic Follow-up Study. *Arch Intern Med* 163, no. 16 (Sep 8, 2003): 1897–904.

13. "Blueberries: Colorful Protection for a Healthier Heart, Sharper Brain and Cancer Defense," Lyon, *Life Extension Magazine* Feb 2009.

14. Kalea, A., F. Lamari, A. Theocharis, et al. Wild blueberry (*Vaccinium angustifolium*) consumption affects the composition and structure of glycosaminoglycans in Sprague-Dawley rat aorta. *J. Nutritional Biochemistry* 17, no. 2 (Feb 17, 2006): 109–116.

15. Medicinal Food, Spring 2005; 8(1):8–13.

16. Nutrition Reviews, May 8, 2001.

17. Penn State Science Blog, May 2001.

18. Kris-Etherton, et al. Nuts and their bioactive constituents. *Am J Clinical Nutrition* 70, no 3, (September 1999): 504S–511S.

19. "Pomegranate Juice Could Benefit Diabetes," Newswise, www.newswise.com/articles/view/522980.

20. Bucco, Gloria. "Kilmer McCully, M.D., Connects Homocysteine and Heart Disease," *Nutrition Science News,* July 1999.

21. Stacey, Michelle. "The Fall and Rise of Kilmer McCully," *The New York Times,* Aug 10, 1997.

22. Rowe, M.D., John and Robert Kahn, Ph.D. *Successful Aging.* New York: Dell, 1998.

23. Stanner, Sara, ed. "Homocysteine" in *Cardiovascular Disease: Diet Nutrition and Emerging Risk Factors: The Report of the British Nutrition Foundation Task Force,* Blackwell Publishing, 2005.

24. SEARCH Study Collaborative Group, L. Bowman, J. Armitage, et al. Study of the effectiveness of additional reductions in cholesterol and homocysteine (SEARCH). *Am Heart J* 154, no. 5 (Nov 2007): 815–23.

25. Spence, J., H. Bang, L. Chambless, et al. Vitamin intervention for stroke prevention trial: An efficacy analysis, original contributions. *Stroke* 36, no. 11 (Nov 1, 2005): 2404-2409.

26. Stampfer, M. J., M. R. Malinow, W. C. Willett, et al. A prospective study of plasma homocyst(e)ine and risk of myocardial infarction in U.S. physicians. *JAMA* 268, no. 7 (Aug 1992): 877–81.

27. Nygård, O., J. Nordrehaug, H. Refsum, et al. Plasma homocysteine levels and mortality in patients with coronary artery disease. *NEJM* 337 (July 24, 1997): 230–237.

28. Koenig, W., M. Sund, M. Frohlich, et al. C-Reactive protein, a sensitive marker of inflammation, predicts future risk of coronary heart disease in initially healthy middle-aged men: results from the MONICA (Monitoring Trends and Determinants in Cardiovascular Disease) Augsburg Cohort Study, 1984 to 1992. *Circulation* 99, no. 2 (Jan 19, 1999): 237–42.

29. Bassuk, S. S., N. Rifai, and P. M. Ridker. High-sensitivity C-reactive protein: Clinical importance. *Current Problems in Cardiology* 29, no. 8 (Aug 2004): 439–93.

30. Cushman, M., A. M. Arnold, B. M. Psaty, et al. C-reactive protein and the 10-year incidence of coronary heart disease in older men and women: The Cardiovascular Health Study. *Circulation* 112, no. 1 (Jul 5, 2005): 25–31.

31. Addison, *Can Med Assoc J*, 18: 281–285, 1928, cited in *Modern Nutrition in Health and Disease*, vol 2, 8th ed. Shils, Olson, Shike, eds. Lea and Febiger, 1994, p 1290.

32. Houston, et al. *What Your Doctor May Not Tell You About Hypertension.* Warner Books, 2003.

33. Hu, et al. Fish and omega-3 fatty acid intake and risk of coronary heart disease in women. *JAMA* 287, no. 14 (2002): 1815–1821.

34. Albert, C., H. Campos, M. Stampfer, et al. Blood levels of long-chain n-3 fatty acids and the risk of sudden death. *NEJM* 346 (April 11, 2002): 1113–1118.

35. Marchioli, R., F. Barzi, E. Bomba, et al. Early protection against sudden death by n-3 polyunsaturated fatty acids after myocardial infarction. *Circulation* 105 (2002): 1897-903.

36. Langsjoen, Peter H. "Introduction to Coenzyme Q10," http://faculty.washington.edu/ely/coenzq10.html.

37. Sinatra, S. *Reverse Heart Disease Now.* Hoboken, NJ: Wiley and Sons, 2007.

38. Breithaupt-Grogler, K., M. Ling, H. Boudoulas, and G. G. Belz. Protective effect of chronic garlic intake on elastic properties of aorta in the elderly. *Circulation* 96 (1997): 2649–55.

39. Kuriyama, S., T Shimazu, K. Ohmori, et al. Green tea consumption and mortality due to cardiovascular disease, cancer, and all causes in Japan: The Ohsaki Study. *JAMA* 296, no. 10 (Sep. 13, 2006): 1255–65.

40. Kim, J. A., G. Formoso, Y. Li, et al. Epigallocatechin gallate, a green tea polyphenol, mediates NO-dependent vasodilation using signaling pathways in vascular endothelium requiring reactive oxygen species and fyn. *J Biol Chem* 282, no. 18 (May 4, 2007): 13736–45.

41. Antonello, M., D. Montemurro, M. Bolognesi, et al. Prevention of hypertension, cardiovascular damage and endothelial dysfunction with green tea extracts. *Am J Hypertens* 20, no. 12 (December 2007): 1321–8.

42. Yang, Y. C., F. H. Lu, J. S. Wu, et al. The protective effect of habitual tea consumption on hypertension. *Arch Intern Med* 164, no. 14 (July 26, 2004): 1534–40.

43. Sato, Y., H. Nakatsuka, T. Watanabe, et al. Possible contribution of green tea drinking habits to the prevention of stroke. *Tohoku J Exp*

Med 157, no. 4 (April 1989): 337–43.

44. Suzuki, M., M. Tabuchi, M. Ikeda, et al. Protective effects of green tea catechins on cerebral ischemic damage. *Med Sci Monit* 10, no. 6 (June 2004): BR166–74.

45. Sutherland, B. A., O. M. Shaw, A. N. Clarkson, et al. Neuroprotective effects of (-)-epigallocatechin gallate following hypoxia-ischemia-induced brain damage: Novel mechanisms of action. *FASEB J* 19, no. 2 (February 2005): 258–60.

46. Choi, Y. B., Y. I. Kim, K. S. Lee, et al. Protective effect of epigallocatechin gallate on brain damage after transient middle cerebral artery occlusion in rats. *Brain Res* 1019, no. 1-2 (Sep. 3, 2004): 47–54.

Chapter 8: How to Keep Your Brain Sharp

1. Colcombe, S. J., K. I. Erickson, P. E. Scalf, et al. Aerobic exercise training increases brain volume in aging humans. *J Gerontol A Biol Sci Med Sci* 61, (2006): 1166–1170.

2. Greendale, G., D. Kritz-Silverstein, T. Seeman, et al. Higher basal cortisol predicts verbal memory loss in postmenopausal women: Rancho Bernardo study. *Journal of the American Geriatrics Society* 48 (2000): 1655–1658.

3. "Mayo Clinic research shows that improving brain processing speed helps memory," *Life Extension Daily*, Feb. 11, 2009.

4. Lupien, S., M. de Leon, S. de Santi, et al. Cortisol levels during human aging predict hippocampal atrophy and memory deficits. *Nature Neuroscience* May 1998.

5. de Quervain, D. J., B. Roozendaal, R. M. Nitsch, et al. Acute cortisone administration impairs retrieval of long-term declarative memory in humans. *Nature Neuroscience* 3 (2000): 313-314.

6. Esch, T., G. B. Stefano, G. L. Fricchione, et al. The role of stress in neurodegenerative diseases and mental disorders. *Neuoro Endocrinology Letters* 23, no. 3 (June 2002): 199–208.

7. Xu, W., C. Qiu, B. Winblad, et al. The effect of borderline diabetes on the risk of dementia and Alzheimer's disease. *Diabetes* 56 (2007): 211–216.

8. "Salk study links diabetes and Alzheimer's disease," Salk Institute, May 15, 2008, www.salk.edu/news/pressrelease_details.php?press_id=221.

9. "Omega-3 fatty acids," University of Maryland Medical Center, www.umm.edu/altmed/articles/omega-3-000316.htm.

10. Scarmeas, N., Y. Stern, R. Mayeux, et al. Mediterranean diet and mild cognitive impairment. *Arch Neurol* 66, no. 2 (2009): 216–225.

11. Shukla, P. K., V. Khanna, M. Khan, et al. Protective effect of curcumin against lead neurotoxicity in rats. *Human & Experimental Toxicology* 22 (2003): 653–58.

12. Ammon, H. P., H. Safayhi, T. Mack, et al. Mechanism of anti-inflammatory actions of curcumine and boswellic acids. *J Ethnopharmacol* 38, no. 2-3 (1993): 113–119.

13. Yang, F., G. P. Lim, A. N. Begum, et al. Curcumin inhibits formation of amyloid {beta}oligomers and fibrils, binds plaques, and reduces amyloid in vivo. *J Biol Chem* 280 (2005): 5892–5901.

14. Ono, K., K. Hasegawa, H. Naiki, et al. Curcumin has potent anti-amyloidogenic effects for Alzheimer's beta-amyloid fibrils in vitro. *J Neurosci Res* 75 (2004): 742–50.

15. Chandra, V., R. Pandav, H. H. Dodge, et al. Incidence of Alzheimer's disease in a rural community in India: The Indo-U.S. study. *Neurology* 57, no. 6 (2001): 985–989.

16. Kedar, N. P. Can we prevent Parkinson's and Alzheimer's disease? *Journal of Postgraduate Medicine* 49, no. 3 (July–September 2003): 236–245.

17. Milgram, N. W., J. A. Araujo, T. M. Hagen, et al. Acetyl-l-carnitine and alpha-lipoic acid supplementation of aged beagle dogs improves learning in two landmark discrimination tests. *FASEB J* 21, no. 13 (2007): 3756–3762.

18. Brooks, J., J. Yesavage, A. Carta, et al. Acetyl-l-carnitine slows decline in younger patients with Alzheimer's disease. *International Psychogeriatric Association* 10 (1998): 193–203.

19. Ames, B. N. and J. Liu. Delaying the mitochondrial decay of aging with acety-l-carnitine. *Ann N Y Acad Sci* 1033 (2004): 108–116.

20. The Hospital for Sick Children, press release. "Canadian kids don't get enough vitamin d," May 4, 2009.

21. Maalouf, J., M. Nabulsi, R. Vieth, et al. Short- and Long-Term Safety of Weekly High-Dose Vitamin D3 Supplementation in School Children. J *Clin Endocrinol Metab* 93, no. 7: 2693-2701.

22. National Osteoporosis Foundation website, www.nof.org/prevention/vitaminD.htm.

23. Cannell, J. "Questions and Answers about Vitamin D supplementation." *Townsend Newsletter*, November 2006.

24. "Vitamin D and your Health: Deficiency," Vitamin D Council, www.vitamindcouncil.org/health/deficiency/am-i-vitamin-d-deficient.shtml.

25. Bone, Kerry. "Amazing New Uses for an Old Herbal Standby," *Nutrition and Healing*, November 2008, www.wrightnewsletter.com.

26. "Dietary Supplement Fact Sheet: Vitamin B12," Office of Dietary Supplements, National Institutes of Health, http://ods.od.nih.gov/factsheets/vitaminb12.asp.

27. Carmel, R. Megaloblastic anemias. *Current Opinion in Hematology* 1 (1994): 107–12.

28. Hendler, Sheldon and David Rorvik. *Physicans' Desk Reference for Nutritional Supplements*, 2nd edition. Physicians' Desk Reference, Inc., 2008.

29. Oudshoorn, C., F. U. Mattace-Rasu, N. van der Velde, et al. Higher serum vitamin D3 levels are associated with better cognitive test performance in patients with Alzheimer's disease. *Dement Geriatr Cogn Disord* 25, no. 6 (2008): 539–43.

30. Perlmutter, David, and Carol Colman, *The Better Brain Book*, Berkley Publishing Group, 2004.

31. Balestreri, R., L. Fontana, and F. Astengo. A double-blind placebo controlled evaluation of the safety and efficacy of vinpocetine in the treatment of patients with chronic vascular senile cerebral dysfunction. *J Am Geriatr Soc* 35, no. 5 (May 1987): 425–430.

32. Witte, A.V., M. Fobker, R. Gellner, et al. Caloric restriction improves memory in elderly humans. *Proc Natl Acad Sci USA 106*, no. 4 (Jan. 27, 2009): 1255-60.

Chapter 9: How to Protect and Maintain Strong Bones, Muscles, and Joints

1. Janssen, I., D. S. Shephard, P. T. Katzmarzyk, et al. The healthcare costs of sarcopenia in the United States. *J Am Geriatr Soc 52*, no. 1 (Dec 24, 2003): 80–85.

2. "Baseball's Money Business on the Upswing," *USA Today*, Nov. 11, 2006.

3. "Orthopaedic Surgery: Hip Fracture," University of Virginia Health System, www.healthsystem.virginia.edu/uvahealth/adult_orthopaedics/hipfract.cfm.

4. Green, C.J., K. Bassett, V. Foerster, et al. Bone mineral density testing: Does the evidence support its selective use in well women? British Columbia Office of Health Technology Assessment, Sep. 1998, *www.chspr.ubc.ca*.

5. "D-bunking the role of vitamin d in bone health," American Medical Women's Association, www.amwa-doc.org/index.cfm?objectid=97141F72-D567-0B25-5E6E71C12C78F497.

6. National and state medical expenditures and lost earnings attributable to arthritis and other rheumatoid conditions—United States, 2003. *Morbidity and Mortality Weekly Report 56*, no.01 (2007): 4–7.

7. Maetzel A., L. C. Li, J. Pencharz, et al. The economic burden associated with osteoarthritis, rheumatoid arthritis, and hypertension: A comparative study. *Ann Rheum Dis 63*, no. 4 (2004): 395–401.

8. "Cox-2 Inhibitors," MedicineNet.com, www.medicinenet.com/cox-2_inhibitors/article.htm.

9. Reginster, J. Y., R. Deroisy, L. C. Rovati, et al. Long-term effects of glucosamine sulfate on osteoarthritis progression: A randomized, placebo-controlled clinical trial. *Lancet 357*, no. 9252 (2001): 251–256.

10. Pavelká, K., J. Gatterová, M. Olejarová, et al. Glucosamine sulfate use and delay of progression of knee osteoarthritis: A three-year, randomized, placebo-controlled, double-blind study. *Arch Intern Med 162*, no. 16 (2002): 2113–2123.

11. McAlindon, T., M. LaValley, J. Gulin, et al. Glucosamine and chondroitin for treatment of osteoarthritis: A systematic quality assessment and meta-analysis. *JAMA 283*, no. 11 (2000): 1469–1475.

12. Coates, Paul, ed. *Encyclopedia of Dietary Supplements*, National Institute of Health, Marcel Dekker, 2005.

13. Ibid.

14. Stenlake, Richard. "How Do Glucosamine and Chondroitin Work," The Arthritis & Glucosamine Information Center.

15. Ibid.

16. Coates, Paul, ed. *Encyclopedia of Dietary Supplements*, National Institute of Health, Marcel Dekker, 2005.

17. Messier, S., D. J. Gutekunst, C. Davis, et al. Weight loss reduces knee-joint loads in overweight and obese older adults with knee osteoarthritis. *Arthritis & Rheum 52*, no. 7 (July 2005): 2026-32.

18. Felson, D., Y. Zhang, J. M. Anthony, et al. Weight loss reduces the risk for symptomatic knee osteoarthritis in women. *Ann Intern Med 116* (1992): 535–539.

Chapter 10: Boost Your Immune System

1. Segerstrom, S., S. Taylor, M. Kemeny, et al. Optimism is associated with mood, coping, and immune change in response to stress. *J of Personality and Soc Psychology 74*, no. 6 (June 1998): 1646–1655.

2. Wachi, M., M. Koyama, M. Utsuyama, et al. Recreational music-making modulates natural killer cell activity, cytokines and mood states in corporate employees. *Med Sci Monit 13*, no. 2 (Feb 2007): CR57–70.

3. "Theraputic Benefits of Laughter," Holisticonline, www.holistic-online.com/Humor_Therapy/humor_therapy_benefits.htm.

4. Head, J. F., F. Wang, R. L. Elliott, et al. *Ann N Y Acad Sci 690* (1993): 340–342.

5. Levy, S. M., R. B. Herberman, M. Lippman, et al. Immunological and psychosocial predictors of disease recurrence in patients with early-stage breast cancer. *Behav Med 17*, no 2 (1991): 67–75.

6. David Serban-Schreiber, *Anti-Cancer: A New Way of Life*, Viking Penguin, 2008.

7. Chandra, R. K. Effect of vitamin and trace-element supplementation on immune responses and infection in elderly subjects. *Lancet 340* (1992): 1124–1127.

8. Chandra, R. K. Nutrition, immunity and outcome: Past, present and future. 11th Gopalan Gold Medal Oration. *Nutr Res 8* (1988): 225–237.

9. Bogden, J. D., A. Bendich, F. W. Kemp, et al. Daily micronutrient supplements enhance delayed-hypersensitivity skin test responses in older people. *Am J Clin Nutr 60* (1994): 437–447.

10. Foote, J., A. Giuliano, and R. Harris. Older adults need guidance to meet nutritional recommendations. *J Am Coll Nutr 19* (2000): 628–640.

11. "Diet, Exercise, Stress and the Immune System," Cleveland Clinic website, accessed March 15, 2009.

12. Institute of Medicine, P.O.M. *Dietary Reference Intakes*, National Academy Press: Washington, DC, 2002.

13. Wintergerst, E. S., S. Maggini, and D. H. Hornig. Contribution of selected vitamins and trace elements to immune function. *Ann Nutr Metab 51* (2007): 303–23.

14. Turner, R. B. and W. E. Cetnarowski. Effect of treatment with zinc gluconate or zinc acetate on experimental and natural colds. *Clin Infect Dis 31* (2000): 1202–8.

15. Yan, Y. S. Effect of Chinese tea extract on the immune function of mice bearing tumor and their antitumor activity. *Zhonghua Yu Fang Yi Xue Za Zhi 26*, no. 1 (Jan 1, 1992): 5–7.

16. Sano, J., S. Inami, K. Seimiya, et al. Effects of green tea intake on the development of coronary artery disease. *Circ J 68*, no. 7 (Jul 2004): 665–70.

17. Giammanco, M., E. Tripoli, G. Tabacchi, et al. The phenolic compounds of olive oil: structure, biological activity and beneficial effects on human health. *Nutrition Research Reviews* 18, no. 1 (June 2005): 98–112.

18. Isolauri, E., Y. Sütas, P. Kankaanpää, et al. Probiotics: Effects on immunity. *Am J Clin Nutrition* 73, no. 2 (Feb 2001): 444S–450S.

19. Gill, H., K. Rutherfurd, M. Cross, et al. Enhancement of immunity in the elderly by dietary supplementation with the probiotic bifidobacterium lactis HN019. *Am J Clin Nutrition* 74, no. 6 (Dec 2001): 833–839.

20. "Diet, Exercise, Stress and the Immune System," Cleveland Clinic website, accessed March 15, 2009.

21. Rountree, Robert, and Carol Colman. *Immunotics*, G T Putnam's Sons, 2000.

22. "Diet, Exercise, Stress and the Immune System," Cleveland Clinic website, accessed March 15, 2009.

23. Meydani, S. N., M. Meydani, J. B. Blumberg, et al. Vitamin E supplementation and in vivo immune response in healthy elderly subjects: A randomized controlled trial. *JAMA* 277 (May 7, 1997): 1380–1386.

24. Life Extension Foundation Interview with Simin Meydani, "Vitamin E: Revitalizing Your Immune System," *Life Extension Magazine*, February 1999.

25. Haaland, D. A., T. F. Sabljic, D. A. Baribeau, et al. Is regular exercise a friend or foe of the aging immune system? A systematic review. *Clin J Sport Med* 18, no. 6 (Nov 2008): 539–548.

26. Burns, E. "Aging and the Immune System," Healthlink.

Chapter 11: What You Should Know about Hormones

1. Marigliano, V., C. Bauco, F. Campana, et al. Normal values in extreme old age. *Ann N Y Acad Sci* 673 (December 22, 1992): 23–28.

2. Gnagnarella, P., S. Gandini, C. La Vecchia, et al. Glycemic index, glycemic load and cancer risk: A meta-analysis. *Am J Clin Nutr* 87, no. 6 (June 2008): 1793–1801.

3. Institute of Functional Medicine, *Textbook of Functional Medicine*, 2005.

4. Canonico, M., Oger E., Plu-Bureau G., et al. Estrogen and Thromboembolism Risk (ESTHER) Study Group. Hormone therapy and venous thromboembolism among postmenopausal women: impact of the route of estrogen administration and progestogens: The ESTHER study. *Circulation* 115 (2007): 840–845.

5. Korenchevsky, V. *Physiological and Pathological Aging*, S. Karger, Basel, 1961.

6. Bland and Jones, "Clinical Approaches to Hormonal and Neuroendocrine Imbalances," *Textbook of Functional Medicine*, Institute of Functional Medicine, 2005.

7. Escobar-Morreale, H. F., M. J. Obregón, F. Escobar del Rey, et al. *J Clinical Invest* 96, no. 6 (Dec 1995): 2828–38.

8. Bunevicius, R., G. Kažanavičius, R. Žalinkevičius, et al. Effects of thyroxine as compared with thyroxine plus triiodothyronine in patients with hypothyroidism. *NEJM* 340, no. 6 (February 11, 1999): 424-429.

9. Shames and Shames, "The Top Five Supplements for Thyroid Support," Thyroid-info.com, http://www.thyroid-info.com/articles/topsupplements.htm.

10. Mariotti, S., P. Sansoni, G. Barbesino, et al. Thyroid and other organ-specific autoantibodies in healthy centenarians. *Lancet* 339 (1992): 1506–8.

11. Vliet, E. *Screaming to Be Heard*, M. Evans & Company, 1995.

12. Greenspan, F.S., et al. "Chapter 7: The Thyroid Gland," *Basic and Clinical Endocrinology*, 5th edition. New York: Appleton and Lange; 1997.

13. Pizzorno and Ferril. "Thyroid," *Textbook of Functional Medicine*, Institute of Functional Medicine, 2005.

14. Barnes, Broda. *Hypothyroidism: The Unsuspected Illness*. HarperCollins, 1976.

15. "Clinical Approaches to Hormonal and Neuroendocrine Imbalances," *Textbook of Functional Medicine*," Institute of Functional Medicine, 2005.

16. Arlt, W., F. Callies, J. van Vlijmen, et al. Dehydroepiandrosterone replacement in women with adrenal insufficiency. *NEJM* 341, no. 14 (1999): 1013–1020.

17. Hunt, P. J., E. M. Gurnell, F. A. Huppert, et al. Improvement in mood and fatigue after DHEA replacement in Addison's disease in a randomized double-blind trial. *J Clin Endocrinol Metab* 85, no. 12 (2000): 4650–4656.

18. Barrett-Connor, E., and D. Goodman-Gruen. The epidemiology of DHEA-S and cardiovascular disease. *Ann NY Acad Si* 774 (1995): 259–270.

19. Trivedi, Khaw. DHEA-S and mortality in elderly men and women. *J Clin Endocrinol Metab* 86, no. 9 (2001: 4171–4177.

20. Greendale, G. A., S. Edelstein, and E. Barrett-Connor. Endogenous sex steroids and bone mineral density in older women and men: The Rancho Bernado Study. *J Bone Miner Res* 12, no. 11 (1997): 1833–1843.

21. Morales, A. J., J. J. Nolan, J. C. Nelson, et al. Effects of replacement dose of dehydroepiandrosterone (DHEA) in men and women of advancing age. *J Clin Endocrinol Metab* 78, no. 6 (1994): 1360–1367.

22. Morales, A. J., R. H. Haubrich, J. Y. Hwang, et al. The effect of six months treatment with a 100 mg daily dose of DHEA on circulating sex steroids, body composition and muscle strength in age-advanced men and women. *Clin Endocrinol (Oxf)* 49, no. 4 (1998): 421-433.

23. Baulieu, E. E., G. Thomas, S. Legrain, et al. Dehydroepiandrosterone (DHEA), DHEA sulfate, and aging: contribution of the DHEAge Study to a sociobiomedical issue. *Proc Natl Acad Sci U S A* 97, no. 8 (2000): 4279-4284.

24. Bland and Jones, "Clinical Approaches to Hormonal and Neuroendocrine Imbalances," *Textbook of Functional Medicine*, Institute of Functional Medicine, 2005.

25. Nakahata, Y., S. Sahar, G. Astarita, et al. Circadian control of the NAD+ salvage pathway by CLOCK-SIRT1. *Science* 324, no. 5927 (March 12, 2009): 654-657.

26. "Body clock regulates metabolism, finds UCI study," NewsRx. com, March 26, 2009, www.lef.org/news/LefDailyNews. htm?NewsID=8058&Section=Aging.

27. Cagnacci, A., M. Cannoletta, A. Renzi, et al. Prolonged melatonin administration decreases nocturnal blood pressure in women. *Am J Hypertens* 18, no. 12 (December 2005): 1614-1618.

Section III: The Secrets of Emotional Intelligence: Underrated and Ignored—Until Now

1. Harrington, Ann. *The Cure Within*, W.W. Norton, 2008.

2. Wolf, Stewart and John Bruhn. *The Power of Clan*, Transaction Publishers, 1992.

3. Kochilas, Diane. "Ikarian Diet a Key to Health and Longevity," AC360°, ac360.blogs.cnn.

4. Buettner, Dan. *The Blue Zones*, National Geographic, 2008.

5. Rowe, J. and Kahn, R. *Successful Aging*, Dell Publishing, 1998.

6. Langer, E. and Rodin, J. The effects of choice and enhanced personal responsibility for the aged: A field experiment in an institutional setting. *J Pers Soc Psychol* 34, no. 2 (1976): 191-198.

7. Rowe, J. and Kahn, R. *Successful Aging*, Dell Publishing, 1998.

8. Ertel, K. A., M. M. Glymour, and L. F. Berkman. Effects of social integration on preserving memory function in a nationally representative US elderly population. *Am J Public Health* 98, no.7 (2008): 1215-20.

9. Berkman, Syme. Social networks, host resistance and mortality: A nine-year follow-up study of Alameda county residents. *Am Journal of Epidemiology* 109, no. 2: 186-204.

10. Snowdon, D. *Aging with Grace: What the Nun Study Teaches Us about Leading Longer, Healthier and More Meaningful Lives*, Bantam, 2001.

11. Rowe, J. and R. Kahn. *Successful Aging*, Dell Publishing, 1998.

12. "Volunteering Produces Health Benefits," press release, AmeriCorps / Corporation for National and Community Service, www.americorps. gov/about/newsroom/releases_detail.asp?tbl_pr_id=687.

13. AM SURV: House, James. Americans' Changing Lives: Waves I, II, III, and IV, 1986, 1989, 1994, and 2002. Inter-University Consortium for Political and Social Research (2008).

14. Buettner, Dan. *The Blue Zones*, National Geographic, 2008.

Conclusion: A Plan for You: The 7 x 3 Matrix of Healthy Aging

1. Gao, Y. T., J. K. McLaughlin, W. J. Blot, et al. Reduced risk of esophageal cancer associated with green tea consumption. *J Natl Cancer Inst* 86, no. 11 (June 1,1994): 855-858.

2. Shrubsole, M. J., W. Lu, Z. Chen, et al. Drinking green tea modestly reduces breast cancer risk. *J Nutr* 139, no. 2 (Feb 2009): 310-316.

3. Alexopoulos, N., C. Vlachopoulos, K. Aznaouridis, et al. The acute effect of green tea consumption on endothelial function in healthy individuals. *Eur J Cardiovasc Prev Rehabil* 15 (2008): 300-305.

4. Hirano, R., Y. Momiyama, R. Takahashi, et al. Comparison of green tea intake in Japanese patients with and without angiographic coronary artery disease. *Am J Cardiol* 90, no. 10 (2002): 1150-1153.

5. Paschka, A. G., R. Butler, and C. Y.-F. Young. Induction of apoptosis in prostate cancer cell lines by the green tea component EGCG. *Cancer Letters* 130, no. 1-2 (Aug 14, 1998): 1-7.

6. Ehrnhoefer, D. E., J. Bieschke, A. Boeddrich, et al. EGCG redirects amyloidogenic polypeptides into unstructured, off-pathway oligomers. *Nature Structural and Molecular Biology* 15 (May 30, 2008): 558-566.

7. Kelly Jr., J. H. and J. Sabaté. Nuts and coronary heart disease: An epidemiological perspective. *Br J Nutr* 96, Suppl 2 (Nov. 2006): S61-7.

8. Villegas, R., Y. T. Gao, G. Yang, et al. Legume and soy food intake and the incidence of type 2 diabetes in the Shanghai Women's Health Study. *Am J Clin Nutr* 87, no. 1 (January 2008): 162-167.

9. Bazzano, L. A., J. He, L. G. Ogden, et al. Legume consumption and risk of coronary heart disease in US men and women. *Arch Intern Med* 161 (Nov. 26, 2001): 2573-2578.

10. Strandhagen, E., P-O Hansson, I. Bosaeus, et al. High fruit intake may reduce mortality among middle-aged and elderly men. *Eur J Clin Nutrition* 54 (2000): 337-341.

11. Joshipura, K. J., F. B. Hu, J. E. Manson, et al. The effect of fruit and vegetable intake on risk for coronary heart disease. *Ann Int Med* 134 (2001): 1106-1114.

12. Liu, S., J. E. Manson, I. M. Lee, et al. Fruit and vegetable intake and risk of cardiovascular disease: The Women's Health Study. *Am J Clini Nutri* 79 (2000): 922-928.

13. Heller, L. "Scientist concerned at plummeting nutrient levels," Food Navigator, foodnavigator-usa.com, 2006.

14. Davis, D. Declining fruit and vegetable nutrient composition: What is the evidence? *J HortScience* 44 (2009): 15-19.

15. Lawrence, Felicity. "Mineral Levels in Meat and Milk Plummet Over 60 Years," *The Guardian*, Feb 2, 2006.

16. Varga, Z. Omega-3 Polyunsaturated fatty acids in the prevention of atherosclerosis. *Orv Hetil* 149, no. 14 (Apr. 6, 2008): 627-37.

17. Simopoulos, Artemis and Jo Robinson. *The Omega Diet: The Lifesaving Nutritional Program Based on the Diet of the Island of Crete.* New York: Harper Paperbacks, 1999.

18. Sears, Barry. *Omega Rx Zone: The Miracle of the New High-Dose Fish Oil.* New York: HarperCollins, 2005.

19. Tribole, Evelyn. *The Ultimate Omega-3 Diet.* New York: McGraw-Hill, 2007.

20. Stoll, Andrew. *The Omega-3 Connection.* New York: Simon & Schuster, 2001.

21. Hoffman, P. R. and M. J Berry. The influence of selenium on immune responses. *Mol Nutr Food Res* 52, no. 11 (Nov. 2008): 1273-80.

22. Templeton, David. "Penn State Study: Selenium Slows AIDS Progression," *Pittsburg Post Gazette*, December 1, 2008.

23. Hurwitz, B. E., J. R. Klaus, M. M. Llabre, et al. Suppression of human immunodeficiency virus type 1 viral load with selenium supplementation: A randomized controlled trial. *Arch Intern Med* 167, no. 2 (Jan. 22, 2007): 148-54.

24. Akbaraly, T. N., J. Arnaud, I. Hininger-Favier, et al. Selenium and mortality in the elderly: Results from the EVA Study. *Clinical Chemistry* 51 (2005): 2117-2123.

25. Akbaraly, T. N., I. Hininger-Favier, I. Carrière, et al. Plasma selenium over time and cognitive decline in the elderly. *Epidemiology* 18, no. 1 (Jan. 2007): 52-58.

26. Clark, L. C. G. F. Combs Jr., B. W. Turnbull, et al. Effects of selenium supplementation for cancer prevention in patients with carcinoma of the skin: A randomized controlled trial. *JAMA* 276 (Dec. 25, 1996): 1957-1963.

27. Hendler, Sheldon and David Rorvik. *Physicans' Desk Reference for Nutritional Supplements*, 2nd edition. Physicians' Desk Reference, Inc., 2008.

28. Melamed M. L., E. D. Michos, W. Post, et al. 25-hydroxyvitamin d levels and the risk of mortality in the general population. *Arch Intern Med* 168, no. 15 (Aug. 11, 2008): 1629-37.

29. Lappe, J. M., D. Travers-Gustafson, K. M. Davies, et al. Vitamin D and calcium supplementation reduces cancer risk: Results of a randomized trial. *Am J Clin Nutr* 85, no. 6 (Jun 2007): 1586-91.

30. Knekt, P., M. Laaksonen, C. Mattila, et al. Serum vitamin D and subsequent occurrence of type 2 diabetes. *Epidemiology* 19, no. 5 (Sep. 2008): 666-71.

31. Giovannucci, E., Y. Liu, B. W. Hollis, et al. 25-hydroxyvitamin D and risk of myocardial infarction in men: a prospective study. *Arch Intern Med* 168, no. 11 (June 9, 2008): 1174-80.

32. Llewellyn, D. J., K. M. Langa, and I. A. Lang. Serum 25-hydroxyvitamin D concentration and cognitive impairment. *J Geriatr Psychiatry Neurol* 22, no. 3 (Dec. 10 2008): 188-95.

33. Houston, D. K., M. Cesari, L. Ferrucci, et al. Association between vitamin D status and physical performance: The InCHIANTI study. *J Gerontol A Biol Sci Med Sci* 62, no. 4 (April 2007): 440-446.

34. Ginde, A.A., J. M. Mansbach, and C. A. Camargo. Association between serum 25-hydroxyvitamin d level and upper respiratory tract infection in the third national health and nutrition examination survey. *Arch Intern Med* 169, no. 4 (Feb. 23, 2009): 384-90.

35. Reinberg, Steven. "Many Americans Fall Short on Their Vitamin D," GoodGuide.com, March 24, 2009.

36. Hendler, Sheldon and David Rorvik. *Physicans' Desk Reference for Nutritional Supplements*, 2nd edition. Physicians' Desk Reference, Inc., 2008.

37. Ibid.

38. Coates, Paul, ed. *Encyclopedia of Dietary Supplements*, National Institute of Health, Marcel Dekker, 2005.

39. Hendler, Sheldon and David Rorvik. *Physicans' Desk Reference for Nutritional Supplements*, 2nd edition. Physicians' Desk Reference, Inc., 2008.

40. Snowdon, D. *Aging With Grace: What the Nun Study Teaches Us About Leading Longer, Healthier, and More Meaningful Lives*. Bantam Books, 2001.

41. Coates, Paul, ed. *Encyclopedia of Dietary Supplements*, National Institute of Health, Marcel Dekker, 2005.

42. Hendler, Sheldon and David Rorvik. *Physicans' Desk Reference for Nutritional Supplements*, 2nd edition. Physicians' Desk Reference, Inc., 2008.

43. Galpern, W. R., and M. E. Cudkowicz. Coenzyme Q10 treatment of neurodegenerative disease of aging. *Mitochondrion* 7, supp.1 (2007): S146-153.

44. Rozen, T. D., M. L. Oshinsky, C. A. Gebeline, et al. Open label trial of coenzyme Q10 as a migraine preventive. *Cephalalgia* 22 (2002): 137-41.

45. Hendler, Sheldon and David Rorvik. *Physicans' Desk Reference for Nutritional Supplements*, 2nd edition. Physicians' Desk Reference, Inc., 2008.

46. Pereira, A. C., D. E. Huddleston, A. M. Brickman, et al. An in vivo correlate of exercise-induced neurogenesis in the adult dentate gyrus. *Proc Natl Acad Sci USA* 104, no. 13 (March 27, 2007): 5638–5643.

47. Colcombe, S. J., K. I. Erickson, P. E. Scalf, et al. Aerobic exercise training increases brain volume in aging humans. *J Gerontol A Biol Sci Med Sci* 61 (2006): 1166-1170.

48. Blumenthal, J. A., M. A. Babyak, K. A. Moore, et al. Effects of exercise training on older patients with major depression. *Arch Intern Med* 159 (1999): 2349-2356.

49. "Greenland's Constant Summer Sunlight Linked to Summer Suicide Spike," *Science Daily*, May 10, 2009.

50. Ferrie, J. E., M. J. Shipley, F. P. Cappuccio, et al. A prospective study of change in sleep duration: Associations with mortality in the Whitehall II cohort. *Sleep* 30, no. 12 (2007): 1659-66.

51. Okinawa Centenarian Study data presented at the American Geriatrics Society annual meeting, 2001. Cited by H. McCord and G. McVeigh, "NutritionNews: 'Magic' Appetite Shutoff from the Orient," *Prevention*, January 2002, pages 52-3.

52. Kagawa, Y. Impact of Westernization on the nutrition of Japanese: Changes in physique, cancer, longevity and centenarians. *Preventive Medicine* 7, no. 2 (June, 1978): 205-17.

53. Okinawa Centenarian Study data presented at the American Geriatrics Society annual meeting, 2001. Cited by H. McCord and G. McVeigh, "NutritionNews: 'Magic' Appetite Shutoff from the Orient," *Prevention*, January 2002, pages 52-3.

Acknowledgments

As every author on the planet knows, a book is a collaborative effort. This one might have my name on it but it wouldn't have been possible if a veritable army of very, *very* smart people had not been willing to take time out of their busy days to answer my questions and generously share their significant intellectual firepower.

To wit: Daniel Amen, M.D.; Suzanne Bennett, D.C.; Ann Knight, D.C.; Mark Houston, M.D.; Dave Leonardi, M.D.; Barry Sears, Ph.D.; and Beth Traynor, M.D. Special thanks are due to Larry McCleary, M.D., who generously read and critiqued the chapter on the brain; Keith McCormick, D.C., who did the same for the section on osteoporosis; and Dan Buettner, whose outstanding work, *The Blue Zones*, inspired much of section III on emotional intelligence. A special thanks goes to Sue Copp, M.S., whose help, always generously available for the asking, is so greatly appreciated. And of course, to Christopher Loch, my marketing director and Web designer who has been the greatest business partner anyone could ask for.

And then there's that amazing team at Fair Winds Press, my publisher since 2005. That would be the same team that takes my dry, black-and-white Word documents and somehow miraculously transforms them into gorgeous books like this one. (Don't ask me how they do it; I don't even know how to change a flat tire.) Ken Fund, Will Kiester, Jill Alexander, Tiffany Hill (project manager extraordinaire), Karen Levy (you don't know how important a good copy editor is until you've worked with Karen), and the absolutely phenomenal design team of Meg Sniegoski, Rosalind Wanke, Luke Herriott, and Rowan Moore-Seifred, as well as photo researcher Janine Blackstock.

Then there's Cara Connors.

This is the fifth book I've done with Cara Connors as editor, and it's hard to imagine doing one without her. Editors are kind of like directors—the public pays attention to the actors on screen, but it's the director's invisible hand that shapes those performances. So it is with Cara. She's the ultimate "Jonny wrangler" (and it ain't an easy job); she's knowledgeable, patient, funny, and smart, and she knows when to leave me alone and when to push for changes. Cara, you have my eternal thanks for everything you do.

A great agent does a lot more than just broker a deal. She nurtures, she cajoles, she suggests book ideas and then helps flesh them out, she "pre-edits," she wrangles, she plays good cop (or bad cop), she's fiercely protective, and she's ultimately the best friend an author can have in the world of publishing. My agent, Coleen O'Shea, of the Allen O'Shea Literary Agency, does all that and more. She is, quite simply, the most perfect agent on the planet. Thank you.

But wait, there's more.

Every writer has his writing heroes, and I'm no exception. Top of the list is William Goldman, who could no more write a boring word than Aaron Copland could write a bad piece of music or Miles Davis could take a bad solo. The writing of the late Ed McBain (Evan Hunter) has been a source of infinite delight to me for decades. I would never think of missing a column by either Peggy Noonan or Gail Collins. And then, of course, there's the greatest science writer in America, Robert Sapolsky, who proves that humor, style, accessibility, and scholarship can coexist in the same package. I may not always achieve that goal, but the fact that Sapolsky does it every single time he sets pen to paper gives me faith that it is in fact attainable on the Planet Earth.

Professor Ernest van den Haag of the New School for Social Research was instrumental in teaching me how to think, always a good thing if you're planning on writing, teaching, and speaking. I never thanked him, but I'm doing it now.

Werner Erhard, wherever you are, my greatest wish is for you to know how much you mean to me and how deeply and profoundly you have altered my life. (And a deep thanks to the film director Robyn Symon for rescuing the reputation of this great man in her incredible film, *Werner Erhard: The Transformation of a Man*. It's out now on DVD. You should see it.)

My friends Jack Canfield, Les Brown, T. Harv Eker, Alex Mandossian, and Mark Victor Hansen—you all make such a difference in the lives of so many.

Thanks to Howard, Robin, Fred, Gary, and Artie for putting a smile on my face each and every single day since 1995. And a special thanks to you guys for staying on the air on September 11, 2001.

My family: my dear brother Jeffrey Bowden, my sister-in-law Nancy Fiedler, and my niece and nephew Cadence Bowden and Pace Bowden. I love you all. Even you, Pace.

And then, finally, my "chosen" family, who have sustained and nourished me, some of them for more than twenty-five years, some of them more recently: My "sisters" Randy Graff and Laurie Dash; my "brothers" Peter Breger and Oz Garcia; my dear friends, the Wood-Duncan family (Susan, Christopher, Charlie Ann, Miles, and Brock), my partner-in-crime for a decade, Sky London; Doug Monas; Liz Neporent; Diana Lederman; Glen Depke; Paul Ruben; Andreas Weyerman; Gina Lombardi and Kevin Sizemore (and Gunnar!); Billy Stritch; Scott Ellis; Oliver Beaucamp and Jennifer Schneider and their beautiful daughter Leslie; Kimberly Wright, the Sushi Goddess; my lifelong spiritual advisor and friend, Jeanette Lee Bessinger; and my newest friend, Ann Knight—thank you for everything.

And, of course, my "person"—Anja Christy.

As Peggy Noonan once said, "Without her, there is no him."

About the Author

Jonny Bowden, Ph.D., C.N.S., a board-certified nutritionist with a master's degree in psychology, is a nationally known expert on nutrition, weight loss, and health. A member of the Editorial Advisory Board of *Men's Health Magazine* and the health columnist for *Forbes Online*, he's also written or contributed to articles for dozens of national publications (print and online) including *The New York Times, The Wall Street Journal, Forbes, Time, Oxygen, Marie Claire, W, Remedy, Diabetes Focus, US Weekly, Cosmopolitan, Family Circle, Self, Fitness, Allure, Essence, Men's Health, Weight Watchers, Pilates Style, Prevention, Woman's World, In Style, Fitness, Natural Health,* and *Shape.* He is the author of *The 150 Most Effective Ways to Boost Your Energy* and *The 100 Healthiest Foods to Eat During Pregnancy* (coauthored with Allison Tannis, R.D.).

A popular, dynamic, and much sought-after speaker, he's appeared on CNN, Fox News, MSNBC, ABC, NBC, and CBS, and speaks frequently around the country.

In addition to the above, he is the author of six books on health and nutrition, including the award-winning *Living the Low Carb Life: Controlled Carbohydrate Eating for Long-Term Weight Loss, The Most Effective Natural Cures on Earth, The Healthiest Meals on Earth* (coauthored with Jeanette Bessinger), and his acclaimed signature best seller, *The 150 Healthiest Foods on Earth.*

You can find his DVDs, *The Truth About Weight Loss* and *The 7 Pillars of Longevity,* his popular motivational CDs, free newsletter, free audio programs, and many of the supplements and foods recommended in this book on his website, www.jonnybowden.com.

He lives in Southern California with his beloved animal companions Woodstock, Emily ll, and (sometimes) Roxy-Emily Christy.

Index

· · · · · · · · · ·

B

back, 163, *163*, 165, *165*, *167*, 167–170, *168*, *169*, *170*, 172, *172*
baked goods, 76
balance, 37–38
Baltimore Longitudinal Study of Aging, 205
bananas, 108, 222
Barnes, Broda, 221
basal temperature test for thyroid, 221
basic abdominal strengthener, *166*, 166
basophils, 182
B-cells, 183, 184, 187
beans, 25, 29, 32, 43, 94, 98, 99, 108, 109, 250. *See also specific beans*
beef, 44, 117. *See also* meat
beet greens, 222
beets, 29
bell peppers, 20, 29, 32, 43, 109
Bennett, Susanne, 213–214
Bensen, Herbert, 131
Berk, Lee, 187
Berkson, Bert, 195
berries, 25, 32, 251. *See also specific berrries*
beta-carotene, 34, 196, 197
bicep curls, 163, *163*
biceps, 163, *163*
biologics, 157
Biotics Research, 113
black beans, 29
blackberries, 25, 28
black currant oil, 44
blackened foods, 50
Bland, Jeffrey, 12, 207, 210, 215, 225
Blatt, Harvey, 19
blood clots, 92
blood pressure, 108, 110–111, *112*, 113, 116, 118
blood sugar, 47, 48, 131–133, 134, 154, 193, 201–207. *See also* glycation
blueberries, 25, 28, 29, 32, 99, 135, 136–137
"Blue Zones", 213, 238, 250, 251
Bone, Kerry, 146
bones, 28, 69, 147, 149–176
    bone density, 153
    bone matrix, 151
    bone mineral density, 153
    bone quality, 153
borage oil, 44
Bowden, Jonny
    The 150 Healthiest Foods on Earth, 25, 98, 138

The 150 Most Effective Ways to Boost Your Energy, 77, 117, 128
The Healthiest Meals on Earth, 30, 96, 97
Living Low Carb, 204
The Most Effective Natural Cures on Earth, 45, 57, 128, 225
"The Relaxation Response", 128
Shape Up, 242
brain cells, 139, 142–143
brain health, 56, 68–69, 120–148
    cortisol and, 127
    exercise and, 125–127, 130
    memory and, 130
    stress and, 55–56
    supplements for, 139–148
bran, 222
brassica vegetables, 25, 32, 43, 220, 222
Brazil nuts, 222
breathing. *See* deep breathing
British Columbia Office of Health Technology Assessment, 153
broccoli, 25, 29, 76, 97, 98, 154
Broiled Salmon with Tamari-Orange Marinade, 31
browning effect, 49–50
brown rice, 222
Brownstein, David, 217
Bruhn, John, *The Power of Clan*, 234
Brussels sprouts, 25, 29
Buckner, Randy, 123
Buddha, 184
Buettner, Dan, 93, 237–238, 241, 250
    The Blue Zones, 10, 237–238
Burns, Edith, 198–199
bursa of Fabricius, 183
butter, 22
B vitamins, 103, 106, 107. *See also specific B vitamins*

C

cabbage, 25, 76
caffeine, 76
calcitriol, 145
calcium, 28, 109, 151, 154–155, 156, 190
calcium elenolate, 194
caloric restriction, 63, 64, 148, 259
Caloric Restriction Society, 63
calories, 63. *See also* caloric restriction
Canadian Pediatric Society, 144
cancer, 11
Candida albicans, 195
Cannell, John, 145

cantaloupe, 222
carbs, 205, 206–207
carcinogens, 19
Carey, Benedict, 68
carmelization, 50
carnosine, 47, 50–51
carotenoids, 26, 28, 34, 197, 199
cartilage, 159
cashews, 109
cat and camel, *167*, 167
celery, 20
cell-mediated immunity, 183
cell membranes, 23
Centers for Disease Control and Prevention, 19, 72
cerebrovascular disease, 89
Chandra, Ranjit, 190
Chang, Michael N., 33
chard, 108, 109, 222
chemical estrogen, 211–214
chemotaxis, 195
Chen, Steve, 247
cherries, 20, 29
chest, *162*, 162, 171, *171*, *172*, 172
chest presses, 162, *162*
chest stretch, 171, *171*
chicken, 222
chili peppers, 222
chocolate, 43
choice, 235
cholesterol, 23, 24, 69, 87, 89, 91–92, 102–103, 118
chondroitin sulfate, 159
chronic inflammation, 36, 38, 39, 103–104, 152
chronic stress, 188
cinnamon, 25, 43
circadian rhythms, 78, 227
clams, 222
Clegg, Daniel O., 158, 159
Cleveland Clinic, 190, 195, 196
cloves, 25, 43
cocoa, 25, 43
coconut oil, 22
coconuts, 22
cod liver oil, 145
coenzyme Q10, 17, 24, 117, 252, 256–257
coffee, 20, 32
cognitive decline, lowering risk of, 137–148
cola, 155
collagen, 33, 153
collard greens, 222

gastrointestinal dysfunction, 156
Geiger, E. Michael, 34
genetics, 11, 59, 60–69
German Commission E monographs, 146
germ theory of disease, 178–179
ghrelin, 80
Ginde, Adit, 253
ginger, 25, 43
ginkgo biloba, 140, 144, 146
GLA (gamma-linolenic acid), 44, 45
glucocorticoids, 187–188
glucosamine, 158–159
glucose metabolism, 127, 129
glutathione, 24, 142
glycated proteins, 49–50
glycation, 15, 45, 46–51, 192, 204
    cooking and, 49–50
    definition of, 47
glycemic index, 93
glycotoxins, 49
goitrogens, 220
Goleman, Daniel, *Emotional Intelligence*, 232
good fats, 93
Gore, Cindy, 81
Gore, Russel, 81
Gorman, Christine, 38, 39
GPC (GlyceroPhosCholine), 140, 143–144
grapefruit, 29
grapes, 20, 29, 32
grapeseed extract, 25
grass-fed meat, 44, 94, 250
gratitude, 245, 262
gray matter, 125
green leafy vegetables, 25, 32
green tea, 118–119, 192–193, 250
green tea extract, 192–193
grilled foods, 50
Grossman, Terry, *Fantastic Journey: The Science Behind Radical Life Extension*, 62
growth hormone, 20
Guarente, Leonard, 62

H

Haas, Elson, 76
haddock, 222
halibut, 136
hamstring, *174*, 174
hamstring stretch, *174*, 174
Hanbury, David, 194
hara hatchi bu, 259
Harman, Denham, 18
Hashimoto's Thyroiditis, 218

Health and Retirement Study, 240
Health Professionals Follow-Up Study, 251
heart, anatomy of the, 88, *90*
heart disease, 11, 42, 85–86, 89, 92, 106. *See also* heart health
    prevention of, 102–107
heart health, 69, 84–119
heart-healthy diet, five principles of a, 93–94
hemoglobin, 48
hemoglobin A1c blood test, 48
herbicides, 19
herbs, 25, 43
herring, 136, 250
high blood pressure, 110–111, *112*
high-glycemic diet, 205
high-sugar foods, 25
hippocampus, 55, 127, 133
Hippocrates, 249
HMG-coenzyme A reductase (HMG-CoA reductase), 204
Holick, Michael, 144, 254
homocysteine, 103, 104–105, 106, 107, 146
homocystinuria, 104
hormonal system, 69
hormone replacement therapy (HRT), 210–214, 219–220
hormones, 53, 54–55, 200–226
Horn, Floyd P., 136
hot peppers, 222
Houston, Mark, 45, 62, 64, 65, 89, 91, 108, 109, 110, 113, 117
hs-CRP (high-sensitivity CRP) test, 42, 43, 107, 110
human growth hormone (HGH), 78, 214–215
humoral immune response, 183
Hurley, Chad, 247
Hurricane Katrna, 81
hydroxyl radicals, 226
hypertension, 110–111, *112*
Hypertension Institute, 111, 113, 118
hypothalamus, 54, 129
hypothyroidism, 215–216, 218–219

I

IGF-1, 214
ikagi, 260
Ikaria, 235–238
imbalance, 57–58
immune system, 21, 69, 152, 177–199, 252–253
    aging and, 198–199

halo effect, 179–180
    stress and, 187–189
    supplements for the, 189–199
indoles, 222
inflammation, 15, 34, 35–45, 152, 156–159, 187–188
    brain health and, 132, 137, 139
    controlling, 43–45
    C-reactive protein (CRP) and, 107, 110
    definition of, 36
    heart health and, 91–93, 99, 103–104
    measurement of, 41, 42, 107, 110
Institute for Functional Medicine, 225
Institute of Medicine of the National Academies of Science, 146
instrinsic factor, 146
insulin, 131–133, 201–207
    exercise and, 205–206
    insulin resistance, 131–133, *133*, 201–207
    insulin sensitivity, 201–207
iodine, 217, 222
Iosol Iodine, 217
isothiocyanates, *26*

J

Jackson, Christopher, 158, 159
Johnny Bowden's four food groups, 77, 206
Joint Food and Agriculture Organization/ World Health Organization Expert Consultation, 72
joint pain, 156–157
joints, 69, 149–176, 156–161
    weight loss and, 159, 160
Jones, David, 12, 13, 207, 215, 225
Jordon, Karin Granstrom, 51
Joseph, James, 251
Joseph, Jim, 136, 137
JUPITER study, 38, 43

K

Kahn, Robert, 105
kale, 28, 76, 108, 109, 222
Kamada, 241
Karim, Jawed, 247
Kawas, Claudia, 68
Kenyon, Cynthia, 12
Khalsa, Dharma Singh, 121, 124, 127, 129
Kidd, Parris, 143, 144
kidney beans, 25, 29, 99
kindness, 262
kiwifruit, 29, 32

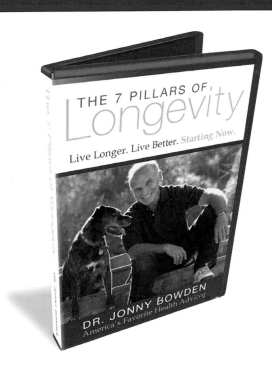

Best-selling books by acclaimed nutritionist Jonny Bowden, Ph.D., C.N.S.

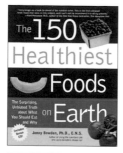

The 150 Healthiest Foods on Earth
The Surprising, Unbiased Truth about What You Should Eat and Why

"*The 150 Healthiest Foods on Earth* is simply delightful! The information is accurate; the presentation is a visual feast. All in all, reading this book is a very satisfying experience."
—CHRISTIANE NORTHRUP, M.D., author of *Mother-Daughter Wisdom*, *The Wisdom of Menopause*, and *Women's Bodies, Women's Wisdom*

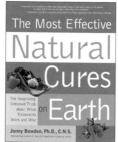

The Most Effective Natural Cures on Earth
The Surprising, Unbiased Truth about What Treatments Work and Why

"I reference this beautifully written and illustrated review of the best cures on the planet so often that it lives on my desk rather than the bookshelf."
—MEHMET C. OZ, M.D., coauthor of *You: The Owner's Manual*

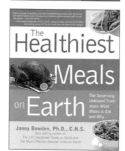

The Healthiest Meals on Earth
The Surprising, Unbiased Truth about What Meals to Eat and Why

"What a simply irresistible book with mouthwatering recipes from all around the world! I plan to use this book as a resource guide and as a gift for all the people I truly care about."
—ANN LOUISE GITTLEMAN, PH.D., C.N.S., author of *The Fat Flush Plan* and *Before the Change*

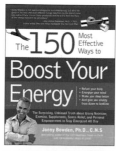

The Most Effective Ways to Boost Your Energy
The Surprising, Unbiased Truth about Using Nutrition, Exercise, Supplements, Stress Relief, and Personal Empowerment to Stay Energized All Day

"Get everyone you love to read my friend Dr. Jonny's brilliance!"
—MARK VICTOR HANSEN, coauthor of *Chicken Soup for the Soul*

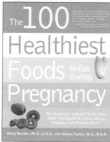

The 100 Healthiest Foods to Eat During Pregnancy
The Surprising, Unbiased Truth about Foods You Should Be Eating During Pregnancy but Probably Aren't

"Another great book from Jonny Bowden! In his signature expert style, Jonny, along with Allison Tannis, recommends the healthiest foods and spices for pregnant women . . . all pregnant women should read this book."
—DEAN RAFFELOCK, D.C.,C.C.N., author of *A Natural Guide to Pregnancy and Postpartum Health*

www.jonnybowden.com